Management of Posttraumatic Spinal Instability

AANS Publications Committee
Paul R. Cooper, MD, Editor

Neurosurgical Topics

American Association of Neurological Surgeons
Park Ridge, Illinois

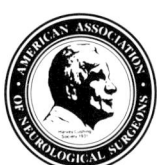

Library of Congress Catalog Number: 90-81239
ISBN: 0-9624246-2-5

Neurosurgical Topics ISBN: 0-9624246-6-8

Copyright © 1990 by American Association of Neurological Surgeons

First Printing — 1990
Second Printing — 1991

All rights reserved. None of the contents of this publication may be reproduced in a retrieval system or transmitted in any form or by any means (electronic, mechanical, photocopying, recording, or otherwise) without prior written permission of the publisher.

This publication is published under the auspices of the Publications Committee of the American Association of Neurological Surgeons (AANS). However, this should not be construed as indicating endorsement or approval of the views presented, by the AANS, or by its committees, commissions, affiliates, or staff.

Robert H. Wilkins, MD, Chairman
AANS Publications Committee

Gabrielle J. Loring, Publications Production Manager

AANS1.5M291

Foreword

Based on the idea that the American Association of Neurological Surgeons should provide neurosurgeons, especially those not located in an academic institution, with periodic publications related to neurosurgery, a Publications Committee was formed by George T. Tindall, MD, in 1987. The Committee first assembled in April 1988 and has met regularly since that time.

The Committee has concerned itself initially with three projects. The first was sponsorship of a collection of essays by Bengt Ljunggren, MD, PhD; this was published in 1989 as *Great Men with Sick Brains & Other Essays*. The second was the organization of a *Neurosurgical Operative Atlas,* which is to be published first in loose-leaf, fascicle form and eventually in case-bound form.

The third project is the Neurosurgical Topics series of monographs dealing with specific topics of interest to neurosurgeons. The first of these books is the present *Management of Posttraumatic Spinal Instability,* edited by Paul R. Cooper, MD. Seven other books in this series are currently in preparation. We are pleased to see this project launched and hope that it will be of value to its intended readership.

Robert H. Wilkins, MD
Chairman, AANS Publications Committee

Forthcoming Books in the *Neurosurgical Topics* Series

1990

Malignant Cerebral Glioma
 Edited by Michael L. J. Apuzzo, MD

Intracranial Vascular Malformations
 Edited by Daniel L. Barrow, MD

Neurosurgical Treatment of Disorders of the Thoracic Spine
 Edited by Edward Tarlov, MD

1991

Treatment of Pituitary Adenomas
 Edited by Paul R. Cooper, MD

Neurosurgical Aspects of Epilepsy
 Edited by Michael L. J. Apuzzo, MD

Complications and Sequelae of Head Injury
 Edited by Daniel L. Barrow, MD

Complications of Spinal Surgery
 Edited by Edward Tarlov, MD

Contents

Chapter 1	Early Assessment, Transport, and Management of Patients with Posttraumatic Spinal Instability *Randall M. Chesnut, MD, and Lawrence F. Marshall, MD*	1
Chapter 2	Imaging and the Determination of Posttraumatic Spinal Instability *Wendy Cohen, MD*	19
Chapter 3	Clinical Assessment of Posttraumatic Spinal Instability *Lawrence F. Borges, MD*	37
Chapter 4	Spinal Orthoses *Mark N. Hadley, MD*	51
Chapter 5	Management of Occipito-cervical Instability *Arnold H. Menezes, MD, and Michael Muhonen, MD*	65
Chapter 6	The Evaluation and Management of Trauma to the Odontoid Process *Craig T. Clark, MD, and Michael L. J. Apuzzo, MD*	77
Chapter 7	Management of Nonodontoid Upper Cervical Spine Injuries *Volker K. H. Sonntag, MD, and Mark N. Hadley, MD*	99
Chapter 8	Stabilization of Fractures and Subluxations of the Lower Cervical Spine *Paul R. Cooper, MD*	111
Chapter 9	Thoracolumbar Spine Injuries *Thomas J. Errico, MD, and R. David Bauer, MD*	135
Chapter 10	Sacral Fractures *Robert G. Watkins, MD, and William H. Dillin, MD*	163
Chapter 11	Special Problems in Patients with Preexisting Spine Disease *Raj Murali, MD*	173
Chapter 12	Special Problems of Spinal Stabilization in Children *Dachling Pang, MD, and Edward N. Hanley, MD*	181

List of Contributors

Michael L. J. Apuzzo, MD
Professor of Neurological Surgery
University of Southern California School of Medicine
Los Angeles, Calif

R. David Bauer, MD
Department of Orthopedic Surgery
New York University Medical Center
New York, NY

Lawrence F. Borges, MD
Neurosurgical Service
Massachusetts General Hospital
Boston, Mass

Randall M. Chesnut, MD
Department of Neurological Surgery
University of California
San Diego Medical Center
San Diego, Calif

Craig T. Clark, MD
Clinical Instructor
Department of Neurological Surgery
University of Southern California School of Medicine
Los Angeles, Calif

Wendy Cohen, MD
Associate Professor of Radiology
University of Washington School of Medicine
Seattle, Wash

Paul R. Cooper, MD
Associate Professor of Neurosurgery
New York University Medical Center
New York, NY

William H. Dillin, MD
Kerlan-Jobe Orthopedic Clinic
Los Angeles, Calif

Thomas J. Errico, MD
Assistant Professor of Orthopedic Surgery
New York University Medical Center
New York, NY

Mark N. Hadley, MD, Maj, USAF, MC
Chief, Division of Neurological Surgery
David Grant U.S. Air Force Medical Center
Travis AFB, Calif

Edward N. Hanley, MD
Associate Professor of Orthopedic Surgery
University of Pittsburgh School of Medicine
Pittsburgh, Pa

Lawrence F. Marshall, MD
Professor of Neurological Surgery
University of California
San Diego Medical Center
San Diego, Calif

Arnold H. Menezes, MD
Professor and Vice Chairman
Division of Neurosurgery
University of Iowa Hospitals and Clinics
Iowa City, Iowa

Michael Muhonen, MD
Resident in Neurosurgery
University of Iowa Hospitals and Clinics
Iowa City, Iowa

Raj Murali, MD
Associate Professor of Clinical Neurosurgery
New York University School of Medicine;
St. Vincent's Hospital and Medical Center of
 New York
New York, NY

Dachling Pang, MD, FRCS(C), FACS
Associate Professor of Neurosurgery
University of Pittsburgh School of Medicine;
Chief of Pediatric Neurosurgery
Children's Hospital of Pittsburgh
Pittsburgh, Pa

Volker K. H. Sonntag, MD, FACS
Director, Spinal Cord Injury Service
Division of Neurological Surgery
Barrow Neurological Institute
Phoenix, Ariz

Robert G. Watkins, MD
Clinical Associate Professor of Orthopedic
 Surgery
University of Southern California School of
 Medicine
Los Angeles, Calif

AANS Publications Committee

Robert H. Wilkins, MD, Chairman
Michael L. J. Apuzzo, MD
Daniel L. Barrow, MD
Paul R. Cooper, MD
Setti S. Rengachary, MD
Thoralf M. Sundt, Jr., MD
Edward Tarlov, MD

Preface

The management of patients with posttraumatic instability of the spine has undergone dramatic changes in the past two decades. Computerized tomography (CT) has enabled us to accurately define the bony anatomy of spinal injuries; magnetic resonance imaging (MRI), because of its ability to accurately define the relationship between the spinal cord and its bony surroundings, has virtually eliminated the need for myelography.

These advances, along with an increased understanding of biomechanics and a critical analysis of past treatment successes and failures, have led to a more rational and effective management of patients with spinal instability. Refinement of well-established operations and the rapid development of a plethora of instrumentation techniques for stabilization of the spine have truly revolutionized the care of patients with posttraumatic instability.

The eminent neurosurgical and orthopedic contributors to this volume discuss these advances in detail and provide the reader with a firm foundation for understanding the state-of-the-art management of patients with spinal instability.

Paul R. Cooper, MD
Editor

CHAPTER 1

Early Assessment, Transport, and Management of Patients with Posttraumatic Spinal Instability

Randall M. Chesnut, MD, and Lawrence F. Marshall, MD

The well-being of the spinal cord injury patient, as with any accident victim, begins at the moment of first contact by the medical team and depends on careful, continuous, and vigilant care from that point through resuscitation and stabilization. Due to the marginal recuperative abilities of the central nervous system, prevention of further insults to the damaged spinal cord plays a crucial role in optimizing the outcome of these patients. While it is notable that recent advances in prehospital trauma care have markedly increased survival from severe trauma,[1,2] 29% of patients suffering spinal cord injury die prior to reaching a hospital.[3] We have addressed this critical period by dividing it into the accident scene itself, transport, and initial hospital resuscitation and address these separately below.

Accident Scene

A primary tool in the recognition of actual or potential spinal cord injury by the responding emergency medical services team is a high index of suspicion. As noted above, motor vehicle accidents, falls, gunshot wounds, and trauma related to water sports commonly result in spinal column injury,[4] but as it is not possible to satisfactorily rule out spinal injury in the field, accident victims of any sort must be assumed to have an unstable spine until proven otherwise. Increased awareness of the need for stabilization prior to mobilization has been associated with a decline in complete spinal cord lesions from 50% to 39%.[5]

In the setting of an automobile accident, if the automobile requires towing, the incidence of cervical spine injury in the victim is 1 in 300. Ejection increases the risk of spinal injury by a factor of 36.[6] For the victims wearing seat belts, the type of restraint may dictate the resultant spinal injury. Lap belts are associated with flexion-distraction fractures at the thoracolumbar junction, often with injuries to adjacent viscera suggested by ecchymosis across the anterior iliac crests and lower abdomen.[7-10] The three-point, lap-shoulder belt is associated with cervical injury via two postulated mechanisms: (1) restraint of the victim's chest with free movement above the cervicothoracic junction allows hyperflexion-distraction vectors to produce cervical spine fractures, dislocations, or subluxations[11]; (2) alternatively, should the victim slide under the cross-chest restraint the chin may be caught and the neck forcibly hyperextended.[12]

The unrestrained motorcycle victim is characteristically thrown over the handlebars, landing on his head or shoulder, resulting in hyperflexion-compression injuries to the thoracolumbar spine. For helmeted victims, face shield models are less frequently associated with cervical spine injury than are open-faced helmets.[13]

A particularly difficult situation is the victim who has suffered concomitant spinal and head injuries.[14,15] The unconscious patient cannot complain of axial skeletal pain or neurological symptoms; the confused, combative patient combines similar diagnostic difficulties but also risks exacerbating the injury by uncontrolled movements. All head-injured patients should therefore be assumed to have spinal cord injuries and be appropriately stabilized until definitive diagnostic studies can be performed.

Initial Evaluation and Treatment

In any emergency response protocol, the primary goal is the preservation of life. The need for a primary ABC survey applies to the suspected spinal cord injury patient as to any other accident victim. Because aspiration and shock are the primary causes of death in spinal cord injury victims before they arrive at the hospital, pulmonary and circulatory management are crucial. If the airway is adequate on initial assessment, the patient should be stabilized and secured "as he lies" and supplemental oxygen administered via face mask or nasal cannula. If the airway is compromised, the chin lift should be substituted for the jaw thrust or neck extension as the initial maneuver aimed at clearing the airway. This minimizes the chance of inadvertently mobilizing an unstable cervical spine injury. If this is inadequate to restore satisfactory ventilation, gentle manual traction should be applied in line with the axial skeleton and intubation performed. Axial traction is used solely for stabilization and must not be overly vigorous; serious vertebral distraction can result from even moderate traction during intubation.[16]

Intubation may be required because of airway compromise, inadequate ventilation from intercostal or diaphragmatic muscular paralysis, or a depressed level of consciousness. In all accident victims and especially in the patient with a cervical spine injury, this must be accomplished with complete stabilization of the head and neck. Nasotracheal intubation is easier than oral intubation, does not require hyperextension, and diminishes the likelihood of aspiration,[17] but the patient must have spontaneous respirations. If such is not the case, laryngoscopically guided orotracheal intubation will be required and should be performed gently, with the head and neck immobilized by an assistant. Cricothyroidotomy should be avoided if possible as the wound compromises later anterior approaches to the cervical spine.

Shock is not only a significant cause of early mortality in patients with spinal cord injury but may decrease the likelihood of optimal outcome.[18] Hypotension associated with spinal cord injury and multiple trauma may be hypovolemic or cardiogenic.[19] Hypovolemic hypotension can be a sequela of hemorrhage or be neurogenic in nature; loss of peripheral sympathetic drive with decreased peripheral vascular resistance results in venous pooling and decreased cardiac preload.[20]

Initial therapy for hypovolemic shock of either etiology should follow routine protocols of intravascular volume expansion, positioning, and military anti-shock trousers (MAST) application. Intravenous access should be rapidly gained and administration of isotonic fluids initiated. The Trendelenburg position will increase central venous return in addition to diminishing the risk of aspiration. Although neurologic deterioration has been associated with inflation of MAST trousers, which include a posterior (thoracolumbar) bladder, newer designs eliminate this compartment, diminishing the likelihood of inadvertently mobilizing the spine during inflation.[21]

Cardiogenic shock is caused by loss of the sympathetic antagonism of descending vagal negative influences, with resultant bradycardia despite concomitant hypotension. Increasing the filling pressure by volume expansion will counteract this to some extent by means of the Starling mechanism. For hypotension accompanied by bradycardia that does not adequately respond to volume expansion, intravenous atropine (0.5–1.0 mg IV) or glycopyrolate (0.1 mg IV) (Robinul; A.H. Robbins, Richmond, Virginia) may be required. Spinal shock should respond to the above measures and lack of such response usually suggests inadequate intravascular volume expansion. The use of intravenous inotropes to treat hypotension associated with spinal cord injury should be a last resort.

A rapid head-to-toe secondary survey should be performed at the accident scene and may provide clues to vertebral or spinal cord trauma. Scalp injuries suggest possible cervical spine injury and its mechanism. The lower abdominal ecchymoses often associated with thoracolumbar seat-belt trauma have been mentioned already. Axial tenderness or deformity are also important, but immobilization must not be compromised during any such examination. Motor or sensory deficits imply neurological damage and are clues to the level of injury. Finally, the patient's temperature should be assessed as sympathetic nervous system damage results in virtual poikilothermia, and external warming or cooling may be necessary to maintain normal body temperature.

Occasionally, patients with acute spinal cord injuries or spinal column injuries who are entirely awake will hold the head in a specific position other than neutral. If patients are comfortable in that position, it is important for prehospital and in-hospital personnel not to attempt to manipulate the neck back into a position of neutrality against the patient's wishes. The patient is obviously splinting against the possibility of further injury and this should not be violated.

Stabilization for Transport

Barring the presence of extreme extenuating circumstances such as fire, no patient should be moved before institution of rigorous spinal stabilization. While still in the vehicle, an intermediate (5-foot) radiolucent backboard can be passed beneath the victim. After immobilization of the thoracic spine, the cervical spine should be similarly restrained prior to moving the patient. Sandbags should be placed alongside the head and neck and then secured by 3-inch tape passed from one edge of the backboard, across the forehead, to the other edge of the backboard.[22] This method allows free motion of the jaw and lower face for airway control, while providing stability equal to rigid, external orthoses.[23] Soft collars do not provide significant immobilization and should not be used.[24,25]

A useful alternative to the backboard is the Kendricks Extrication Device, a close-fitting jacket with extensions behind and on both sides of the neck, allowing rigid stabilization of the entire spinal column. It also may be applied in the vehicle and can be attached to a hoist for use in extrication. Other devices used in extrication are the scoop-sled stretcher and the Stokes litter. The scoop-sled stretcher breaks apart longitudinally in the midline and can be assembled underneath a patient without mobilizing the spine. Care must be taken in its application, however, to ensure proper midline support before lifting the patient. The Stokes litter is a meshwork metal basket that comes up around the sides of the patient, affording some protection during difficult extrications such as may occur during helicopter evacuations. Spinal immobilization must be carried out prior to placing the patient inside the basket.

Prior to extrication and transport, the patient must be securely fastened to the transport device and able to withstand complete inversion without loss of immobilization. Either cloth tape or nylon seat-belt webbing should be employed to prevent loosening due to difficulties in transport or a combative patient.

Transport

In most cases, the initial response team will arrive via ambulance and must be equipped and prepared for evaluation, stabilization, extrication, and transportation. In many systems the team will have the option of calling in a helicopter and mobilizing primary air evacuation. This is particularly useful when distance or special technical difficulties mitigate against successful ground transportation.

In either case, during transportation the patient will be contained in a confined space, which will make many medical maneuvers more difficult and some nearly impossible. Therefore, although time is certainly at a premium, difficulties must be anticipated and prevented prior to transportation. In the case of the spinal cord injured patient, several special circumstances must be addressed. Since the patient is fully immobilized, it is necessary to prevent any possibility of the immobilization device breaking free within the transportation vehicle in the event of an accident or unstable transport conditions.

Given the frequency of occurrence and high morbidity of early pulmonary problems in such patients, facilities for treatment of regurgitation and prevention of aspiration should be available at all times. Finally, if there is a question about the adequacy of the airway or of respiratory mechanics, intubation should be performed prior to loading the patient into the carrier to avoid the necessity of a difficult and hazardous emergency intubation en route.

Hospital Course

Initial Evaluation and Resuscitation

Upon arrival at the trauma center, the patient with a suspected or confirmed spinal injury must be subjected to the same thorough trauma evaluation afforded any multiple trauma patient, regardless of the time since the accident. A period of stable vital signs following trauma does not imply absence of serious injury, particularly in a patient with damage to the central nervous system. It is important to avoid focusing exclusively on the spinal cord injury until other injuries have been diagnosed or ruled out. The primary goal during the initial hospital resuscitation is preservation of life. Although the potential of spinal injury must be kept in mind, the strict rules of immobilization must not prevent lifesaving maneuvers from being expeditiously carried out. In an attempt to facilitate such resuscitations, a series of algorithms have been constructed to serve as guidelines (Figures 1-4).

The procedures performed during the initial resuscitation will combine maneuvers applicable to trauma patients in general and spinal cord injured patients in particular. Reassessment of the airway and of respiratory function, with intubation, if necessary, is a first priority. The same guidelines followed in the field apply to the trauma receiving team. Strict immobilization is critical and the nasotracheal route of intubation is preferred. If difficulties arise, intubation over a flexible fiberoptic bronchoscope is very useful.

Maintenance of blood pressure within normal limits is crucial.[26] The legs should be wrapped to increase central venous return, Trendelenburg position should be maintained as required until blood pressure is stabilized, bradycardia should be treated if it is contributory, and the adequacy of fluid replacement should be determined by central venous pressure monitoring. If the blood pressure remains low, a pressor such as dopamine should be started and titrated to effect. If pressors are required, a Swan-Ganz catheter should be inserted to monitor left-sided filling pressure and cardiodynamics.

A Foley catheter should be placed to monitor urine outflow and to prevent bladder distention in patients with neurogenic urinary retention. A thoracic sensory deficit will block painful stimuli arising from intraabdominal injuries and spinal shock will prevent the development of abdominal muscular rigidity. Diagnostic peritoneal lavage or abdominal computed tomography (CT) scanning should be performed in any confused or unconscious patient, or in any patient whose neurologic dysfunction may mask intraabdominal pathology. A trauma skeletal x-ray series should be performed as indicated. This is particularly important in the presence of a neurological deficit as 11% of fractures associated with a head or spinal cord injury are missed.[27] Finally, euthermia should be restored, if absent, by external warming, warmed IV fluids, and heated inspired air if the patient is mechanically ventilated.

In the worst case scenario, the patient must be rapidly transported to the operating room for emergent, lifesaving surgery. In this situation, anteroposterior and lateral radiographs of the cervical spine should be obtained as soon as possible. The thoracolumbar area should also be imaged in the emergency area or the operating room. Further diagnostic studies such as oblique films or CT scanning are performed after the patient is medically stabilized.

In the less emergent situation, the patient can be rapidly assessed from a multi-systems viewpoint and the axial skeleton and spinal cord investigated in an orderly manner. If the patient is alert and oriented, a full neurological examination can be carried out with his cooperation and the presence or absence of spinal cord injury can be definitively assessed. However, if the patient is combative or unconscious a spinal injury must be assumed to be present until specifically ruled out. Such patients, as well as those with significant sensory deficits, also present special hazards during transportation and positioning for special studies due to the difficulty of diagnosing subtle neurological changes in the absence of patient feedback. A systematic approach should allow most, if not all, diagnostic studies to be carried out with the patient still secured in the initial immobilization device. In such a case, the spinal injury patient will require only one early transfer from the backboard to the bed designated for further care.

Nursing and General Care

From the time of admission through the patient's discharge, it is important to provide proper and thorough medical and nursing care to the spinal cord injured patient. These patients are uniquely susceptible to pulmonary, genitourinary, hematologic, and dermatologic complications. Early efforts at prevention are very important in facilitating subsequent mobilization and rehabilitation.

Choice of Bed

A basic but important aspect of treatment is the choice of the bed for immobilization and nursing. The two most commonly used specialized beds are the Stryker Frame (Stryker Corporation, Kalamazoo, Michigan) and the kinetic therapy bed (Rotobed, Roto-Rest Kinetic Treatment Table, Kinetic Concepts, Inc., San Antonio, Texas). Although both have seen extensive use, there have been significant questions raised recently about the adequacy of the Stryker Frame in immobilizing unstable injuries of the cervical or lumbar spine.[28,29] We now employ the Rotobed exclusively and find its stability and simplicity greatly facilitate immobilization, pulmonary toilet, and nursing care. It facilitates chest physiotherapy and reduces the incidence of pulmonary complications.[30] The slow rotation is well tolerated in the majority of patients and the arc is adjustable as required.

Pulmonary Care

Aggressive pulmonary care of the spinal cord injured patient is critical, particularly for the patient with injury to the cervical spinal cord. Mobilization of secretions, adequate lung expansion, and avoidance of ventilation-perfusion mismatching must be facilitated by patient positioning without compromising immobilization of the unstable spine. Use of the Rotobed must be supplemented by adequate hydration, incentive spirometry, avoidance of aspiration, and close monitoring for signs of ventilatory compromise, atelectasis, or pneumonia.

Transcutaneous oxygen saturation should be monitored during the early course of all high spinal cord injury patients. Frequent monitoring of peak expiratory flow rate (PEFR) and vital capacity by bedside spirometry are useful monitoring adjuncts in the patient with cervical spinal cord injury. Any deterioration in the ability to perform these tasks should be immediately investigated. The altered ventilatory mechanics often present in spinal cord injured patients may result in poor or unevenly distributed lung expansion or the inability to effectively clear the airway by coughing. Atelectasis is therefore a constant threat and, when discovered, should be treated with respiratory therapy, increased incentive spirometry, and flexible bronchoscopy if necessary.

Pneumonia is also a serious risk, particularly in the intubated or mechanically ventilated patient, and should be diagnosed and treated early and rapidly when it occurs. Finally, deterioration in respiratory function may result from ascension of the spinal cord injury itself and, in this setting, requires both pulmonary therapy and investigation into the mechanism of this ascension.

The Gastrointestinal System

During the early post-spinal cord injury period, a nasogastric tube and low, constant suction are routinely used to decompress the stomach until gastrointestinal function has returned. This minimizes the risk of vomiting and aspiration. Gastric pH is monitored and maintained above 5.0 with antacids and/or H_2 receptor blockers.

The Urinary System

A Foley urinary drainage catheter is generally inserted upon admission for monitoring of fluid output and prevention of bladder distention from retained urine. The indwelling catheter is later removed and replaced by intermittent catheterization each 4 to 6 hours to keep bladder volumes less than 200 cc. Urinary acidification is accomplished by administration of 500 mg of vitamin C every 6 hours. Prophylactic antibiotic treatment is not employed; with careful attention to the urinary tract of the spinal cord injured patient, urinary tract infections are no longer the major source of morbidity and mortality that they once were.

Venous Thromboembolism

Deep venous thrombosis occurs in approximately 15% of paralyzed patients and is accompanied by pulmonary embolism in about half that number.[31] Although optimally treated by low-dose heparin administration, anticoagulation is less desirable when there is acute trauma and anticipated surgery. Frequent movement of the lower extremities, early physical therapy, and pneumatic anti-embolism stockings (Venodyne Stockings, Kendall Co., Boston, Massachusetts) offer a useful alternative to heparinization during this early period.

Skin Care

Careful attention to skin integrity will prevent the development of decubitus ulcers during the period of immobilization. Use of the Rotobed to redistribute pressure is helpful, but frequent movement of the patient, and vigilance on the part of the nursing staff for early signs of pressure injury, are also necessary.

Nutrition

Inactivity, the stress of trauma, loss of muscle mass, and the caloric demands of associated injuries make the spinal cord injured patient prone to nutritional deficiency. Early nutritional assessment and institution of caloric replacement are important to weaning from the ventilator and maintaining the patient's ability to withstand subsequent surgery and rehabilitation. Total parenteral nutrition should be initiated early and be replaced by enteral nutrition via a feeding tube or oral intake after the resolution of gastric atony and intestinal stasis.

Autonomic Dysfunction

The potential for autonomic dysfunction arises after the disappearance of spinal shock. Seventy percent of patients with injuries above T7 are at risk.[32] Autonomic dysfunction occurs because the sympathetic reflexes below the level of injury are disconnected from descending control. It is manifested as significant hypertension with reflex bradycardia, profuse sweating, flushing of the skin, and severe headache. Hypertension can reach systolic levels of 300 mm/Hg and may lead to myocardial infarction or hypertensive intracerebral hemorrhage. It is frequently stimulated by bladder overdistention and, in such cases, is effectively treated by prompt bladder evacuation. If this is ineffective, sympatholytic antihypertensive agents should be administered.

Physical and Occupational Therapy

During the period of immobilization and acute treatment, flexibility and function must be maintained to facilitate rehabilitation later. Exercise and range of motion exercises may also diminish the risk of venous thromboembolism and boost patient morale. Well before the anticipated time of discharge from the acute care setting, the rehabilitation team should work with the patient to ease the transition to this important phase of treatment. This is particularly important if rehabilitation is to be carried out at a separate institution.

Patient Emotional Support

Drastic changes in lifestyle are inevitable in patients with spinal cord injuries. The patient and family members should be helped to understand the injury, treatment, and prognosis from the earliest opportunity. Given the shock and denial common during this period, ensuring their understanding often requires numerous and repetitive interactions between patient, family, and the medical staff. Patience and understanding are needed from all care-givers. In addition, sufficient communication must exist between members of the patient care team to assure that they all have a similar understanding of the situation and are unified in their presentations to the patient and family. A social worker and psychologist or psychiatrist should be available to the patient and his family early in the treatment. Emotional rehabilitation should begin immediately, as it will influence all subsequent aspects of patient care.

Timing of Imaging Studies

In a patient with a suspected or proven injury to the vertebral column or spinal cord, the diagnosis must be made and therapy instituted in the most expeditious manner consistent with the safety of the patient. Initial plain radiographs are easily obtained with the patient remaining on the backboard used for transport. The patient should also undergo CT scanning while still on the backboard in order to minimize the number of transfers. Gardner-Wells tongs (Ruggles Corporation, North Quincy, Massachusetts) can be applied and traction initiated on the backboard. In many cases, this approach can limit the transfers to the single instance of placing the patient in his hospital bed. Tomography can also be performed on the backboard, as can MRI scanning if the backboard is completely nonferrous. The latter two studies, however, are rarely as important as the CT scan in establishing the initial diagnosis. In general, following an expeditiously performed CT study, further imaging should be deferred in the interest of initiating definitive patient immobilization.

MRI, Myelography, and Early Surgery

If the neurological deficit is unexplained by radiographic findings, further studies should be considered to rule out compression of the spinal cord from a disc herniation, extra-axial hematoma, or bony spicule. Myelography requires significant patient manipulation, introduction of contrast material into the subarachnoid space around an injured spinal cord, and time to perform. Myelography should usually be reserved for patients who retain some neurological function below the level of the injury, whose CT scan does not reveal neural compression, and in those patients who experience neurological deterioration while being well immobilized.

The role of MRI in acute spinal cord injury remains undefined. Preliminary reports suggest that MRI will demonstrate all of the lesions sensitive to myelography,[33] as well as intramedullary pathology such as edema and hematomyelia.[34] MRI is noninvasive and involves significantly less patient manipulation than myelography. Unfortunately, it is not usually readily available for immediate use and is difficult if not impossible to perform safely on patients requiring intensive care or metallic life-support devices. Therefore in the immediate postinjury period MRI is best considered investigational and should be performed only if immediately available to a patient with a stable injury and an unexplained or progressive neurological deficit.

Stabilization is generally easily achieved by immobilization in bed; surgical stabilization is rarely necessary as an emergency procedure. The major indication for early surgical intervention in spinal cord trauma is the hope of restoring or preserving function. However, there is little substantive evidence that early decompression is accompanied by better outcome and there is an increased incidence of postoperative pulmonary and neurologic complications in spinal cord injury patients operated upon within the first week.[35,36]

We feel that the optimal treatment for these patients is immobilization in a Rotobed with attentive nursing and close observation for the first 7 to 10 postinjury days. After this period of observation, any planned operative stabilization, with or without concomitant decompression, may be carried out on a medically stabilized patient with less risk of coincident pulmonary or neurologic complications. The utility of early surgery for decompression and stabilization is controversial and no controlled clinical trials have been performed comparing early and late decompression and stabilization.

Although we feel that acute decompression is generally not indicated, there are patients who may benefit from elective decompression: those with an incomplete lesion who "plateau" in their recovery phase, or those who show neurological deterioration despite satisfactory immobilization and care. These patients should be studied by MRI or by myelography with water soluble contrast material if MRI is not available. If a compressive lesion or hematomyelia is disclosed, the patient should undergo decompression.

Patient Transfers

Patient transfers are hazardous when there is an unstable spinal column injury. Strict axial alignment without rotation must be maintained at all times. Mechanical devices such as slider-boards maintain a rigid undersurface and facilitate stable patient movement. If manual transfer is performed, there must be adequate manpower to prevent any possibility of violating skeletal immobilization. It is often best to place one person at the head of the bed to manage the cervical spine, and four sturdy people on one side of the patient to all work their hands completely under the patient and then lift in concert from the one side. This allows a sixth party to remove the gurney or other device from underneath the suspended patient and replace it with the bed, without requiring the group holding the patient to move.

Tongs and Traction Reduction of Cervical Spine Injuries

Following the initial general and cervical radiographic evaluation of the patient with an unstable cervical vertebral injury, Gardner-Wells tongs should be applied and traction initiated. Pin placement should be just above the pinnae of the ears on an imaginary plane connecting the mastoid processes and the external auditory canals. Once the tongs have been applied under local anesthesia, traction should be initiated in the plane passing through the cervical articulations and the pin sites, and an initial tong-placement lateral cervical radiograph obtained.

The amount of weight to be applied varies with the level of injury and the amount of suspected ligamentous disruption. When there is significant ligamentous damage, minimal weight should be used initially to avoid overdistraction and potential neurological deterioration. This is particularly true when the actual or suspected fracture is located at a high cervical level. When any uncertainty exists, it is best to start with 5 lbs for upper cervical levels and 10 lbs for lower levels, and await the initial radiograph. Following the application of traction, manipulations of weight or traction axis should be guided by serial radiographs.

After traction has been applied, the timing of further studies may be considered. If the patient requires reduction, he should be transferred directly to a Rotobed (or Stryker Frame if this is the only alternative) using the tongs to assist in stable transfer. If reduction is not required and CT scanning is readily available, tong-traction should be maintained while the patient is scanned on the backboard and subsequently transferred to the nursing bed (Rotobed or Stryker Frame). The need for further studies and the transfers involved can then be determined and performed as necessary.

Traction strategies may be altered to treat a specific fracture/dislocation. For hyperextension injuries where the anterior longitudinal ligaments are disrupted, application of a traction axis posterior to the plane described above may be required to regain normal anatomic alignment. Pin placement slightly behind that recommended above may be used to maintain an attitude of slight flexion. Management of unilateral or bilateral locked facets also may require posterior (flexion) movement of the traction vector during reduction, and is the second instance where posterior pin placement may be appropriate.

Considerable controversy exists as to the optimal methods for traction-reduction in these circumstances. Traction is initially applied in line with the cervical spine and, with careful and frequent radiographic monitoring, the weight is increased until reduction occurs or a maximum weight is reached. The general guideline is a maximum of 5 lbs/vertebral level above the fracture/dislocation. As one approaches this weight, consideration should be directed to alteration of the traction axis with radiographic guidance. The amount of weight that may be used in attempting closed reduction of cervical vertebral dislocations is the subject of considerable controversy. In general, 60 to 80 lbs, depending on the build of the patient, would be a reasonable absolute limit.

The use of muscle relaxants such as diazepam is common during such procedures, but carries the hazards of (1) clouding patient feedback and the neurological examination, and (2) precipitously dropping the paraspinous muscle tension and allowing overdistraction to occur without a change in the applied weight. Therefore, muscle relaxants must be administered slowly and cautiously. Manipulation of the spine has also been advocated, but its utility has not been well established and, in the absence of well-defined techniques and guidelines, cannot be generally recommended. Finally, as the upper levels of weight are approached, or the amount of weight is limited by patient discomfort or radiographic evidence of excessive distraction, the possibility of operative reduction should be addressed. If reduction is accomplished using traction, the weight should be slowly reduced to or slightly below 5 lbs/level to maintain alignment.

Multiple Level Spinal Column Injuries

Radiographic evaluation of the patient with suspected or proven spinal axis injury must include the entire vertebral column. For the entire spine, multiple noncontiguous fractures separated by an area of normal spine have been reported to occur in 4% to 5% of cases.[37-40] Preliminary data from the National Collaborative Spinal Cord Injury Study suggest that this is an underestimate; that study demonstrated an incidence of approximately 13%. Calenoff et al studied 30 patients with spinal cord injury with multiple noncontiguous vertebral fractures.[40] They reported that for patients whose neurological level identifies and focuses attention on a select region of the vertebral axis (primary injury), a significant number of secondary injuries are missed at the time of the initial evaluation. One clue to the likelihood of a secondary injury was the presence of a primary injury at the T2-T7 level, which although comprising less than 5% of all spinal column injuries, accounted for almost 50% of primary injuries in one series of spinal cord injured patients with multiple level fractures. They identified three patterns of multiple level injury and pointed out the importance of careful attention to the distal ends of the vertebral column, as almost half of the secondary injuries in their series occurred at C1, C2, L4, or L5.

Combined Head and Spinal Cord Injury

Minor head injury occurs in a minimum of 25% and perhaps as many as 50% of patients suffering acute spinal cord injury, particularly when the cervical spine is involved. The combination of spinal cord injury and severe head injury, defined as a Glasgow Coma Scale score of 8 or less, is less common, with a frequency of 2% to 3%. This is probably in part a reflection of the extremely high prehospital mortality of the two injuries when combined. Nevertheless, the cognitive deficits that complicate head injury are often severely exacerbated by the motor deficits that result from the spinal cord injury. These factors need to be taken into account in the initial assessment of such patients. Documentation of the level of brain function is very important, as it sometimes becomes a significant issue later.

Pharmacologic Treatment of Spinal Cord Injury

The role of induced hypertension in the treatment of spinal cord trauma is an unresolved issue. Spinal cord injury results in severe focal ischemia and loss of autoregulation.[37-39] Models of spinal cord injury have demonstrated that blood flow and oxygen content of damaged tissue could be increased by elevation of systemic arterial pressure, although it has not proven possible to restore normal perfusion parameters by this method.[40-42] In light of such evidence and given the well-known adverse effect of hypotension on injured cerebral nervous tissue, it has been advocated by some that mild hypertension be maintained in spinal cord injury patients during their early postinjury course. We generally employ adequate volume replacement supplemented by dopamine or Neo-Synephrine (Winthrop-Breon Laboratories, New York, New York) to keep the patient's mean arterial pressure at 100 mm/Hg for the initial 72 hours. Although this has not been well studied in the clinical setting, we have seen cases in which neurological function seemed to be sensitive to the increased perfusion pressure. Given its unproven status, however, it is important to avoid jeopardizing the patient in any way by such treatment. High doses or stronger pressors are not employed, and the presence of advanced age, cardiac disease, or other risk factors are felt to be an absolute contraindication at this point.

Early Assessment, Transport, and Management

A considerable interest has been generated in the possibility of pharmacologic manipulation of the injured spinal cord by reports that glucocorticoids[43,44] and the opioid antagonist naloxone[45-47] are beneficial in experimental spinal cord trauma. However, there are now other studies that show that glucocorticoids[48-50] or naloxone[51-53] is ineffective.

The National Collaborative Spinal Cord Injury Study has just concluded a prospective, randomized, double-blind trial employing three arms of treatment: placebo, high-dose naloxone, and high-dose methylprednisolone. The results of this study have not yet been published, and although treatment with naloxone was ineffective, high-dose methylprednisolone administration was associated with improved outcome. The degree of improvement in individual patients has not been determined, so that the actual clinical applicability of these data is as yet undefined.

Treatment Specific to Vertebral Column or Spinal Cord Injury

The algorithms presented in Figures 1-4 are partitioned into cervical and thoracolumbar injuries, and further divided into spinal column injuries and spinal cord injuries. Two or more different axial injuries may coexist and this will necessitate combining protocols.

Suspected Cervical Spine Injury

For the neurologically intact patient with symptoms related to the neck, immobilization of the cervical spine should be maintained and plain radiographs taken in the lateral, anteroposterior, and odontoid views (Figure 1). If these are normal, oblique and pillars views should be obtained. If these additional studies reveal no fracture, the patient should be maintained in a hard collar for 24-48 hours or until paraspinous muscle

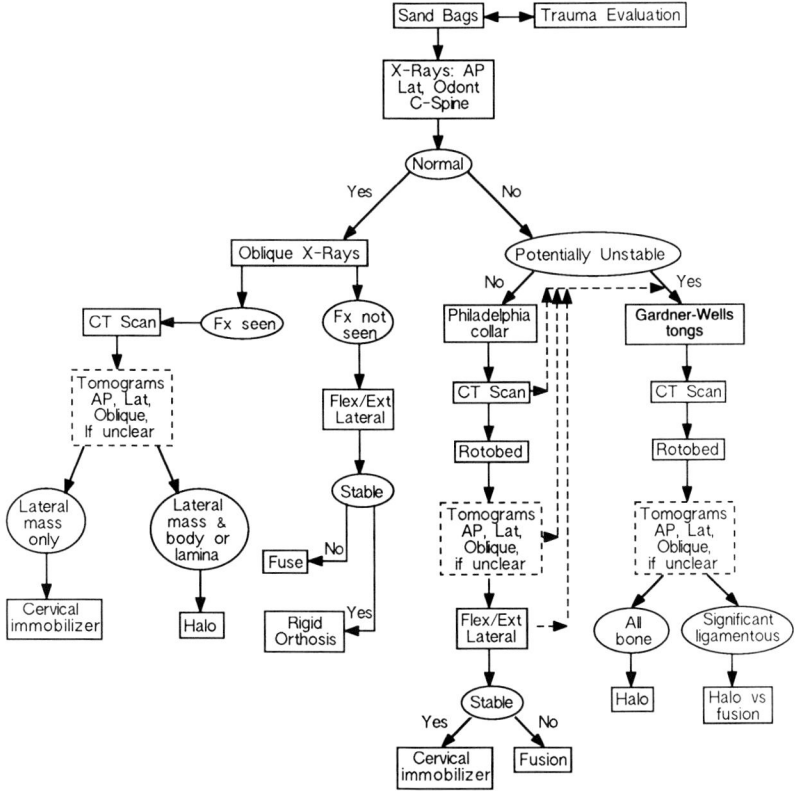

Figure 1. Algorithm for management of the patient with suspected cervical spine injury without neurological deficit.

spasm diminishes and flexion-extension films are taken. If this interval is not allowed the patient with cervical spinal pain, the physiologic "splint" afforded by the spasm in the cervical paraspinals will prevent adequate flexion and extension and these studies will not be sufficient to rule out instability. In contrast, the patient with protracted pain and muscle spasm is not infrequently physiologically splinting a painful instability. This patient must be kept immobilized and observed until the spasm abates or diagnosis is made.

If a high level of suspicion remains despite adequate, negative flexion-extension views, a White-Panjabi stretch test may be performed.[24] If no instability is demonstrated, the patient may be treated with cervical immobilization using a hard collar. If instability is revealed, despite the absence of a proven fracture, the injury is ligamentous and will usually require fusion.

If a fracture or subluxation is found, the anatomy must be adequately defined and stability determined prior to deciding on therapy. If anatomical abnormalities suggestive of instability are revealed by CT, the patient should be placed in Gardner-Wells tongs and traction, and nursed on a Rotobed or Stryker Frame with complete cervical spine immobilization. If further studies such as tomography are indicated, they can be performed under less duress at a later date, after the patient is medically stable.

Suspected Thoracolumbar Spine Injury

The initial evaluation of a patient with a suspected thoracolumbar spinal injury consists of anteroposterior (AP) and lateral

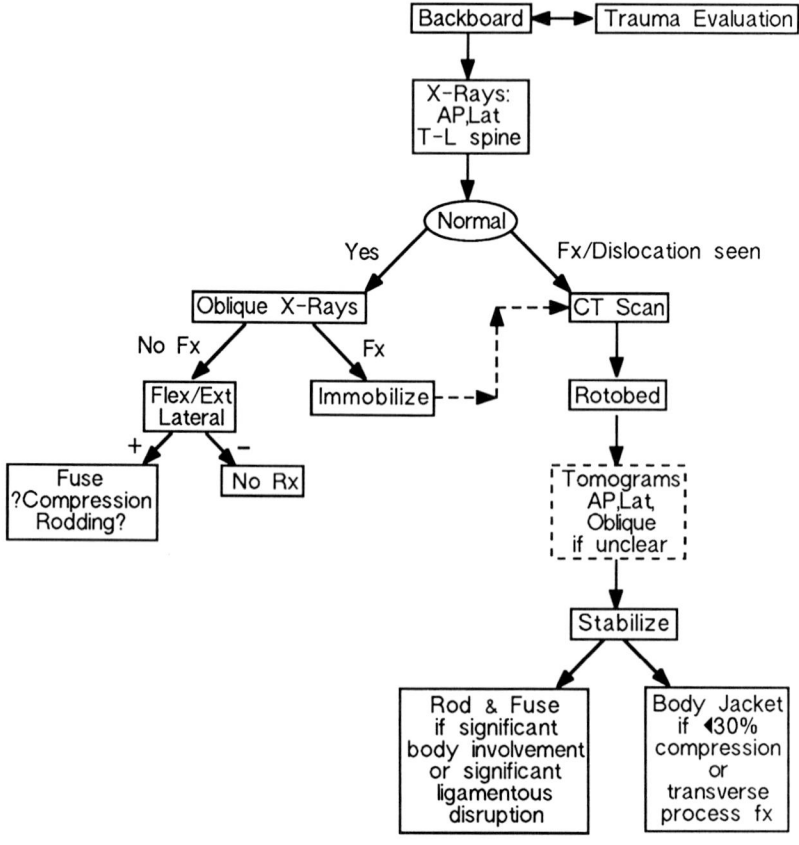

Figure 2. Algorithm for management of the patient with suspected thoracolumbar spine injury without neurological deficit.

radiographs (Figure 2). If no fracture or dislocation is disclosed, oblique views should be performed. If these too are negative, the patient should be nursed on a hard bed with thoracolumbar spine precautions until muscular spasm abates and flexion-extension lateral radiographs should then be obtained.

If a fracture or dislocation is discovered, the goals are again definition of anatomy, determination of stability, and prevention of further injury. The most revealing study at present is the CT scan, which can often be performed with the patient still on the transporting backboard, prior to transfer to bed. The CT scan, in conjunction with the plain radiographs, is generally sufficient to allow determination of stability and planning of the therapeutic approach. In those instances where this is not the case, tomography may be useful.

Cervical Spinal Cord Injury

In the patient with a neurological deficit, the emphasis changes from determining the presence of a bony lesion and preventing possible injury to defining the skeletal damage and minimizing or reversing the deficit. For the patient with a cervical spinal cord injury, the entire body must be maintained immobile during the diagnostic and prestabilization therapeutic period (Figure 3), utilizing a backboard and sandbags or a hard cervical collar plus forehead tape during evaluation, and a Rotobed or Stryker Frame with Gardner-Wells tongs and traction for nursing.

A thorough initial trauma evaluation must be carried out; concomitant with this, the baseline axial skeleton radiographs can be obtained, to include AP, lateral, odontoid, and oblique views of the cervical spine, and AP and lateral views of the thoracic and lumbar spine. Following the initial general physical and radiographic evaluation of the patient with a cervical spinal cord injury, Gardner-Wells tongs should be applied and traction initiated according to the principles discussed above. If the injury does not require reduction, a CT scan should be directly obtained with the patient still on the backboard. Following the scan, the patient is transferred to the nursing bed. If the injury does require reduction, a CT scan should be deferred unless it can be accomplished immediately. Such patients should be transferred to the nursing bed and undergo reduction as expeditiously as possible. Once reduced, the need for further imaging may be assessed by reviewing the studies already performed. Because we believe that surgery should be delayed for 7 to 10 days after injury in the case of spinal cord or unstable vertebral injuries at the cervical level, any supplemental imaging required for planning of stabilization may also be deferred in the interest of maintaining maximum immobilization during this critical early period.

Thoracolumbar Spinal Cord Injury

Like the patient with cervical cord damage, a victim of thoracolumbar spinal cord injury should remain immobilized on a backboard and receive a thorough admission trauma evaluation prior to evaluating the neurological injury (Figure 4). This should include diagnostic peritoneal lavage, if indicated, and x-rays of all skeletal elements distal to the neurological level.[27] If fracture or dislocation is disclosed by the initial radiographic studies, the patient should have a CT scan while still on the backboard and then be transferred to the Rotobed or Stryker Frame for further care. If indicated, further studies may be obtained subsequently under stable and controlled conditions.

If no fracture is found on initial evaluation, the patient should have a CT scan over the region suggested by his neurological deficit. If no lesion is demonstrated by CT, the patient should be placed in the Rotobed or Stryker Frame and arrangements made for myelography or MRI scanning. If no bony lesion or neural compression is discovered, flexion-extension films should be obtained 7 to 10 days following the injury. If this demonstrates significant ligamentous instability, fusion will be required; if no instability is re-

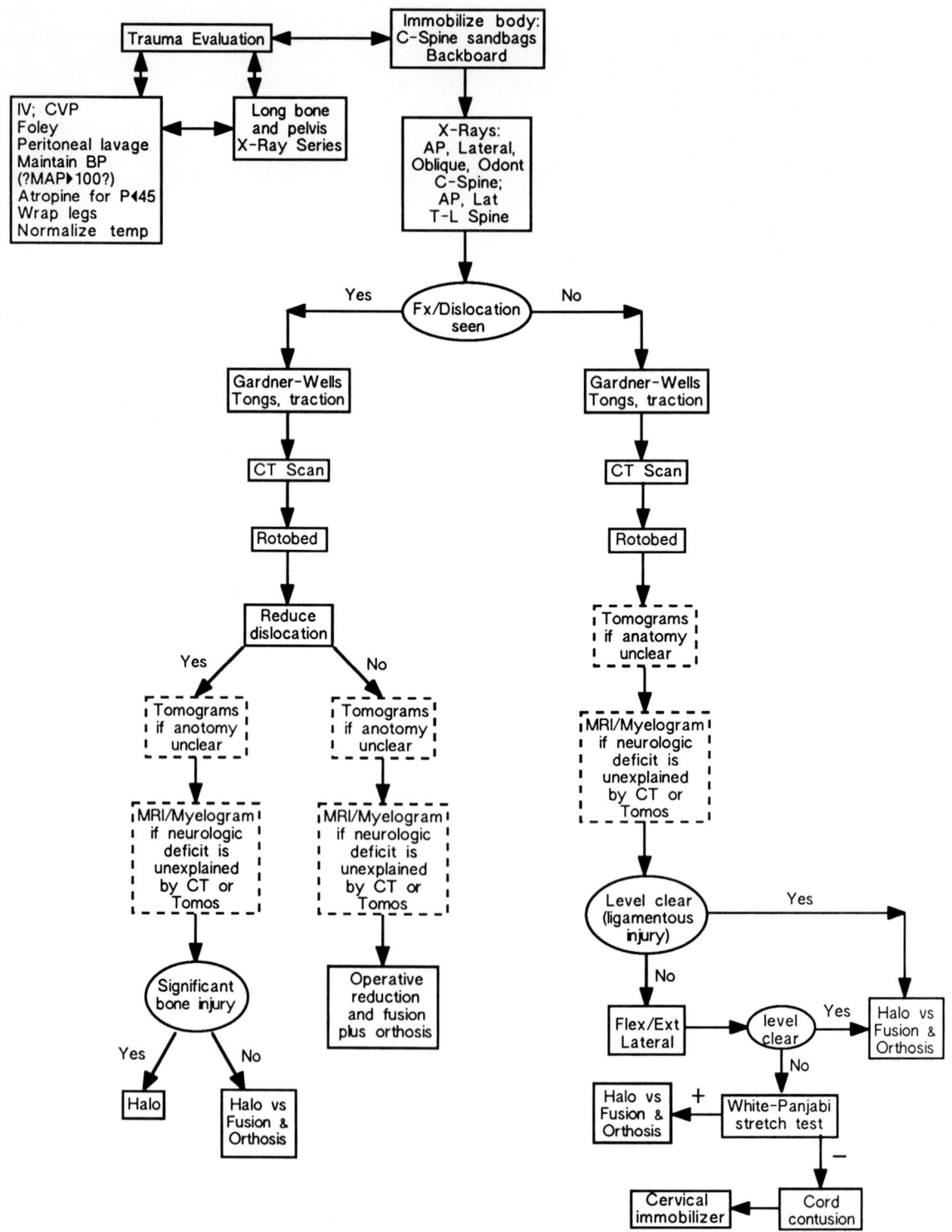

Figure 3. Algorithm for management of the patient with cervical spinal cord injury with neurological deficit.

Early Assessment, Transport, and Management

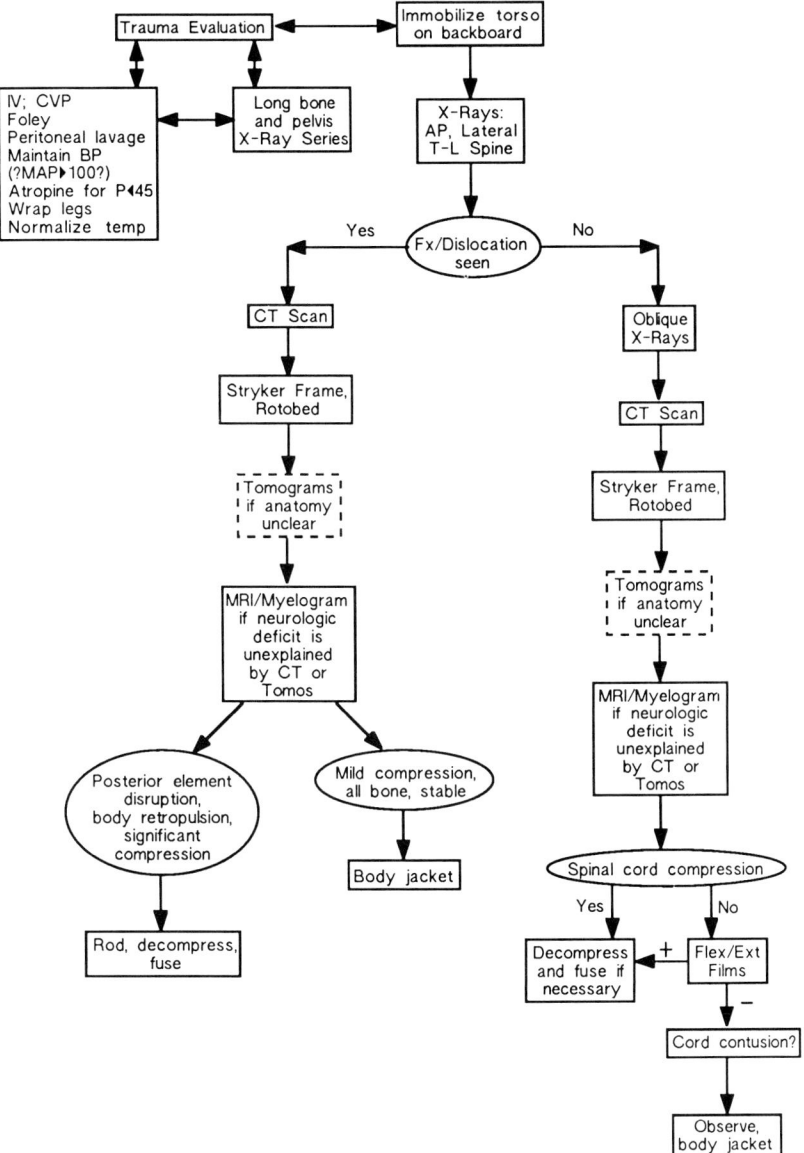

Figure 4. Algorithm for management of the patient with thoracolumbar spinal cord injury with neurological deficit.

vealed, observation in a body jacket is suggested.

References

1. Fortner GS, Oreskovich MR, Copass MK, Carrico CJ. The effects of prehospital trauma care on survival from a 50-meter fall. *J Trauma*. 1983;23:976-981.
2. Shackford SR, Mackersie RC, Hoyt DB, Baxt WG, Eastman AB, Hammill FN, Knotts FB, Virgilio RW. Impact of a trauma system on outcome of severely injured patients. *Arch Surg*. 1987;122:523-527.
3. Mesard L, Carmody A, Mannarino E, Ruge D. Survival after spinal cord trauma: a life table analysis. *Arch Neurol*. 1978;35:78-83.
4. Interdisciplinary, clinical, education, and research aspects of a regional center for the rehabilitation of spinal cord injured persons. Attending Staff Association for the Rancho Los Amigos Hospital, Los Angeles, 1969.
5. Gunby P. New focus on spinal cord injury. *JAMA*. 1981;245:1201-1206. Medical News.
6. Huelke DF, O'Day J, Mendelsohn RA. Cervical injuries suffered in automobile crashes. *J Neurosurg*. 1981;54:316-322.
7. Smith WS, Kaufer H. Patterns and mechanisms of lumbar injuries associated with lap seat belts. *J Bone Joint Surg Am*. 1969;51A:239-254.

8. Chance GQ. Note on a type of flexion fracture of the spine. *Br J Radiol.* 1948;21:452-453.
9. Rogers LF. The roentgenographic appearance of transverse or chance fractures of the spine: the seat belt fracture. *AJR.* 1971;111:844-849.
10. Pavlov H. Radiology for orthopaedic surgeons. *Contemp Orthop.* 1983;7:67-70.
11. Taylor TKF, Nade S, Bannister JH. Seat belt fractures of the cervical spine. *J Bone Joint Surg Br.* 1976;588:328-331.
12. Saldeen T. Fatal neck injuries caused by use of diagonal safety belts. *J Trauma.* 1967;7:856-862.
13. Yeo JD. Five-year review of spinal cord injuries in motorcyclists. *Med J Austr.* 1979;2:381.
14. Kraus JF, Franti CE, Riggins RS, Richards D, Borhani NO. Incidence of traumatic spinal cord lesions. *J Chronic Dis.* 1975;28:471-492.
15. Irving MH, Irving PM. Associated injuries in head trauma patients. *J Trauma.* 1967;7:500-511.
16. Bivins HG, Ford S, Bezmalinovic Z, Price HM, Williams JL. The effect of axial traction during orotracheal intubation of the trauma victim with an unstable cervical spine. *Ann Emerg Med.* 1988;17:25-29.
17. Sellick BA. Cricoid pressure to control regurgitation of stomach contents during induction of anaesthesia. *Lancet.* 1961;2:404-406.
18. Meguro K, Tator CH. Effect of multiple trauma on mortality and neurological recovery after spinal cord or cauda equina injury. *Neurol Med Chir Tokyo.* 1988;28:34-41.
19. Meyer GA, Berman IR, Doty DB, Moseley RV, Gutierrez VS. Hemodynamic responses to acute quadriplegia with or without chest trauma. *N Neurosurg.* 1971;34:168-177.
20. Troll GF, Dohrmann GJ. Anaesthesia of the spinal cord-injured patient: cardiovascular problems and their management. *Paraplegia.* 1975;13:162-171.
21. Rockwell DD, Butler AB, Keats TE, Edlich RF. An improved design of the pneumatic counter-pressure trousers. *Am J Surg.* 1982;143:377-379.
22. Dunford JY Jr. Spinal column trauma. In: Baxt WG, ed. *Trauma: The First Hour.* Norwalk, Conn: Appleton-Century-Crofts;1984:171-219.
23. Podolsky, Baraff LJ, Simon RR, et al. Efficacy of cervical spine immobilization methods. *J Trauma.* 1983;23:687-690.
24. White AA, Panjabi MM. *Clinical Biomechanics of the Spine.* Philadelphia, Pa: Lippincott;1978:345-359.
25. Johnson RM, Hart DL, Simmons EF, Ramsby GR, Southwick WO. Cervical orthoses: a study comparing their effectiveness in restricting cervical motion in normal subjects. *J Bone Joint Surg Am.* 1977;59A:332-339.
26. Bohlman HH, Ducker TB, Lucas JT. Spine and spinal cord injuries. In: Rothman RH, Simeone FA, eds. *The Spine.* 2nd ed. Philadelphia, Pa: WB Saunders Co; 1982;2:661-757.
27. Garland DE, Rhoades ME. Orthopedic management of brain-injured adults, part II. *Clin Orthop.* 1978;131:111-122.
28. McGuire RA, Green BA, Eismont FJ, Watts C. Comparison of stability provided to the unstable spine by the kinetic therapy table and the Stryker Frame. *Neurosurgery.* 1988;22:842-845.
29. Slabaugh PB, Nickel YL. Complications with use of the Stryker Frame. *J Bone Joint Surg Am.* 1978;60A:2222-2223.
30. Brackett TO, Condon N. Comparison of the wedge turning frame and kinetic treatment table in the acute care of spinal cord injury patients. *Surg Neurol.* 1984;22:53-56.
31. Casas ER, Sánchez MP, Arias CR, Masip JP. Prophylaxis of venous thrombosis and pulmonary embolism in patients with acute traumatic spinal cord lesions. *Paraplegia.* 1976;14:178-183.
32. Kurnick NB. Autonomic hyperreflexia and its control in patients with spinal cord lesions. *Ann Intern Med.* 1956;44:678-686.
33. Mirvis SE, Geisler FH, Jelinek JJ, Joslyn JJ. Acute cervical spine trauma: evaluation with 1.5-T MR imaging. *Radiology.* 1988;166:807-816.
34. Chakeres DW, Flickinger F, Bresnahan JC, Beattie MS, Weiss KL, Miller C. MR imaging of acute spinal cord trauma. *AJNR.* 1987;8:5-10.
35. Heiden JS, Weiss MH, Rosenberg AW, Apuzzo MLJ, Kurze T. Management of cervical spinal cord trauma in Southern California. *J Neurosurg.* 1975;43:732-736.
36. Marshall LF, Knowlton S, Garfin SR, Klauber MR, Eisenberg HM, Kopaniky D. Deterioration following spinal cord injury. *J Neurosurg.* 1987;66:400-404.
37. Bentley G, McSweeney T. Multiple spinal injuries. *Br J Surg.* 1968;55:565-570.
38. Blahd WH Jr, Iserson KY, Bjelland JC. Efficacy of the posttraumatic cross table lateral view of the cervical spine. *J Emerg Med.* 1985;2:243-249.
39. Kewalramani L, Taylor RG. Multiple non-contiguous injuries to the spine. *Acta Orthop Scand.* 1976;47:52-58.
40. Calenoff L, Chessare JW, Rogers LF, Toerge J, Rosen JS. Multiple level spinal injuries: importance of early recognition. *AJR.* 1978;130:665-669.
41. Sandler AN, Tator CH. Effect of acute spinal cord compression injury on regional spinal cord blood flow in primates. *J Neurosurg.* 1976;45:660-676.
42. Senter HJ, Yenes JL. Loss of autoregulation and posttraumatic ischemia following experimental spinal cord trauma. *J Neurosurg.* 1979;50:198-206.
43. Smith AJK, McCreery DB, Bloedel JR, Chou SN. Hyperemia, CO_2 responsiveness, and autoregulation in the white matter following experimental spinal cord injury. *J Neurosurg.* 1978;48:239-251.
44. Brodkey JS, Richards DE, Blasingame JP, and Nulsen FE. Reversible spinal cord trauma in cats: additive effects of direct pressure and ischemia. *J Neurosurg.* 1972;37:591-593.
45. Dolan EJ, Tator CH. The effect of blood transfusion, dopamine, and gamma hydroxybutyrate on posttraumatic ischemia of the spinal cord. *J Neurosurg.* 1982;56:350-358.
46. Hukuda S, Mochizuki T, Ogata M. Effects of hypertension and hypercarbia on spinal cord tissue oxygen in acute experimental spinal cord injury. *Neurosurgery.* 1980;6:639-643.
47. Ducker TB, Hamit HF. Experimental treatments of acute spinal cord injury. *J Neurosurg.* 1970;33:554-563.
48. Black P, Markowitz RS. Experimental spinal cord injury in monkeys: comparison of steroids and local hypothermia. *Surg Forum.* 1971;22:409-411.
49. Faden AI, Jacobs TP, Holaday JW. Opiate antagonist improves neurologic recovery after spinal injury. *Science.* 1981;211:493-494.
50. Faden AI, Jacobs TP, Mougey E, Holaday JW. En-

dorphins in experimental spinal injury: therapeutic effects of naloxone. *Ann Neurol.* 1981;10:326-332.
51. Faden Al. Opiate antagonists and thyrotropin releasing hormone. *JAMA.* 1984;252:1452-1454.
52. Ducker TB. Experimental injury of the spinal cord. In: Yinken PJ, Bruyn GW, eds. Handbook of Clinical Neurology. New York, NY: American Elsevier Publishing Co: 1976;25:9-26.
53. Ducker TB, Salcman M, Daniell HB. Experimental spinal cord trauma, III: therapeutic effect of immobilization and pharmacologic agents. *Surg Neurol.* 1978;10:71-76.
54. Young JS, Northrup EN. Statistical information pertaining to some of the most commonly asked questions about SCI. *SCI Dig.* 1979;1:11-31.
55. Gehweiler JA Jr, Clark WM, Schaaf RE, Powers B, Miller MD. Cervical spine trauma: the common combined conditions. *Radiology.* 1979;130:77-86.
56. Guttman L. History of the National Spinal Injuries Centre, Stoke Mandeville Hospital, Aylesbury. *Paraplegia.* 1967;5:115-126.
57. Guttman L. Spinal Cord Injuries: Comprehensive Management and Research. Oxford, England: Blackwell Scientific Publications; 1973.
58. Cheshire DJE. The complete and centralised treatment of paraplegia. *Paraplegia.* 1968;6:59-73.
59. American College of Surgeons. Techniques of helmet removal from injured patients. *Bull Am Coll Surg.* October 1980;65:19-21.
60. Kakulas BA, Bedbrook GM. Pathology of injuries of the vertebral column with emphasis on the macroscopical aspects. In: Yinken PJ, Bruyn GW, eds. *Handbook of Clinical Neurology.* New York, NY: American Elsevier Publishing Co.; 1976; 25 (pt 1):27-42.
61. Tarlov IM. *Spinal Cord Compression.* Springfield, Ill: Charles C Thomas; 1957.
62. Bracken MB, Collins WF, Freeman DF, Shepard MJ, Wagner FW, Silten RM, et al. Efficacy of methylprednisolone in acute spinal cord injury. *JAMA.* 1984;251:45-52.
63. Wallace MC, Tator CH. Failure of naloxone to improve spinal cord blood flow and cardiac output after spinal cord injury. *Neurosurgery.* 1986;18:428-432.
64. Black P, Markowitz RS, Keller S, Wachs K, Gillespie J, Finkelstein SD. Naloxone and experimental spinal cord injury, part 1: high dose administration in a static load compression model. *Neurosurgery.* 1986;19:905-908.
65. Black P, Markowitz RS, Keller S, Wachs K, Gillespie J, Finkelstein SD. Naloxone and experimental spinal cord injury, part 2: megadose treatment in a dynamic load model. *Neurosurgery.* 1986;19:909-913.

CHAPTER 2

Imaging and the Determination of Posttraumatic Spinal Instability

Wendy Cohen, MD

Introduction

Imaging of the patient with a presumed spinal injury should aim to diagnose the full extent of injury. Once diagnosed, the following questions will arise: Will a proposed treatment correct for the injury or is there a likelihood of worsening the patient's condition? Can the neurologic function of the patient be improved and can the spinal column be better aligned or rendered more stable? The answer to these questions requires evaluation of neurologic function and of skeletal anatomy. Prior to magnetic resonance imaging (MRI), imaging studies demonstrated anatomic disruptions of the bony spinal column. MRI now adds information about neural tissue and soft tissues of the spinal column. Although neurologic status is most significant, the type and severity of the injury to the vertebra, disc, and ligament will determine the necessity for stabilization as well as the likelihood that either acute progression or late deterioration of neurologic and spinal column function might occur.

A number of spinal imaging techniques are available. The use of any one of these techniques, the order of implementation, the reliability, and the accessibility varies with both modality and patient. The diagnostic difficulty may lie in choosing the most appropriate modality to help answer questions of fracture extent and stability. A component of this problem is an appreciation of the appropriate time to use any specific type of imaging modality. For example, plain radiographs might show an acute cervical fracture-dislocation with subluxation. The extent of the fracture would indicate ligamentous as well as bone injury. Flexion-extension films would be obviously contraindicated. The same patient, following an interval in a halo vest, may need to be evaluated for fracture healing. Now tomograms may be the best study to look for callus formation, but a flexion-extension study showing absence of motion across the fracture would more securely confirm functional healing. The imaging modalities currently available are well known: plain radiographs, flexion-extension films, fluoroscopic/cine motion examinations, computerized tomography (CT), myelography without or with CT, and MRI.

Stability Defined

The definition of "stability" varies among authors. White et al[1] defined "clinical stability" as the ability of the spine under physiologic loads to prevent displacements which would injure or irritate neural tissue. In the clinical setting they suspected that there would be potential instability if cord or root damage were present with a fracture-dislocation.[2] More recently, Denis separated instability into mechanical, neurologic, and combined types.[3] Mechanical instability implied that the spine could buckle or angulate. Neurologic instability meant that neural tissues were at risk for the development of an injury at any time following the initial trauma, including the late development of neural dysfunction. The combined form of instability occurred when there was a high risk for increased mechanical and neurologic dysfunction in a patient who presented with posttraumatic neurologic symptoms. Common to these definitions is an attempt to clarify the conditions necessary to keep the spine from slipping from an aligned position into a less favorable one.

The three-column model proposed by Denis to classify thoracolumbar injuries has become widely accepted, to some extent replacing the two column model proposed by White et al.[1] In this model the anterior longitudinal ligament, the anterior annulus fibrosus, and the anterior vertebral body form the anterior column; the posterior longitudinal ligament, posterior wall of the vertebral body, and posterior annulus fibrosus form the middle column; and, the posterior bony arch, posterior ligamentous structures (ligamentum flavum, supraspinous ligament, interspinous ligament), and facet joints (capsules and facets) form the posterior column. Failure (injury) of two of the three columns implies that there will be spinal instability.[3]

To decide if a patient has an unstable injury, it is necessary that all of the areas of disruption be appreciated. The identification of fractures through the vertebral body or posterior arch are basic observations easily made with most imaging techniques. Disc disruption, most common with subluxation, and disc herniation are also observed; however, the diagnosis may require more invasive studies (myelography or CT with intrathecal contrast).

More recently the diagnosis of disc herniation has been made with MRI.[4] Ligamentous injury and injury to the capsules of the facet joints remain a somewhat difficult diagnosis.

Prior to MRI, the diagnosis was presumptive, based on the extent of displacement seen on initial radiographic examinations, on the final position of the facet joints following reduction, or upon obvious motion present at the time of flexion-extension films. With MRI it is now possible to image ligamentous disruption directly.[5]

Techniques of Imaging

Plain Radiographs

Plain films are the mainstay of spinal trauma imaging. The initial characterization of a fracture-dislocation of the spine is usually made from a lateral and an anteroposterior (AP) radiograph. Often acquired using portable x-ray machines to avoid moving the patient, these initial films can demonstrate the presence, extent, and severity of injury.

Examination of the cervical spine requires the most complex radiographic techniques. Visualization of the odontoid process requires an open-mouth view, while clearing C7-T1 interspace frequently requires depressing the patient's shoulders or a swimmer's view lateral. Other projections, such as trauma obliques (rotating the tube 30 degrees around the patient) and pillar views (25-30 degrees of caudal angulation) can be used to more fully show the extent of cervical injury.[6] However, the availability and resolution of CT, which should be used whenever a significant fracture or neurologic injury is present, may make obtaining the full six films unnecessary.

One study compared the accuracy of a single lateral cervical spine film vs. a three-film series (AP, open-mouth, and lateral) as the initial screening studies for cervical spine injury. CT was limited to patients with questionable plain film findings. A single lateral film had a sensitivity of 0.85 and a negative predictive value for fracture of 0.97 compared to a sensitivity of 0.92 and a negative predictive value of 0.99 for the three-film series. Adding CT changed the negative predictive value of the study to 1.0. These authors thus advocated CT for patients with questionable plain film findings because their aim was avoidance of a "missed fracture."[7] Another study of missed diagnoses found, in a prospective review of 274 injuries in 253 patients, 41 initially missed injuries in 38 patients. In 17 patients initial radiographs were not obtained, four patients did not seek medical aid, and in 20 the fracture was missed on the initial radiographs, usually as a result of inadequate examination.[8] Yet another retrospective study of cervical spine injury found that 84% of 257 awake patients with proven cervical spine fractures had neck pain or tenderness when initially examined and 8% had subjective symptoms with motor or sensory signs. The 8% in whom the injury was initially missed had painful additional injuries which were felt to mask the cervical trauma.[9] This implies that a higher suspicion of spine fracture may be required in patients who are not awake or who may have multiple injuries.

Another use of plain films occurs during closed reduction of cervical injuries. In particular, lateral films can demonstrate the effectiveness of the reduction, the amount of distraction, and the alignment of the vertebral bodies. If a patient is managed in traction, plain films will confirm that reduction has been maintained. In the thoracolumbar region AP and lateral films are frequently adequate to document injury and, in many cases, to assess stability. Oblique films may be required for evaluation of spondylosis. The CT study is essential to define the full extent of actual or suspected injury in this region.[10]

Flexion-Extension Films

At the time of an acute injury flexion-extension films are commonly used to assess the integrity of the ligamentous structures in patients with suspected injury but no evidence of neurologic dysfunction or fracture.[11] In the patient who has sustained a fracture or subluxation and has been treated, flexion-extension films can prove that the spine is stable.

Most flexion-extension films are obtained in a lateral projection. The patient is instructed to voluntarily flex and extend his spine as far as he can. The physician should not try to increase the patient's range of motion. Using the anterior and posterior margins of the vertebral bodies, the extent of subluxation can be measured. In many cases evaluation is expedited by superimposing two views, one in extension and one in flexion. The distance of a shift and its direction become immediately apparent (Figures 1a-d).

Although flexion-extension studies commonly employ plain radiographs, similar "motion" examinations can be obtained using fluoroscopic and cine techniques. The disadvantage of fluoroscopy is the impermanence of the image. Cine recordings solve this problem but in many cases appreciation of subtle motion is easier with radiographs than with a video image.

Computerized Tomography

Computerized tomography (CT) has become the mainstay for imaging of spinal injury. The advantages and disadvantages have been well described.[10,12] Bone is imaged in exquisite detail with clear demonstration of even small cortical disruptions. The configuration of the spinal canal and the extent of bone encroachment on the canal are immediately obvious. Nevertheless there are difficulties and pitfalls in the CT examination of the spine. Fractures parallel to the scan plane, involving facets, or through the pedicles can be missed on axial sections.[13] Spinal canal contents cannot be assessed without intrathecal contrast agents.[11,14] Rotational alignment is easily evaluated but other subluxations are only appreciated if sagittal and coronal reconstructions are obtained.

Ligamentous injury is inferred by the extent of malalignment because the ligament cannot be imaged directly. Long segment imaging is difficult. Nevertheless, it is easy to perform a CT scan in a patient with severe acute injuries without producing excessive motion. Most available traction devices have

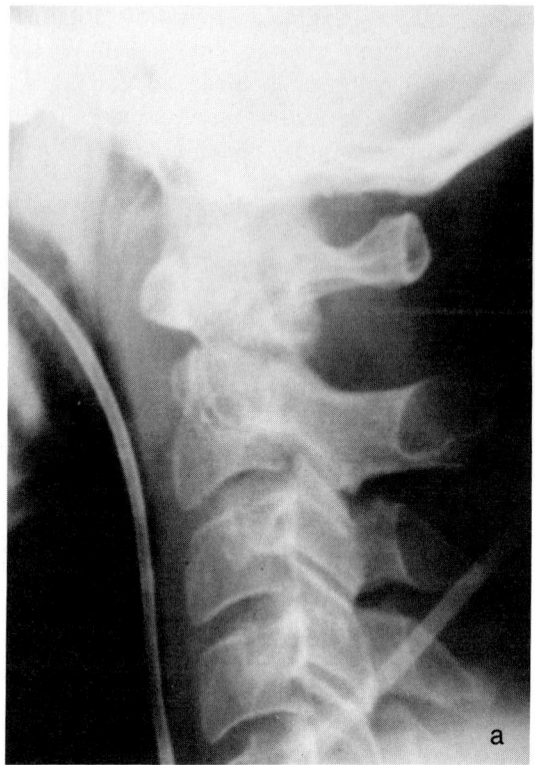 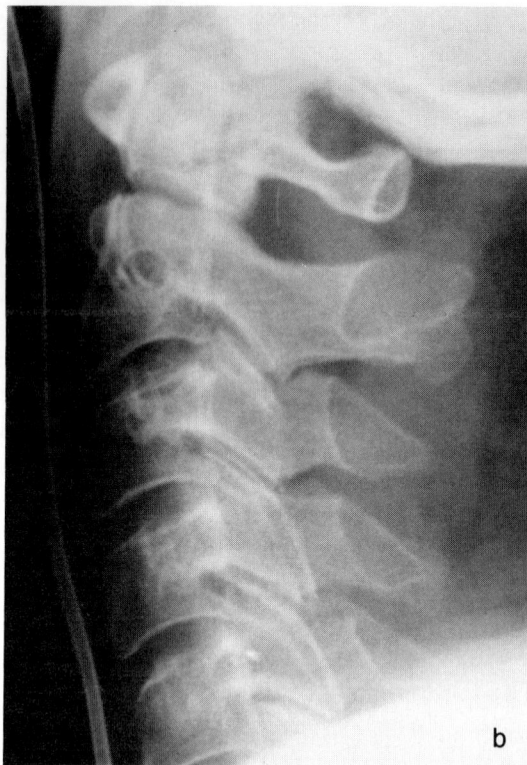

Figure 1a,b. This patient had a history of a prior neck injury. Nonunion of the old odontoid base fracture was suspected. Instability is most clearly shown with flexion-extension films. In flexion (**a**) the odontoid slips posteriorly on C2 while in extension (**b**) the fracture line opens up anteriorly.

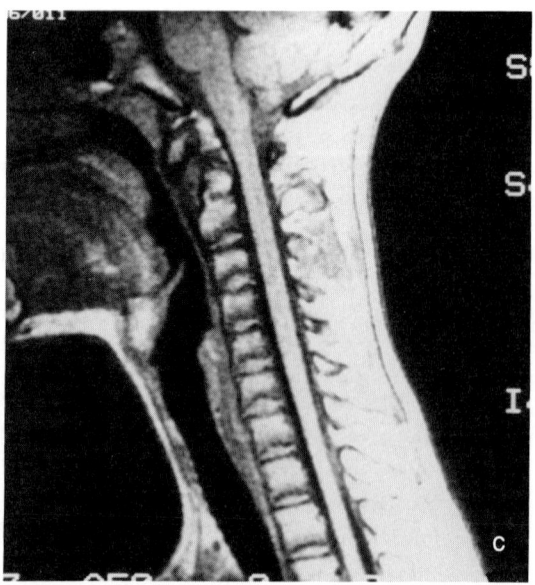 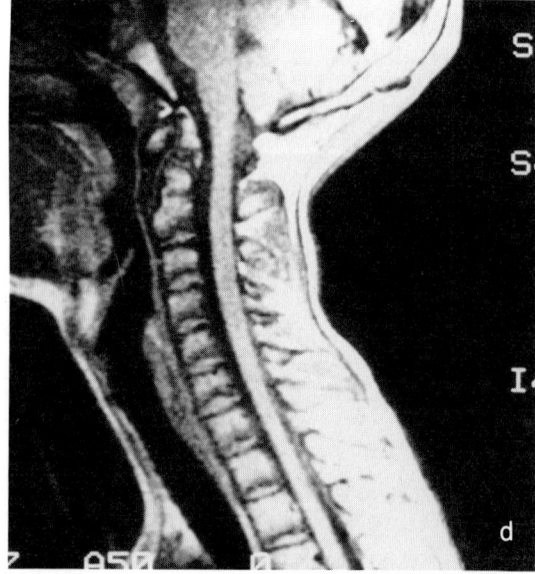

Figure 1c,d. To evaluate compression of neural tissue with motion flexion-extension MRI can be performed. These two sequences were obtained in flexion (**c**) and extension (**d**) in a patient with a history of an inadequately stabilized odontoid fracture. Posterior subluxation of the odontoid on C2 in extension can be appreciated on this T1 weighted sequence. There is no compression of neural tissue.

been adapted to the CT scanners. The scanning is rapid and most bony disruption of the spine is well seen.

Sagittal, coronal, and in some cases oblique reconstructions of the spine are advocated for demonstration of fractures in the plane of section and for evaluation of alignment. There are now a few who advocate three-dimensional reconstructions for spinal injury. In one small series of four complex cervical fractures, the anatomic arrangement of the spine was better appreciated on the three-dimensional reformatted images than on the initial CT.[15] A major limitation of this procedure remains the calculation times, generally on the order of several hours.

Myelography/CT-Myelography

Myelography and CT-myelography, although useful for evaluation of the contents of the spinal canal,[11,14] are less helpful in determining stability. In the presence of a dural tear, which can only be shown with intrathecal contrast, there may be a leak of contrast through a disrupted facet or ligamentous structure. Although this indicates their disruption, it may not imply instability. Similarly, the type of spinal cord injury may suggest a type of treatment and predict the potential for recovery of function, but again not define spinal axis instability.

Tomography

Tomography, whether linear or complex motion, has largely been discarded in favor of CT. With CT the patient remains supine for the entire study, while with lateral tomography, the patient assumes a lateral decubitus position. Tomographic parasite shadows from adjacent sections are more difficult to avoid than are the partial volume averaging effects of CT. The very real problem of the decreasing number of tomographic units also has spurred the switch to CT.

Only in the evaluation for fusion and fracture healing does tomography remain superior to CT. It is not possible to accurately evaluate for small foci of callus formation with plain films. Unfortunately, sagittal CT reconstructions are prone to inaccuracies if there is any patient motion. Motion may produce "pseudofractures" or may not show an area of residual nonunion. Tomographic parasite shadows are less of a problem than CT reconstruction artifacts if the question being explored is the presence of callus formation.

Magnetic Resonance Imaging

Magnetic resonance imaging (MRI) of the spine is advantageous because long vertebral segments can be imaged, tissue characterization is possible when pulse sequences are varied, and multiple imaging planes are routine.[4] The disadvantage of MRI for the patient with a spine injury derives from the relatively long scan time compared to CT and the absolute contraindication to placing any ferromagnetic material in a strong magnetic field. A variety of nonferromagnetic halo rings, vests and traction devices have recently been developed, but it remains difficult to monitor patients requiring life support equipment within a high field magnet.

Although MRI in spinal trauma is usually obtained to delineate abnormalities of neural tissue or disc, it is also possible to show disruption of the relatively lower signal ligamentous structures.[5,16] The difficulty of this diagnosis arises if the ligaments are poorly seen. A tear of the ligament might then be missed. There are no clear evaluations of the sensitivity of MRI in diagnosing ligamentous disruption. However, because confirmation of this diagnosis can only be made with flexion-extension films or surgical evaluation, this information may be difficult to obtain. Also seen with an MRI examination are the longitudinal alignment of facet joints, the alignment of the vertebral bodies, and the position of the intervertebral disc. The use of plain films, CT, and MRI for the complete delineation of a typical cervical spine injury is seen in Figures 2a-d.

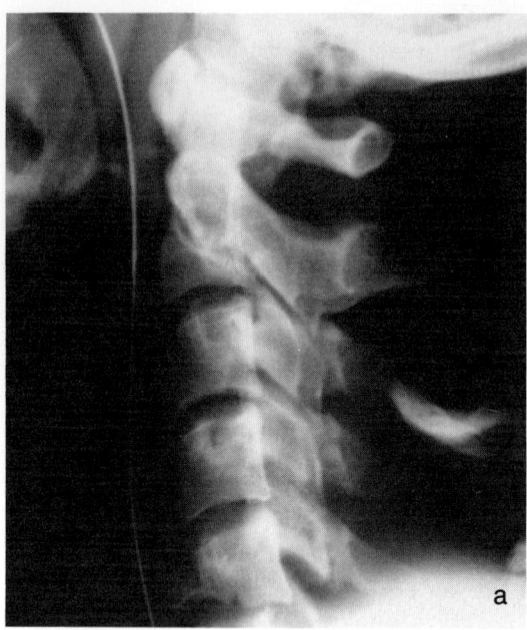

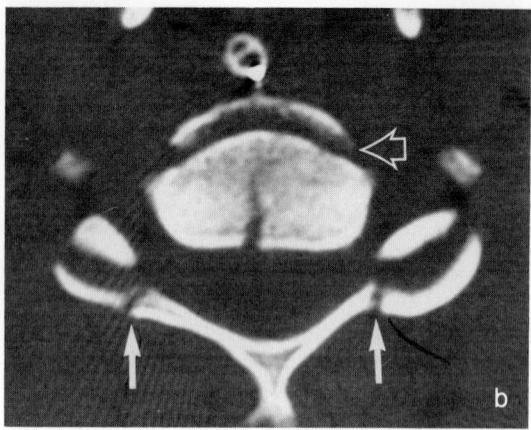

Figure 2a. Lateral radiograph obtained using portable equipment during the initial evaluation and attempt at reduction. C5 is posteriorly displaced on C6, the facet joint is widened, and there is a fracture through the anterior margin of the vertebral body. Subluxation appears to be greater than 3 mm with minimal angulation between the vertebral bodies.

Figure 2b. Axial CT image at the level of injury shows the fracture of the anterior margin of vertebral body (open arrow). Both facet joints are markedly widened and there are fractures extending into the lamina (arrows). There is also a midsagittal fracture through the vertebral body. This suggests that all three columns of the spine are disrupted. Evaluation of ligaments is difficult with plain films and more difficult with CT. Ligamentous disruption is a presumptive diagnosis based upon the extent of subluxation.

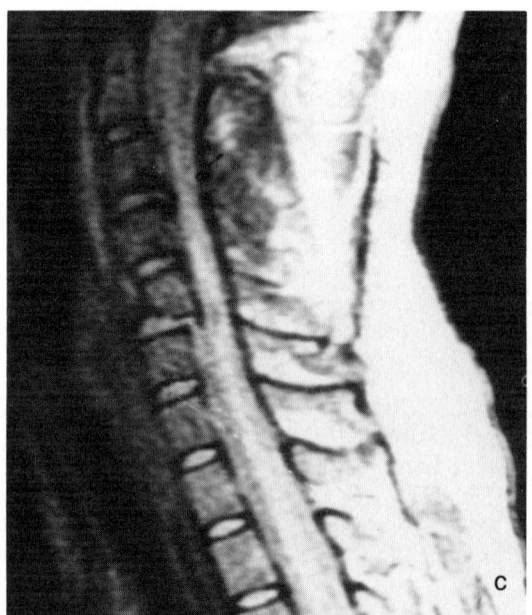

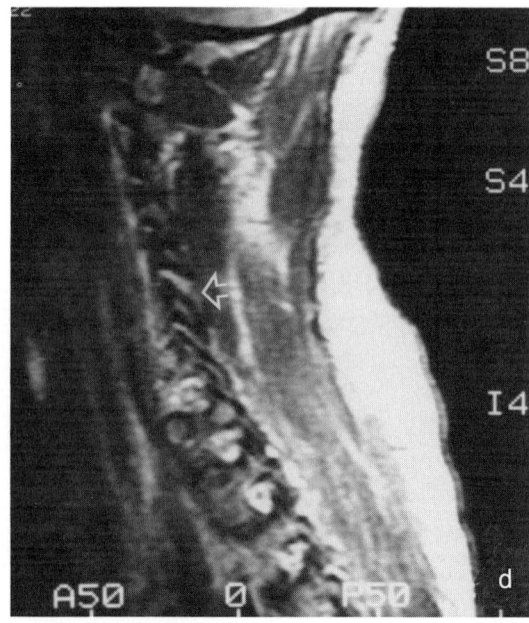

Figure 2c,d. Two lateral MRI sections in the same patient. With this proton density weighted sequence the discs are relatively higher signal than the vertebral bodies and the ligaments are relatively lower signal. The disruption of the posterior longitudinal ligament is seen on the sagittal MR image (arrow). Widening of the facet joint (open arrow) is visible on a more lateral section. This latter finding suggests injury to the capsule of the facet joint.

Acute Injuries

Lower Cervical Spine

Fractures involving the lower cervical spine occur through a variety of mechanisms:

1. *Flexion*—These injuries are caused by anterior forces displacing the vertebral body forward. There is compression of the vertebral body and distraction of posterior elements which can cause injury to soft tissues, bone, or both.
2. *Flexion-rotation injuries*—These tend to disrupt the posterior ligamentous complex. When less severe, compression of the vertebral body ensues. With more severe injury dislocation of facet joints occurs, sometimes accompanied by vertebral body fractures.
3. *Extension injuries*—These fracture the posterior bony structures and may disrupt the anterior longitudinal ligament. Hyperextension can cause a variety of fractures, including hyperextension-dislocation, laminar fractures, and C1-C2 injuries.
4. *Compression*—This occurs from axial loading. If injury is in the lower cervical spine, a burst fracture occurs; if at C1, a Jefferson fracture is produced.[17]

As noted, the plain film evaluation of the lower cervical spine consists of AP, lateral, and possibly a swimmer's lateral projection. A normal lateral film of the cervical spine should have the following characteristics:

1. All vertebral bodies to the top of T1 can be evaluated (Figures 3a,b).
2. There is less than 3.5 mm of subluxation in an anterior-posterior direction. White et al., using cadavers, found that failure of some component insuring spinal stability occurred with 2.7 mm of translation. They felt that 3.5 mm of subluxation was the radiographic correlate that corrected for magnification present in a routine

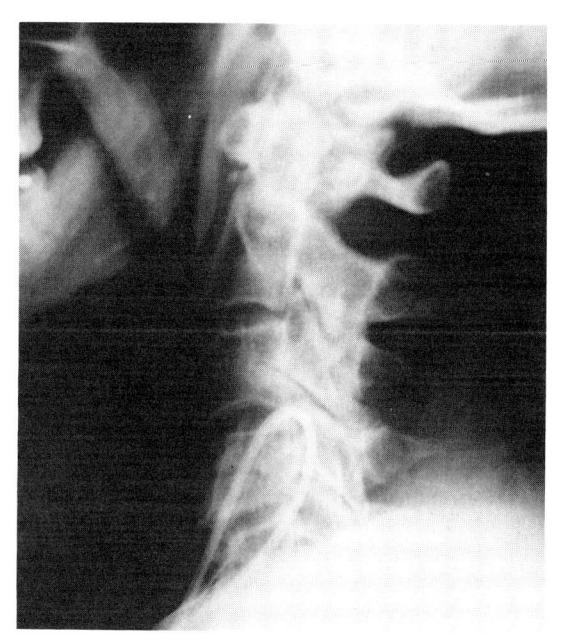

Figure 3a. This elderly patient presented with quadriplegia following a fall from his roof. The initial lateral cervical spine radiograph showed only five vertebral bodies. Degenerative changes were present at C4-C5. This alone is an inadequate study because of failure to visualize the entire cervical spine.

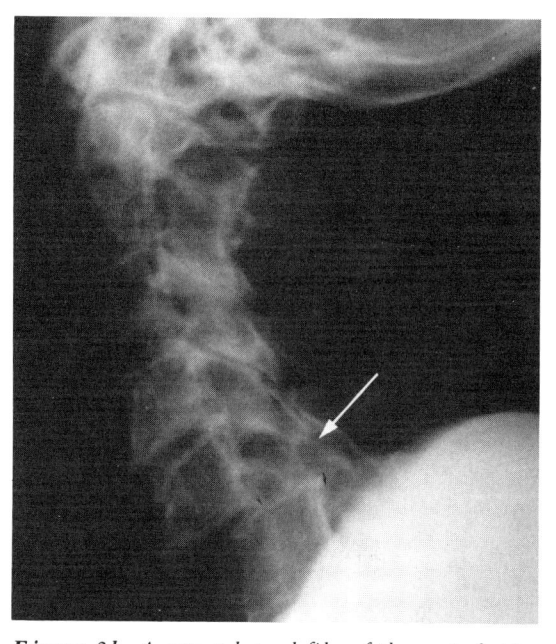

Figure 3b. A repeat lateral film of the cervical spine with greater penetration and caudal displacement of the patient's shoulders now shows six vertebral bodies. There is severe anterior subluxation of C5 on C6 with perching of the facets (arrow). This study exemplifies the problems if the entire spine is inadequately imaged.

lateral film.[1] With a unilateral facet dislocation, the subluxation should be less than half of the diameter of the vertebral body on the lateral projection and the lateral masses should no longer superimpose.[17] Unilateral facet dislocations with significant neural, especially spinal cord, damage, may be unstable because of the presumed greater displacement of the vertebra.[2]

3. Bilateral facet dislocations may be seen with perching or overriding of facet joints and/or angulation of greater than 11 degrees between adjacent vertebral bodies (Figure 4). Without angulation, the displacements may approach 50% of the width of the vertebral body on a lateral x-ray.[1]

4. Widening of the intervertebral disc space without extension of the patient's head or the application of traction suggests tearing of anterior and/or posterior ligamentous complex with disruption of the disc. Other signs of disc disruption include vacuum disc or narrowing of the disc space without preexisting disc disease.[18,19]

5. Prevertebral soft tissue swelling has been postulated to be a sign of bone or ligamentous injury. Penning advocates 1-8 mm as a normal width for prevertebral soft tissues at C4, while Gehweiler used 7 mm as an upper limit of normal.[6,20] A more recent study suggests that prevertebral soft tissue thickening may be a relatively insensitive measurement because many normals will be included in the group. Soft tissue changes may require a number of hours to develop or may not be present with posterior fractures.[21]

6. Wider separation of adjacent spinous processes at the level of injury when compared to the remainder of the spine is a sign of injury to the interspinous ligaments. No clear numbers have been established, although angulation greater than 11 degrees between two vertebral bodies or subluxation anteriorly greater than 3.5 mm should suggest interspinous ligament injury.

Similar comments can be made regarding the normal AP radiograph:

1. The vertebral bodies should be aligned with uniform distances between the vertebral endplates.
2. The spinous processes should be in a straight line and evenly spaced. Uneven spacing suggests disruption of the interspinous ligament and lateral displacement suggests a unilateral facet dislocation.
3. The endplates of the vertebrae and uncinate processes should be clearly seen.

CT, commonly used to fully evaluate the extent of spinal injury, can aid analysis of potential instability. To completely understand the CT it is necessary to place injuries in the appropriate anatomic "column." For example, the flexion-teardrop fracture which usually involves the anterior column has an inferior fracture fragment passing through the vertebral body in a coronal plane (anterior column), multiple fracture fragments extending through the posterior annulus (middle column), and fractures through the lamina and facets (posterior column). This suggests instability, although failure of the posterior column may not be diagnosed unless there is greater than 2.7 mm of anterior subluxation on CT.

The configuration of the facet joints can be evaluated with axial sections; however, the alignment is sometimes better appreciated using sagittal reconstructions. Lateral displacement of the facets, fractures into the facets, marked widening of the facet joint, or a "naked facet" will suggest that the joint capsule, which forms part of the posterior column, has been disrupted.[13] These changes can be appreciated even after reduction has been obtained (Figures 4, 5a-c). Perched

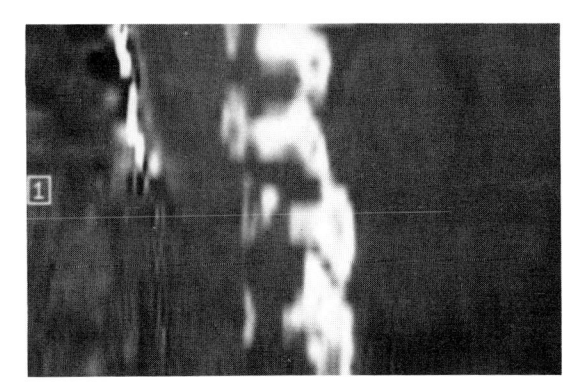

Imaging and Posttraumatic Spinal Instability

Figure 4. A single sagittal reconstruction shows perching of the C4-C5 facets. The normal C5-C6 facet is inferior. At times the alignment of the facet joints may be more easily evaluated using reconstructions.

facets show only minimal continuity between the facet joints on the axial section, while true overriding facets will have the rounded outer surfaces of the facets rather than the flat, articulating surfaces apposed. This may occur at levels above or below the major injury.

Subluxation in an anterior-posterior or in a lateral direction is more easily evaluated using plain films or sagittal and coronal reformatted CT images than with axial CT. To make the diagnosis of a subluxation using axial sections, it is first necessary that the scanning plane be parallel to the intervertebral disc space. If this criterion is not met, the scans will be obtained in a "partial" coronal plane, which will appear subluxed even in a normal spine.

The diagnosis of subluxation then rests upon visualization of adjacent sides of the spinal canal or of the anterior margins of adjacent vertebral bodies on a single slice (double ring). This is better appreciated on slightly thicker (4-5 mm) sections than on the 1.5 mm high resolution sections, because the diagnosis is based on the presence of partial volume averaging of adjacent vertebral endplates. Rotational disruption is more easily evaluated with CT than with standard plain films. In this case the major axes of adjacent vertebral bodies will be offset. Diagnosis of subluxation on reformatted images would follow the guidelines for plain films.

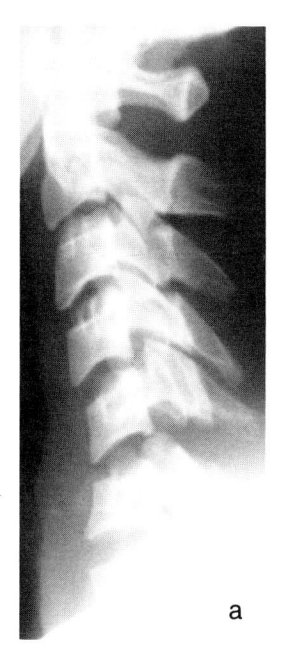

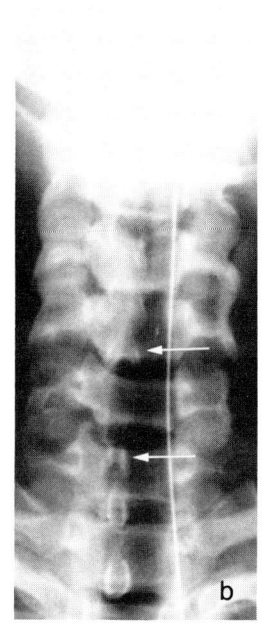

Figure 5a,b. This patient has complete ligamentous disruption at C5-C6 easily diagnosed with the lateral (a) and AP (b) plain films. The disc space and facet joints are markedly widened with separation of the spinous processes on the lateral projection. There is angulation without subluxation. The AP film (b) shows separation of spinous processes without rotational displacement off midline (arrow). This is a highly unstable injury, difficult to hold in traction.

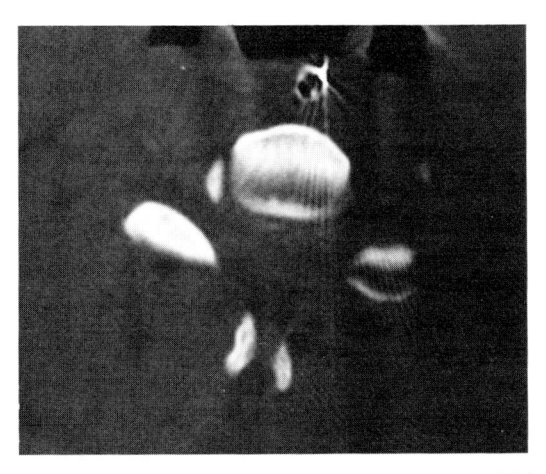

Figure 5c. Axial CT section demonstrates a widened left facet joint space and a "naked" superior facet on the right. Normally the flat surface of the facets are apposed. Widening of the joint space suggests disruption of the joint capsule, while a "naked" facet suggests severe distraction. No bony injury occurred in this patient.

Ligamentous disruption still requires flexion-extension films for diagnosis. Motion greater than 3-4 mm is believed to indicate potential instability regardless of the presence or absence of fractures.[22]

Upper Cervical Spine

The structures from the occiput to C2 have different ligamentous and joint configurations and should be considered separately from the lower cervical spine. The specific injuries at this level include the following:

1. Occipito-atlantal dislocation
2. Transverse ligament rupture with subluxation of C1-C2
3. Traumatic spondylolisthesis (hangman's fracture)
4. Jefferson fracture
5. Odontoid base fractures (I = tip, II = base, III = body of C2)
6. Rotatory subluxation C1-C2

Adequate imaging of any of these fractures may necessitate a combination of plain films, flexion-extension films, axial CT, and reformatted CT images. Despite the potential of MRI to demonstrate ligamentous disruption, there are, as yet, no published series confirming that ligaments which appear intact on MRI are functionally normal.

Plain films of the upper cervical spine consist of lateral, open-mouth, and, if necessary, caudally angled views centering on C1 to confirm the integrity of the atlanto-axial complex (Figures 6a-c). Observations must include the following:

1. The odontoid base should be without fracture.
2. The odontoid should lie equidistant between the two lateral masses of C1. This position may be artifactually displaced on the films if the patient's head is rotated. The lateral masses of C1 should not extend beyond the lateral margins of C2. Displacement greater than 7 mm suggests transverse ligament rupture.
3. The occipital condyles should be in contact with the upper margin of C1.
4. In adults, the distance between the anterior ring of C1 and the odontoid

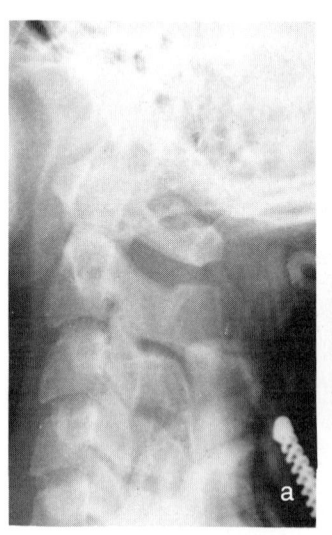

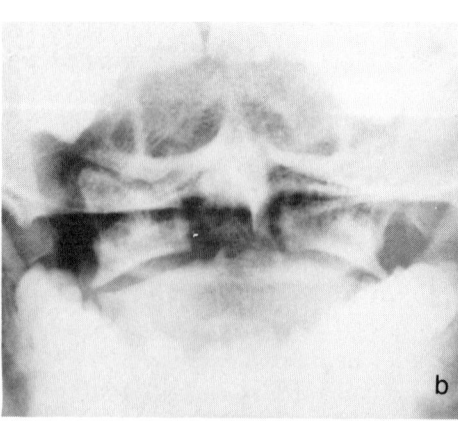

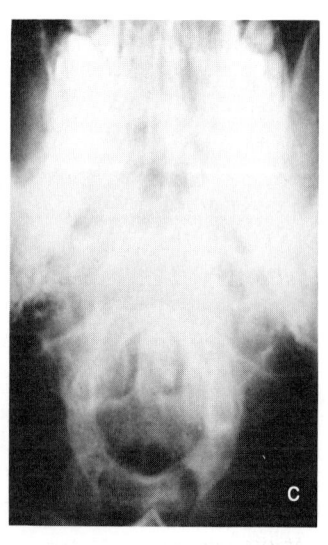

Figure 6a,b,c. The patient presented with neck pain following a fall. Three plain films demonstrate a fracture at the base of the odontoid. On the lateral projection (a) there is faintly seen disruption of the posterior margin of the odontoid with minimal, focal prevertebral soft tissue swelling. The anterior ring of C1 and the odontoid maintain a normal relationship. Both the open mouth (b) and angled odontoid (c) projections suggest a fracture of the base of the odontoid (right is reversed on the open-mouth film). If the patient cannot achieve an open-mouth projection, a caudally angled film, centered on C1, may enable examination of the odontoid and body of C2.

should be less that 2 mm; in children, it should be less than 3-5 mm.
5. Retropharyngeal soft tissues are sometimes difficult to evaluate, but they should be less than 7 mm at C2. Focal enlargement in the absence of other disease may also be significant.[6]

CT of this region, more than in other areas of the spine, requires high resolution routine sagittal and coronal reconstructions calculated from thin (1.5-2.0 mm) axial sections. Odontoid fractures comprise 7-14% of all cervical fractures and may occur parallel to the scanning plane.[23] In particular, odontoid type II fractures may only be seen using reconstructions.

Jefferson fractures are best seen on axial sections, however, because the entire ring of C1 can be seen on a single image. The configuration of C1 is easiest to appreciate if the scanning plane lies parallel to the C1 ring. If software limitations or the patient's anatomy requires that the scan angle lie in a different plane from the plane of the vertebrae, paraoblique reconstructions derived from a midline sagittal image can produce an image in the desired axial plane. The difficulty with misangled slices lies in the possible obscuration of subtle fracture lines as the scan section passes through adjacent sections of the vertebral body.

At C1-2 assessment of stability may require flexion-extension views, especially if there is no fracture line to suggest potential instability. Even with a traumatic spondylolisthesis of C2, commonly taken to be unstable, there are those who feel that only a motion study will fully assess stability.[22] The extent of displacement necessary to diagnose instability is again difficult to quantitate. Levine, when classifying traumatic spondylolisthesis, used 3 mm of translation as the cut-off between a stable and unstable injury. He proposed that a type I hangman's fracture with this minimal subluxation was stable. Type II and type III, both with greater subluxation and/or severe angulation, proved to be unstable, even in halo vests.

Odontoid base fractures (type II) are problematic because of the high incidence of late nonunion ranging from 5-88% depending upon the series. The patient with nonunion is potentially unstable.[24] Either CT with reformatted images or tomography can be used to confirm the presence of corticated bone around the fracture line, but proof of instability requires flexion-extension films (Figures 1a-d, 7a,b).

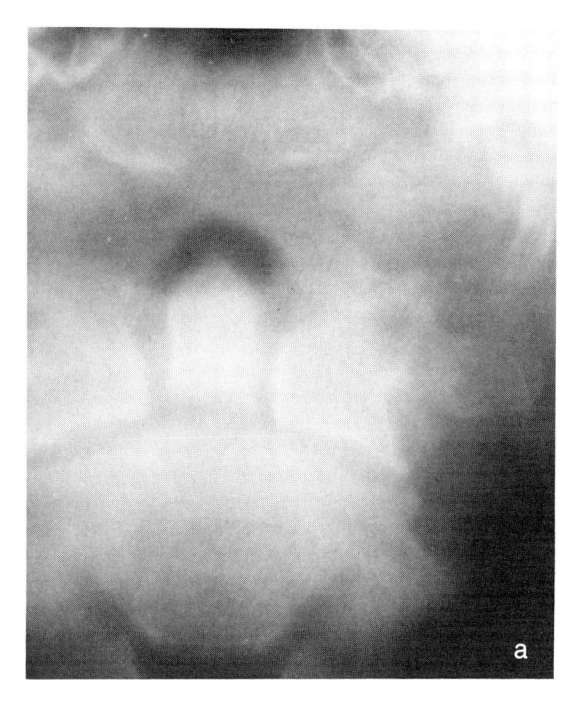

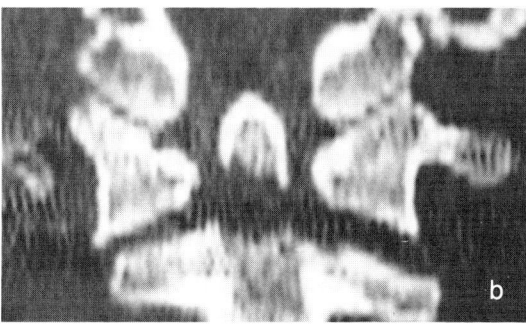

Figure 7a,b. If diagnosis of an odontoid fracture cannot be made on the basis of the plain film examination several options are open: (**a**) AP tomogram; (**b**) coronal reformatted CT at the level of the odontoid in a different patient. Highly detailed reconstruction can be obtained from contiguous 1.5 mm axial CT sections. These are useful in the diagnosis of horizontally oriented fractures and of alignment, both difficult to appreciate with axial CT.

Thoracolumbar Spine

Acute Injuries

Thoracolumbar fractures, less variable in configuration than cervical injuries, have been classified by Denis. This schema helps to clarify the probability of instability in a specific injury. Instability results from the failure (disruption) of the middle column in addition to either the anterior or posterior column. This is the schema to use:

1. Compression fractures involve only the anterior column and are stable. The middle column, in particular, is intact. This injury is caused by flexion rather than axial loading.
2. Burst fractures commonly arise from failure of the anterior and middle columns under axial loads and are considered unstable.
3. Seat-belt type injuries are included as flexion-distraction injuries in mechanistic classifications and are unstable because they consist, at a minimum, of failure of posterior and middle columns. Anterior column components may be involved.
4. Fracture-dislocation injuries. These will disrupt all three columns. There are potentially multiple types of forces involved: flexion-rotation, shear, and flexion-distraction.[3]

As in other regions, the function of any imaging procedure is the diagnosis of the injury and confirmation of its extent. The choice of modality will depend upon the extent of injury, the clinical condition of the patient, and the information required.

Plain films remain the mainstay of the imaging in the thoracolumbar region. Thoracic injuries, because of the presence of the rib cage, are a specific problem. Major observations on the AP film are as follows:

1. Asymmetry of the distances between the spinous processes
2. Offsetting of the spinous processes or pedicles
3. Tilting of the disc space
4. Loss of height of a vertebral body, especially if asymmetric
5. Lateral translation of one vertebral body with respect to another

The lateral film can be difficult to interpret, especially if the patient remains supine, because of problems seeing the vertebral bodies through the rib cage and the scapulae in the upper thoracic region. It is usually necessary to resort to sectional imaging techniques if there is any question of injury. By the same token, neurologic dysfunction frequently accompanies significant injury to thoracic levels and, irrespective of the severity of the injury, the question of acute instability may be less significant because the rib cage tends to act as a stabilizing influence.

In the lower thoracic and upper lumbar region lateral plain films are more informative. Signs to observe on the lateral film, include the following:

1. Loss of height of a vertebral body
2. Loss of height of a disc space in the absence of degenerative changes
3. Injury to the posterior margin of the vertebral body (seen as discontinuity of the line of the vertebra)
4. Disruption/perching/overriding of the facet joints

Rotational and lateral injuries are better appreciated using the AP projection. CT in these cases serves as a confirmation of the extent of injury and a more precise evaluation of the condition of the facets and spinal canal (Figures 8a-c). The need for CT is more obvious if instability is not apparent because extension of the fracture into the middle column with minimal interpedicular widening may be appreciated only on CT. Oblique plain films will not clarify the problem of bone retropulsed into the spinal canal.

Compression fractures by definition involve only the endplate of the vertebral body. They may look fragmented on the CT, but should not involve the posterior margins or pedicles of the vertebral body. There should be no bone retropulsed into the spinal canal and no displacements of the facet joints. Burst fractures are a separate entity and have a potential for late instability.[25] This is particularly true if there are translational components, compression greater than 50% of the vertebral body height, fracture of the posterior elements, or increased interpedicular distance on the AP radiograph. Using CT, the loss of height of a vertebral body and translational components of the fracture are best evaluated on the reformatted images. Injury to the facet joints with disruption or override, and fractures of the laminae or facets may be better appreciated with axial CT.[26-28] The configuration of the spinal canal is also best seen with axial CT sections; however, reformatted images may better demonstrate canal narrowing if angulation is severe.

In lap belt injuries, CT is more difficult to interpret than either the plain radiographs or reformatted images (Figures 9a-c, 10a-c). CT is most helpful with subtle fractures if a horizontal fracture line through the vertebral body, posterior elements, and/or disc space is not obvious on the lateral radiograph. Because the fracture line lies within the plane of the CT section, the absence of normal vertebral elements is the main sign of injury on axial sections. For this fracture, CT demonstration of the extent of injury is easily seen only on reformatted images. These may clarify the precise location of the fracture in relation to the vertebral body and the posterior elements.

The rotational and translational components of thoracolumbar injuries require close attention to the direction of the main axis of each of the vertebral bodies. The signs are similar to those in the cervical spine. Using an AP radiograph, the spinous process in a rotational injury is seen to shift off midline. Subluxations, either lateral or dorsal/ventral are also easily diagnosed using plain films. CT imaging of a translational injury is difficult, requiring the presence of both sides of the vertebral body or of the spinal canal on a single nonangled slice. Rotational injuries are somewhat easier to diagnose with CT, requiring only an awareness of the direction of the main axis of the vertebral body.

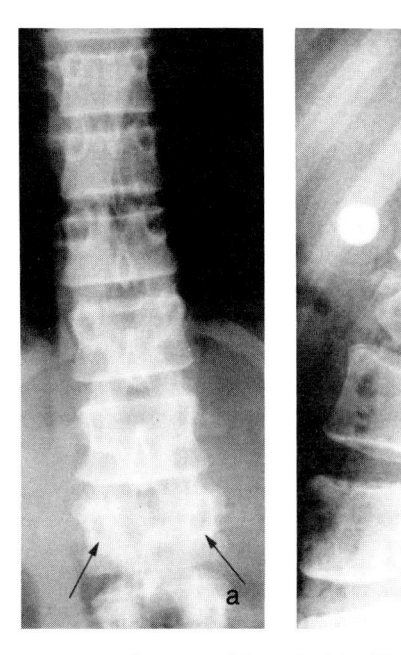

Figure 8a,b. AP and lateral plain films show compression of the vertebral body at T12-L1 with retropulsion of bone fragments into the spinal canal. On the AP projection there is widening of the interpediculate distance (arrows) as well as a suggestion of facet disruption. The fracture appears to involve all three columns.

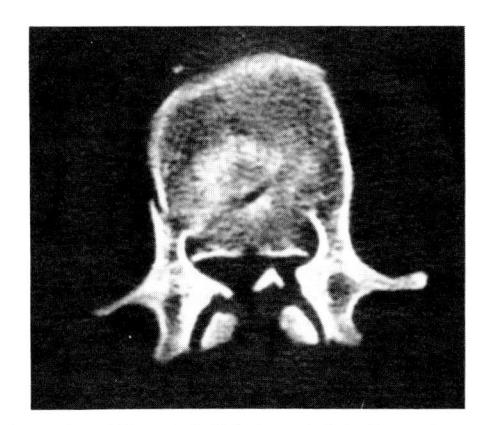

Figure 8c. The axial CT through L1 shows the components of the fracture. There is fragmentation of the anterior and posterior margins of the vertebral body, retropulsion of bone fragments, and lateral displacement of the pedicles. The facet joints are widened with presumed disruption of the joint capsule. The injury to multiple columns of the spine suggests instability.

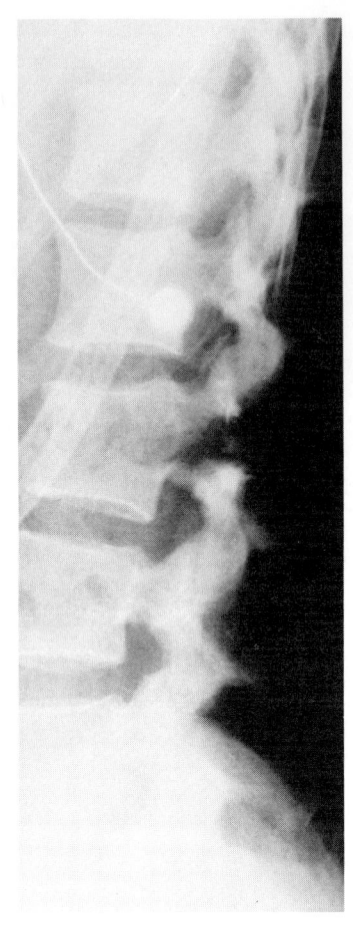

Figure 9a. The female patient was a back seat passenger during a motor vehicle accident. A lateral plain film shows an unstable flexion-distraction injury. The fracture line extends through the vertebral body, the pedicle, and into the facet joints of L3.

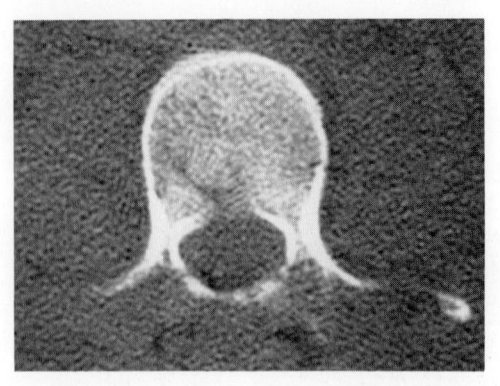

Figure 9b. Axial CT images through L3. The clue to the type of fracture arises from the absent structures. Everything posterior to the transverse processes and pedicles is missing, suggesting a horizontal fracture passing through the pedicles.

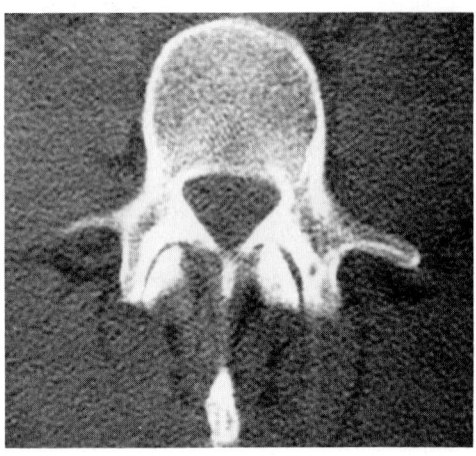

Figure 9c. The comparison slice from the L2 vertebral body shows a normal axial CT at the level of the pedicles.

MRI has no clear role in the assessment of thoracolumbar spinal stability. Injury to the conus, however, should prompt evaluation with MRI rather than postmyelography CT scanning in order to identify disc protrusion or injury to the conus medullaris.

Subacute Injuries

Once the components of the injury have been identified and treatment has begun, the clinical concerns involve recovery of neurologic function and maintenance of reduction. A usual problem is loss of reduction, a potentially dynamic process which has to be evaluated by static studies obtained at a single point in time. Usually plain films are the study of choice. The optimum time interval between films is open to question. In some cases the need for more detailed information will suggest the use of sectional imaging methods. It is convenient to consider this imaging in relation to the time course of the injury rather than to anatomic areas.

Early Treatment

Patients in weighted traction usually have a cervical injury. Traction may be used prior to other stabilization or as a primary treat-

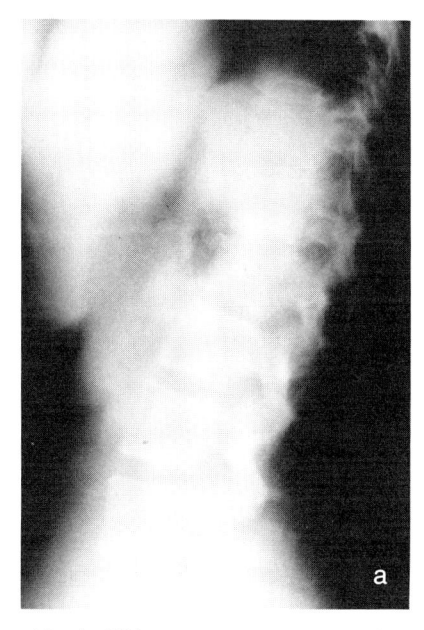

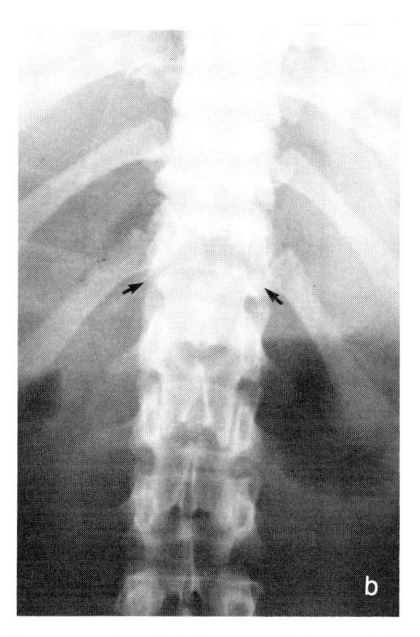

Imaging and Posttraumatic Spinal Instability

Figure 10a,b. This woman was a passenger in a vehicular accident. She presented with back pain. The lateral plain film (**a**) shows the angulation of T12 on L1 with compression of the superior endplate of L1, extension into the middle column at T12-L1, and involvement of the posterior elements of T12. The AP projection (**b**) suggests widening of the T11-T12 facet joint with a fracture line through the lamina (arrow) and dislocation of the left twelfth rib. The extent of bone disruption seen with these plain films is relatively unclear compared to the patient whose imaging studies are seen in Figure 9.

ment. Any fracture which can be considered unstable (i.e. likely to have excessive motion) has a potential to displace in weighted traction (Figures 11a,b). This would suggest that frequent lateral films of the neck are required to reassess alignment. Any suspicion that the fracture has displaced or that the patient's neurologic status has changed should suggest

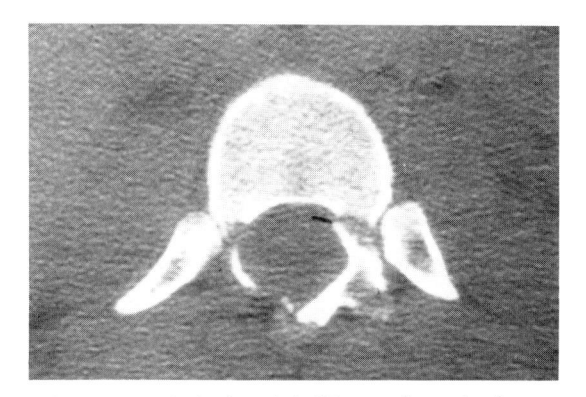

Figure 10c. A single axial CT scan shows the elements suggesting a flexion-distraction injury. The structures normally posterior to the pedicles at T12 are absent with minimal visible injury of anterior structures at this level.

the necessity for this examination. In most cases a portable lateral radiograph is obtained because the process of moving the patient to the x-ray suite may cause loss of reduction. Essential to this evaluation is the presence of a baseline study to serve as a comparison for all subsequent examinations.

A patient in a halo vest also has the potential for displacement or fracture nonunion or displacement. Purely ligamentous injuries and those fractures with a relatively greater degree of ligamentous as compared to bone injury are most likely to remain unstable after nonoperative treatment.

The decision to remove the patient from an immobilization device usually rests upon the demonstration of healing and "stability," an absence of motion when the orthosis is removed. Bony healing implies callus formation or, in a somewhat older injury, the presence of continuity of the bone over the region of the fracture. Because a significant component of this will occur across a fracture line which tends to parallel the disc space, tomography may be more helpful than CT. Plain films rarely have enough resolution to allow identification of small amounts of early callus formation. If CT is used, reformatting techniques are required, because there is a significant potential for missing nonunion of a fracture which lies in the plane of the CT section. Even after callus formation has been demonstrated, there is a reasonable argument for the use of flexion-extension films to confirm that there is no motion across the injury site. For most cervical or thoracolumbar injuries this would be performed as a set of lateral radiographs. Only if there were sufficient concern over rotational components would frontal films, with turning of the head or body, be indicated.

Imaging of patients following surgical stabilization has a different set of difficulties. In most cases, motion at the level of the fracture is not a concern unless there is a failure of a plate, screws, or wires. In those cases, once the disruption of the internal stabilization apparatus is diagnosed or suspected on plain films, flexion-extension films would again be helpful. The other problems concern the position of the wires, plates, and screws. Their relation to the spinal canal, the vertebral body, and the extent of reduction of displaced spinal elements can be difficult to evaluate.

Because of the more frequent use of operative stabilization and instrumentation in the thoracolumbar spine compared to the cervical region, most experience relates to thoracolumbar and lumbar fractures. Although plain films are used to evaluate position of the stabilization device,[31] a more recent study examined the reliability of plain films to show the position for a screw and plate combination. Segmental pedicle screw fixation was performed in cadaver spines. Two observers agreed only 74% of the time on the position of the screw as seen on AP and lateral films. Agreement upon examination of the specimen was on the order of 90%.[32] One alternative would be the use of CT scans, which can demonstrate the relationship between bone and metal stabilization devices if

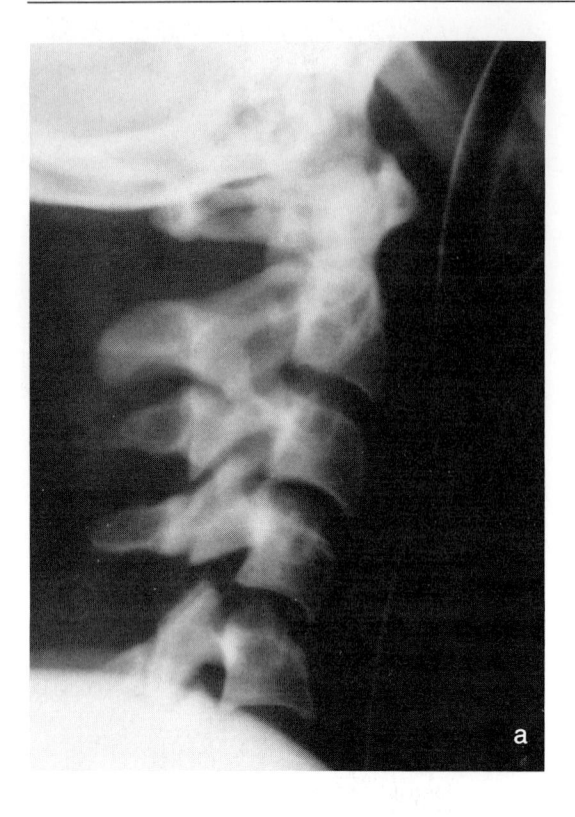

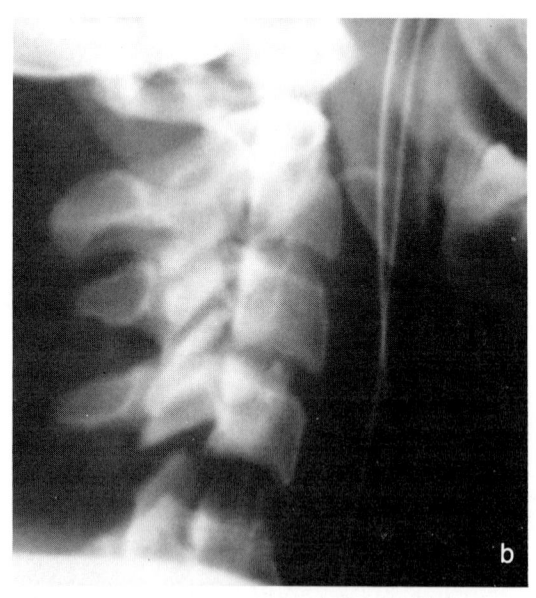

Figure 11a,b. Two lateral films were obtained two days apart while the patient was in traction. A severe ligamentous injury is present. On the earlier film (**a**) there is only widening of the intervertebral disc at C4-5. On the film obtained two days later (**b**) with the patient still in traction, there is a marked increase in distraction. This points up the need for repeated and potentially frequent evaluations of patients in traction who may be unstable.

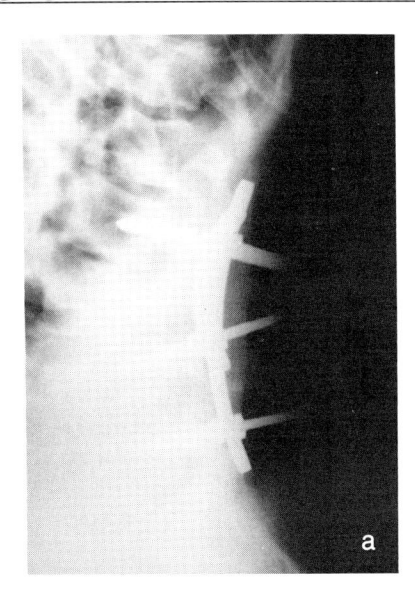

Imaging and Posttraumatic Spinal Instability

Figure 12. This patient underwent internal fixation of an L4 fracture dislocation. Lateral plain film (a) following placement of screws and plates shows the screws lying within the pedicles. The relation to the spinal canal is difficult to appreciate on either this film or the AP projection. (b,c.) These two axial CT sections from a study designed to evaluate screw placement differ only in the windows chosen for imaging. Using the narrower window width (2000 HU) (b) although standard for normal bone imaging, there is enough artifact from the metallic screws to preclude evaluation of relationship of the fixation screw to the spinal canal. With a wider window (4000 HU) (c) the position of the screw within the bone is better seen. If only plain films are used it is difficult to evaluate the position of the fixation screws.

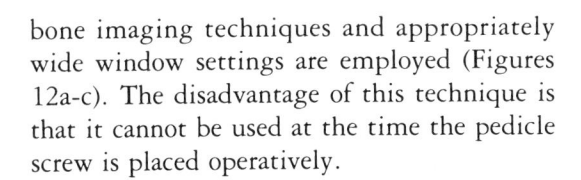

bone imaging techniques and appropriately wide window settings are employed (Figures 12a-c). The disadvantage of this technique is that it cannot be used at the time the pedicle screw is placed operatively.

Conclusion

The radiologic focus in any discussion of spinal stability is an extension of the most basic concerns for any injury. Has the extent of the trauma been completely shown? Are all potential variables which can affect treatment, and thus future function, fully elucidated? If care is taken to observe all of the signs of injury, then the purpose of the imaging studies has been fulfilled, ensuring that the patient receives the most appropriate treatment.

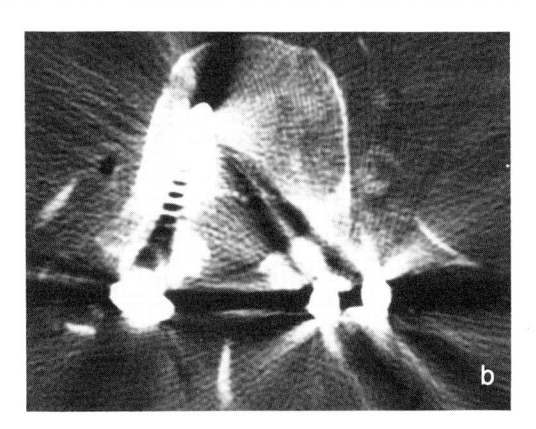

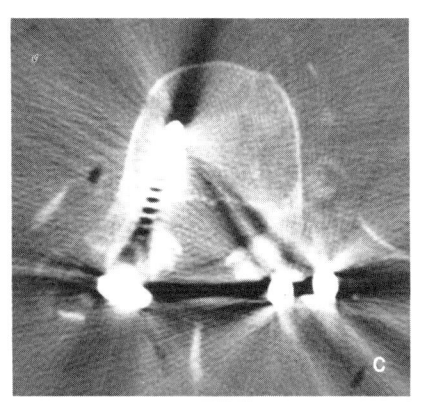

References

1. White AA III, Johnson RM, Panjabi MM, Southwick WO. Biomechanical analysis of clinical stability in the cervical spine. *Clin Orthop.* 1975;109:85-95.
2. White AA, Southwick WO, Panjabi MM. Clinical instability in the lower cervical spine: a review of past and current concepts. *Spine.* 1976;1:15-27.
3. Denis F. The three column spine and its significance in the classification of acute thoracolumbar spinal injuries. *Spine.* 1983;8:817-831.
4. Modic MT, Masaryk T, Paushter D. Magnetic resonance imaging of the spine. *Radiol Clin N Am.* 1986;24:229-245.
5. McArdle CB, Crofford MJ, Mirfakhraee M, Amparo EG, Calhoun JS. Surface coil MR of spinal trauma: preliminary experience. *AJNR.* 1986;7:885-893.
6. Gehweiler JA, Osborne RL Jr, Becker RF. *The Radiology of Vertebral Trauma.* Philadelphia, Pa: WB Saunders Co; 1980.
7. Ross SE, Schwab CW, David ET, Delong WG, Born CT. Clearing the cervical spine: initial radiologic evaluation. *J Trauma.* 1987;27:1055-1060.

8. Reid DC, Henderson R, Saboe L, Miller JDR. Etiology and clinical course of missed spine fractures. *J Trauma*. 1987;27:980-986.
9. Ringenberg BJ, Fisher AK, Urdaneta LF, Midthun MA. Rational ordering of cervical spine radiographs following trauma. *Ann Emerg Med*. 1988;17:792-796.
10. Brant-Zawadzki M, Miller EM, Federle MP. CT in the evaluation of spine trauma. *AJR*. 1981;136:369-375.
11. Cooper PR, Cohen W. Evaluation of cervical spinal cord injuries with metrizamide myelography-CT scanning. *J Neurosurg*. 1984;61:281-289.
12. Keene JS, Goletz TH, Lilleas F, Alter A, Sackett JF. Diagnosis of vertebral fractures: a comparison of conventional radiography, conventional tomography, and computed axial tomography. *J Bone Joint Surg Am*. 1982;64A:586-595.
13. Pech P, Kilgore DP, Pojunas KW, Haughton VM. Cervical spine fractures: CT detection. *Radiology*. 1985;157:117-120.
14. Allen RL, Perot PL Jr, Gudeman SK. Evaluation of acute nonpenetrating cervical spinal cord injuries with CT metrizamide myelography. *J Neurosurg*. 1985;63:510-520.
15. Wojcik WG, Edeiken-Monroe BS, Harris JH Jr. Three-dimensional computed tomography in acute cervical spine trauma: a preliminary report. *Skeletal Radiol*. 1987;16:261-269.
16. Goldberg AL, Rothfus WE, Deeb ZL, Daffner RH, Lupetin AR, Wilberger JE, et al. The impact of magnetic resonance on the diagnostic evaluation of acute cervicothoracic spinal trauma. *Skeletal Radiol*. 1988;17:89-95.
17. Harris JH, Edeiken-Monroe B, Kopaniky DR. A practical classification of acute cervical spine injuries. *Orthop Clin North Am*. 1986;17:15-30.
18. Miller MD, Gehweiler JA, Martinez S, Charlton OP, Daffner RH. Significant new observations on cervical spine trauma. *AJR*. 1978;130:659-663.
19. Edeiken-Monroe B, Wagner LK, Harris JH Jr. Hyperextension dislocation of the cervical spine. *AJR*. 1986;146:803-808.
20. Penning L. Prevertebral hematoma in cervical spine injury: incidence and etiologic significance. *AJR*. 1981;136:553-561.
21. Templeton PA, Young JWR, Mirvis SE, Buddemeyer EU. The value of retropharyngeal soft tissue measurements in trauma of the adult cervical spine. *Skeletal Radiol*. 1987;16:98-104.
22. Levine AM, Edwards CC. The Management of traumatic spondylolisthesis of the axis. *J Bone Joint Surg Am*. 1985;67A:217-226.
23. Schiess RJ, DeSaussure RL, Robertson JT. Choice of treatment of odontoid fractures. *J Neurosurg*. 1982;57:496-499.
24. Dunn ME, Seljeskog EL. Experience in the management of odontoid process injuries: an analysis of 128 cases. *Neurosurg*. 1986;18:306-310.
25. Benson DR. Unstable thoracolumbar fractures, with emphasis on the burst fracture. *Clin Orthop*. 1988;230:14-29.
26. Lindahl S, Willén J, Nordwall A, Irstam. The crush-cleavage fracture: a "new" thoracolumbar unstable fracture. *Spine*. 1983;8:559-569.
27. McAfee PC, Yuan HA, Fredrickson BE, Lubicky JP. The value of computed tomography in thoracolumbar fractures. *J Bone Joint Surg Am*. 1983;65A:461-473.
28. Atlas SW, Refenbogen V, Rogers LF, Kim KS. The Radiographic characterization of burst fractures of the spine. *AJR*. 1986;147:575-582.
29. Lind B, Sihlbom H, Nordwall A. Halo-vest treatment of unstable traumatic cervical spine injuries. *Spine*. 1988;13:425-432.
30. Trent G, Armstrong GWD, O'Neil J. Thoracolumbar fractures in ankylosing spondylitis: high risk injuries. *Clin Ortho*. 1988;227:61-66.
31. Dodd CAF, Fergusson CM, Pearcy MJ, Houghton GR. Vertebral motion measured using biplanar radiography before and after harrington rod removal for unstable thoracolumbar fractures of the spine. *Spine*. 1986;11:452-455.
32. Weinstein JN, Spratt KF, Spengler D, Brick C, Reid S. Spinal pedicle fixation: reliability and validity of roentgenogram-based assessment and surgical factors on successful screw placement. *Spine*. 1988;13:1012-1018.

CHAPTER 3

Clinical Assessment of Posttraumatic Spinal Instability

Lawrence F. Borges, MD

Two major goals must be realized in the treatment of spinal injuries to achieve optimal outcome: the neural elements must be decompressed and the spine must be stabilized. This chapter will focus on the second goal by reviewing the criteria used to determine stability or instability in the spine, and by correlating pertinent clinical literature with relevant laboratory investigations.

Spinal instability can be defined as the loss of the ability of the spine to tolerate physiological loading without incurring neurological deficit, pain, or progressive structural deformity. Since the vertebral column is not a homogeneous structure, the precise combination of factors that determines stability in the spine will vary. Similarly, the criteria used to make a determination of instability must take into account the precise region of the spine under investigation.

Recommendations in the literature regarding spine instability are based upon normal premorbid spines; that is, these spines were free of intrinsic disease prior to the traumatic event. These criteria may not reflect accurately the degree of instability that may occur in an abnormal spine subjected to trauma.

Cervical Spine

Atlanto-Occipital Instability

Stability at the atlanto-occipital junction is provided by an inner and outer set of ligamentous structures. The inner ligaments include the paired alar ligaments, the apical ligament, the vertically oriented cruciform ligament, and the tectorial membrane. The outer ligaments are the articular capsules, the anterior and posterior atlanto-occipital membranes, and the ligamentum nuchae.[1] Working together these ligaments allow approximately 13° of flexion-extension, 8° of lateral bending, and prohibit rotation at the occiput-C1 articulation.[2,3,4,76] In a detailed analysis of the stability of this region, Werne[4] concluded that hyperflexion is prevented by skeletal contact between the anterior margin of the foramen magnum and the odontoid, while hyperextension and vertical translation are controlled by the tectorial membrane. Lateral bending was felt to be limited by the alar ligaments. He also concluded that the tectorial membrane and alar ligaments were the structures most important for maintaining stability, since sectioning of these ligaments led to atlanto-occipital dislocation. Bucholz and Burkhead[5] attempted to assess this problem further by performing postmortem examinations on nine patients who died after motor vehicle accidents and had atlanto-occipital dislocations. They observed that the majority of these patients had disruptions of most, if not all, atlanto-occipital ligaments.

Most traumatic injuries of the atlanto-occipital junction are believed to be fatal. However, survivals have been reported with this injury and it is likely that improvements in prehospital care will increase the number of patients seen with this injury.[6-13] Since stability at this level is directly related to intact ligaments, atlanto-occipital dislocation, which must be the result of ligamentous disruption,[5] is a priori an unstable injury.

Several criteria have been proposed to identify atlanto-occipital dislocation. Wholey et al[14] studied 600 lateral cervical radiographs from normal persons and concluded that there was a constant relationship between the rostral tip of the mid dens and the basion. This distance measured 5 mm in adults and up to 10 mm in children. Powers et al[13] applied these criteria to 150 randomly selected cervical spine radiographs and found that 85% of the normal radiographs fell outside the measurements proposed by Wholey. Powers et al proposed that a more accurate measurement, and one independent of x-ray magnification artifacts, was the BC/OA ratio (Figure 1). Atlanto-occipital dislocation can be defined as a BC/OA ratio greater than 1.0, while the normal population had BC/OA ratios below .9. This ratio was felt to be unreliable in patients with fracture of the C1 arch or congenital anomalies of the foramen magnum.

Dublin et al[15] proposed another method of determining atlanto-occipital dislocation based upon the distance between the anterior border of C1 to the posterior mandible, compared to the distance of the anterior dens to the posterior mandible. Unfortunately, the posterior mandible is in a different sagittal plane than mid-C1 and the dens, and this makes the measurement more difficult to assess when rotation is present on the radiograph. Although these authors proposed ways to overcome this disadvantage, other investigators have preferred the technique suggested by Powers et al.[13]

Atlanto-Axial Instability

Stability at the atlanto-axial articulation is dependent upon the integrity of both ligamentous and osseous structures. The most important ligamentous structure is the tough transverse ligament of the atlas. This ligament passes behind the dens, from which it is separated by a synovial joint, and inserts into tubercles on the medial aspects of the lateral masses of the atlas. The alar ligaments, accessory atlanto-axial ligaments, and tectorial membrane assist the transverse ligament in maintaining stability. The osseous structures important for stability at this level are the dens and anterior arch of the atlas. These structures permit 47° of axial rotation, 10° of flexion-extension, and prohibit lateral bending.[3] Excessive physiologic flexion is limited by the tectorial membrane, while excessive rotation is prevented primarily by the alar ligaments.[16] Excessive extension is prevented by the anterior arch of C1 abutting against the odontoid. The transverse ligament does not play a large role in limiting physiological motion, but it is the major ligamentous structure limiting anterior translation.

Biomechanical studies of the transverse

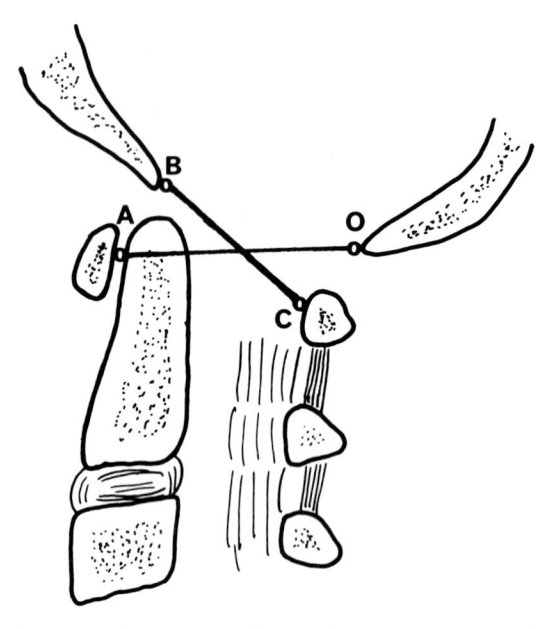

Figure 1. Measurement of the BC/OA ratio as suggested by Powers et al.[13] If BC/OA is greater than 1.0 atlanto-occipital dislocation is present. A ratio less than .9 is normal. Since this measurement is a ratio, it is a dimensionless quantity and knowledge of radiograph magnification is not needed.

ligament performed on cadaver spines by Fielding[17] have demonstrated that this ligament prevents more than 3 mm of anterior displacement between the atlas and the axis, when measured from the posterior cortex of the anterior arch of the atlas to the anterior cortex of the odontoid. The amount of force required to disrupt the transverse ligament varied between specimens. In most specimens ligamentous failure occurred in the body of the ligament, but in 25% of the specimens there was osteoperiosteal failure at the insertion of the ligament into the bone tubercle. Failure of the transverse ligament in these experiments was not associated with failure of the alar ligaments. However, once the transverse ligament failed, remaining ligaments could not prevent lesser forces from producing anterior displacements of C1 on C2 up to 12 mm. Therefore, a distance of greater than 3 mm in adults or 4.5 mm in children, between the posterior cortex of the anterior arch of C1 and anterior border of the odontoid, when measured on a standard lateral radiograph is diagnostic of transverse ligament disruption and instability. This rule holds regardless of the degree of flexion or extension of the spine at the time the radiograph is made.

In assessing displacement between C1 and C2, it is important to remember Steele's "rule of thirds." At the level of the atlas there is 1/3 odontoid, 1/3 spinal cord, and 1/3 space.[18] It is also important to remember that the posterior arch of the atlas can be found in any position between the occiput and the spinous process of C2. Therefore widening of the C1-C2 interspinous distance is not a reliable sign of ligamentous injury.

Since the transverse ligament inserts into the lateral mass of the atlas, it is important to consider which atlas fractures might be unstable. Fractures of the atlas can be classified into three types. The first is the isolated posterior arch injury in which fractures are found on either side of the lamina of C1, often near the groove over which the vertebral artery passes. As an isolated fracture, it is stable. The second fracture is the lateral mass fracture. Fracture lines are found ventral and dorsal to the lateral mass of C1, effectively disconnecting it from the remainder of the ring. The Jefferson fracture, or bursting fracture of C1, is the third type.[19,20] This fracture commonly involves fracture lines through four separate areas of C1 causing total disconnection of both lateral masses. Since the transverse ligament inserts into the lateral mass, any fracture involving the lateral mass at C1 raises the possibility of instability as a result of secondary disruption of the transverse ligament.

Stimulated by a patient with this problem, Spence et al[21] undertook a cadaver study to determine how much lateral displacement of the lateral masses of C1 was needed before the transverse ligament failed. Using 10 cadaver specimens obtained within 24 hours of death, they surgically cut C1 in four places to create a "burst" fracture and then separated the lateral mass fragments until the transverse ligament failed while measuring the transverse diameter of C1. The total excursion of the lateral masses from resting width to ligament rupture ranged from 4.8 to 7.6 mm (mean 6.3 mm). They concluded that if the spread of the lateral mass is less than 5.7 mm on the AP radiograph then there is a high probability that the transverse ligament is intact. Conversely, if the spread is greater than 6.9 mm, the ligament has probably been disrupted (Figures 2a,b). These measurements are important for the neurosurgeon managing atlas fractures.

Levine and Edwards[22] argue that patients manifesting more than 5 mm lateral displacement should be managed in halo traction for six to eight weeks to allow optimal healing of the bony ring of C1 in as correct an anatomical position as possible. Once the bony ring is healed, flexion-extension x-rays are necessary to determine whether or not the transverse ligament is intact.

Odontoid fractures have been classified into three types by Anderson and D'Alonzo.[23] Type I fractures are oblique fractures through the upper part of the odontoid process alone. While rare, they are stable and may be managed with an orthosis of limited stability. The type II fracture occurs at the junction of the odontoid process and the axis body, while in the type III fracture, the fracture lines enter into the axis body itself. Both type II and type III fractures eliminate the odontoid as a stabilizing element at the atlanto-axial junction. Therefore, these are unstable fractures, which need to be managed in a stable orthosis (i.e. halo) or with internal wiring and fusion. In managing these fractures it is important to obtain flexion-extension x-rays after healing so that a restoration of stability can be documented.

Rotary subluxation or dislocations at the atlanto-axial junction are substantially less common in adults than are other injuries to the atlanto-axial joint.[24-26] Levine and Edwards[22] found only two patients with this problem from among their 133 patients with C1-C2 injuries collected over a seven-year period. Because they are a more common problem for the pediatric patient, they are discussed more fully in Chapter 12. Fielding has classified these injuries into four types based upon the amount of displacement between C1 and C2.[25] The most significant issues regarding stability in these injuries revolves around whether or not the transverse ligament is intact. With an intact transverse ligament, complete bilateral dislocation does not occur until 65° of rotation is attained. However, with a deficiency of the transverse ligament, complete dislocation can occur at 45° of rotation.[27] Rotary subluxation of types II-IV that do not have an intact transverse ligament are unstable lesions and should be managed accordingly. Type I rotary subluxations which have less than 3 mm displacement between C1-C2 should be more stable because of the intact transverse ligament. However, if recurrent subluxation occurs after conservative management of type I lesions, fusion is probably indicated.

Fractures of the Neural Arch of the Axis

Fractures of the neural arch of the axis are usually caused by hyperextension and axial loading between C2 and C3, although hyperflexion may be involved in some cases.[22,28-31] Because of their association with judicial hanging, the appelation hangman's fracture has been attached to them.[16] Structurally

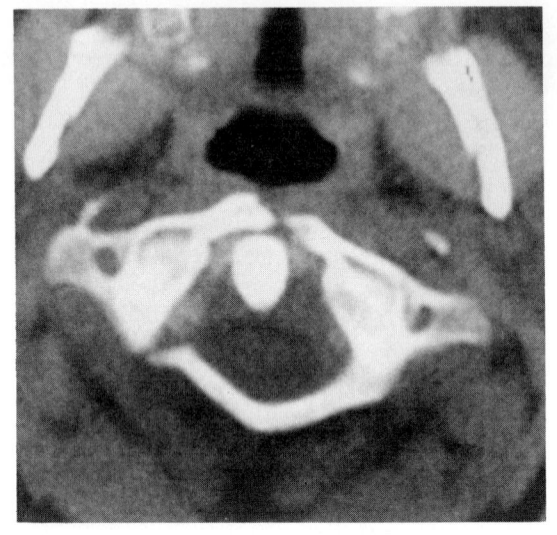

Figure 2a. Fracture of lateral mass of atlas seen on CT scan. Since the transverse ligament inserts into the lateral mass, such a fracture raises the possibility of a transverse ligament disruption.

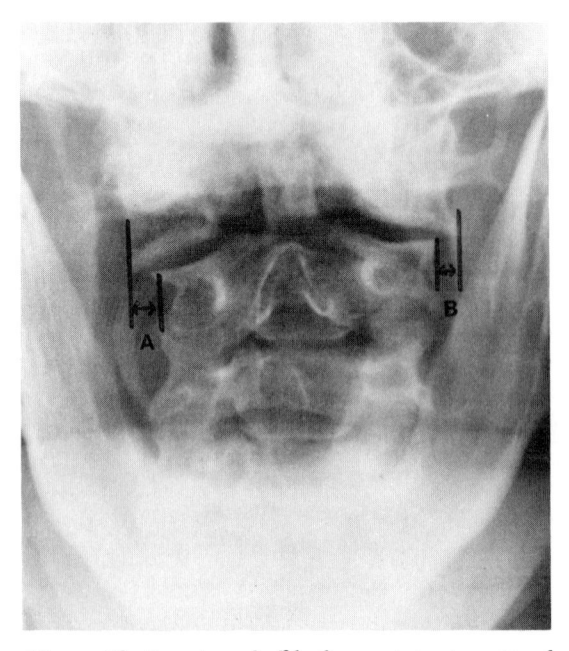

Figure 2b. Spence's method[21] of ascertaining integrity of the transverse ligament. If A + B > 6.9 mm the transverse ligament has probably been disrupted.

these fractures involve a bilateral arch fracture at C2 and a variable degree of displacement between C2 and C3. Various classification schemes have been proposed based on the degree of displacement and angulation between C2 and C3.[22,31-34,78] Effendi[32] has suggested that 65% of these fractures may be stable acutely as defined by being nondisplaced and not showing motion on flexion-extension radiographs.

Successful fusion has been obtained in many of these patients with a limited orthosis alone. Grady et al[35] treated eight patients who had up to 4 mm of subluxation with a combination of cervical traction followed by a Philadelphia collar and suggested this approach as an alternative to halo immobilization in some patients. These fractures should be considered stable only when the integrity of the C2-C3 disc has been preserved as defined by normal alignment of the C2 and C3 bodies across the disc and no displacement on flexion-extension radiographs.

Middle and Lower Cervical Spine

Various anatomical structures have been implicated in maintaining stability within the lower cervical spine. The disc and associated anterior and posterior longitudinal ligaments were believed to be the structures most important for stability by Bedrock[36] and Bailey.[37,38] The experimental work on human cadaver spines done by Roaf[39] provided additional support for this concept. Roaf demonstrated that increasing axial compression, hyperflexion, or hyperextension forces led to osseous failure within the vertebral body while the disc remained intact. However, the discs, joints, and ligaments were found to be more vulnerable to rotation and horizontal shearing forces than were the osseous structures. Munro's experimental work on cadaver spines also supported these observations.[40] Bailey also emphasized the role of the cervical spine muscles in maintaining stability. The importance of interspinous and supraspinous ligaments and the ligamentum nuchae was discussed by Holdsworth.[41] Other investigators have attributed less significance to these structures since they may be attenuated or absent in some segments in normal spines.[42,43]

The experimental work of White and Panjabi has provided additional perspective on the role played by ligaments in maintaining cervical spine stability.[44,45] Using eight cadaver spines, they analyzed 17 different motion segments (two adjacent vertebrae and the intervening soft tissue) in a high humidity chamber. With the lower vertebral body mounted on a firm base, the upper vertebral body was subjected to graded forces of flexion or extension using physiologic loads. Angular and horizontal displacement was measured between vertebral bodies as the load was applied. The anterior ligaments were defined as all the soft tissue structures ventral to and including the posterior longitudinal ligament. The ligaments were cut sequentially from anterior to posterior or from posterior to anterior in different experiments. Failure of the motion segment was defined by the upper vertebra suddenly rotating 90° or flying across the experimental table. Conversely, the posterior ligaments were all the soft tissues posterior to the posterior longitudinal ligaments.

These studies demonstrated failure of the motion segment in three of nine specimens in which all the anterior ligaments had been sectioned and in one of eight specimens in which all the posterior ligaments had been sectioned. From these observations the authors concluded that the loss of either all the anterior or all the posterior elements of the spine could render the lower cervical spine unstable. Furthermore, these investigators determined that the horizontal and angular displacements between vertebrae did not exceed 2.67 mm and 10.7°, respectively, prior to complete failure of the motion segment.

After analyzing this experimental data and correlating it with other concepts of stability White et al[46] proposed a checklist system for determining instability in the lower cervical spine (Table 1). The method of measuring the relative sagittal plane translation or an-

TABLE 1
Diagnosis of Instability in the Lower Cervical Spine

Criteria	Point Value
Anterior Elements Not Functional	2
Posterior Elements Not Functional	2
Relative Sagittal Plane Translation > 3.5 mm	2
Relative Sagittal Plane Angulation > 11°	2
Positive Stretch Test	2
Spinal Cord Injury	2
Nerve Root Injury	1
Abnormal Disc Narrowing	1
Dangerous Loading Anticipated	1
Clinical Instability If > 5	

Adapted from Reference 46.

gulation is illustrated in Figure 3. It should be noted that the translational measurement (>3.5 mm) given in Table 1 and Figure 3 is based on the figure 2.67 mm noted above, but takes into account the magnification likely to be found on standard lateral radiographs. For maximal accuracy it should be applied to lateral cervical radiographs taken with a standard tube to film distance of 183 cm. These measurements for angulation and translation are valid for radiographs obtained with the neck in neutral, flexion, or extension.

White et al[46,47] recognized that flexion-extension x-rays may be very hazardous for patients with significant ligamentous instability and suggested the "stretch test" as a safer alternative. This test is performed by applying increasing traction to the cervical spine via a head halter or skeletal fixation device. The traction is increased until ⅓ of body weight or 30 kg is reached, or evidence of instability is found. Lateral cervical spine radiographs are taken after each weight increase and examined for evidence of instability, which is defined as an increase in disc space height greater than 1.7 mm over the pretraction height or greater than 7.5° change in angulation between pretraction and posttraction vertebral body position. These numbers are based upon a cadaver study and eight normal persons.

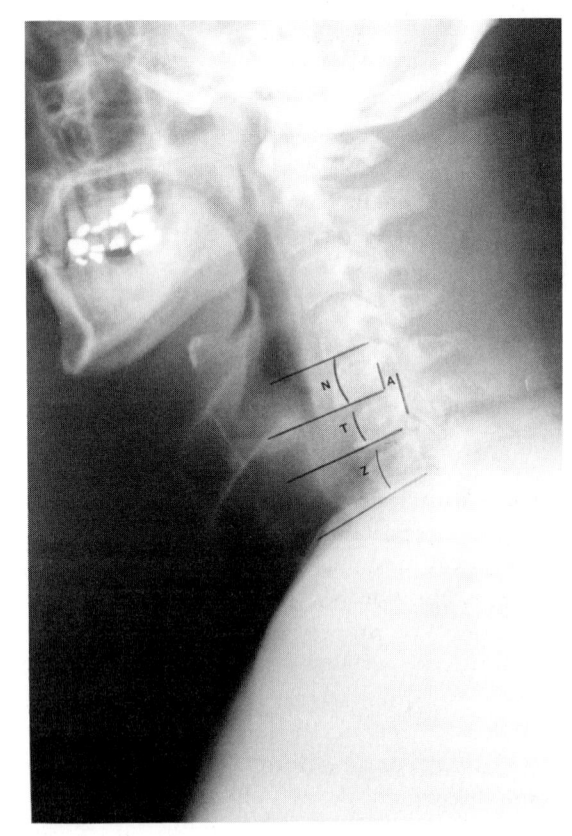

Figure 3. Method of measuring sagittal plane translation and angulation in the lower cervical spine.[46] If the sagittal translation distance is > 3.5 mm, ligamentous instability may be present. Sagittal plane angulation is measured by drawing lines along the bottom of each adjacent vertebral body. If the angle at the level of concern (T) differs from the angles of the adjacent levels N or Z by greater than 11°, instability may be present.

The checklist provided by White et al provides an excellent conceptual framework with which to approach the analysis of spinal stability. As with any system of this type, however, it must not be taken too literally. It is often difficult for the clinician to know about the intactness of all the anterior or all the posterior elements early in the evaluation of these patients.

Stability after facet dislocation has been evaluated experimentally by Beatson.[48] Using the cervical spine from a fresh young adult cadaver, he placed small pieces of Kirschner wire into the inferior articular facets at C4 and the superior articular facets at C5 and studied the spine with radiographs after a variety of maneuvers. He demonstrated that a unilateral facet dislocation was only possible if the corresponding interspinous ligament and joint capsule of the dislocated side were completely ruptured. Such a dislocation could be produced with only minimal damage to the annulus and posterior longitudinal ligament. However, a bilateral facet dislocation was possible only if all the posterior ligamentous structures, including the capsules of both facet joints, interspinous ligaments, annulus, and posterior longitudinal ligament, were ruptured.

These observations have been cited by most subsequent authors as evidence that these injuries are acutely unstable. Another equally important question is whether these injuries will stabilize as a result of ligamentous healing or whether they will require arthrodesis to prevent redislocation. In 1963 Holdsworth stated "when the posterior ligament complex has been ruptured, healing such as to restore the original strength does not occur" and recommended arthrodesis of such injuries.[49]

A recent experimental study in the dog can be cited in support of the aforementioned notion.[50] Whitehill et al divided the anterior longitudinal ligament, annulus fibrosus, and all posterior ligamentous structures in 18 mongrel dogs. After three months elapsed to allow healing of the ligamentous structures, the mechanical stability of these segments was compared to segments from normal dogs. After ligamentous healing, only 455-500 Newtons of force were necessary to induce flexion failure in the motion segments as compared to the 700 Newtons required in C4-C5 motion segments from normal dogs.

The late stability of these injuries has been assessed in several clinical series. While acquiring a series of 257 conservatively managed cervical spine injuries between 1959 and 1968, Cheshire[51] followed 41 patients with unilateral facet dislocations and 35 patients with bilateral facet dislocations. Only three (7.3%) of the unilateral dislocations and two (5.7%) of the bilateral dislocations were found to have late instability. A similar low incidence of late instability was noted by Braakman and Vinken[52] and by Rorabeck et al[53] after conservative care of unilateral facet dislocations. O'Brien[54] reported that three of 18 patients (17%), two with unilateral dislocations and one with bilateral facet dislocation, were unstable after 12 weeks immobilization in a halo brace. Sonntag found that external stabilization was as effective as operative arthrodesis in achieving late stability after bilateral facet dislocation.[55] However, Maiman et al[56] have, for the most part, used an operative approach to this problem.

A biomechanical analysis of compression injuries of the cervical spine has been done by Maiman et al[77] using three intact cadavers and 10 isolated cervical spinal columns. They demonstrated that flexion and extension injuries were produced at approximately 50% of the loads necessary to produce axial compression failure. Most importantly they pointed out that the resulting injuries correlated only partially with the direction of force delivery and they cautioned against overinterpretation of postinjury radiographs. These words of caution are emphasized further in the clinical literature.[57,58] Seemingly simple compression fractures, which are inherently stable injuries, may in fact involve major disruption of posterior ligamentous structures. Posterior ligament disruption would convert these fractures into unstable injuries with the potential for serious trauma to the spinal cord or late instability. Spasm of the cervical paraspinous muscles, immediately after injury, may mask the ligamentous instability during the initial evaluation. Therefore, all patients who are believed to have a simple compression fracture should be managed in an external orthosis initially. After the paraspinal spasm has subsided (usually 1-2 weeks after injury), repeat cervical spine radiographs with flexion-extension views should be obtained to evaluate for ligamentous instability.

It is of some interest to consider why late instability develops in cervical spine injuries. A survey of several reviews of conservatively treated cervical spine injury suggests that late instability is a clinical problem for 6-12% of patients.[46] It is difficult to blame this small incidence of late instability on ligamentous injury alone, since ligamentous injuries are present in a much higher proportion of cervical spine injuries.

In fact Cheshire,[51] who considered this problem carefully, was able to document stable healing of ligamentous injuries in most of his patients. He observed more late instability in patients with anterior subluxations (21%) compared to patients with bilateral facet dislocations (5.7%). In analyzing this problem he stated that the patients with bilateral facet dislocations probably had more posterior ligamentous disruption than the patients with anterior subluxation. He attributed the higher rate of late instability in the latter group to the inadequacy of the conservative management in the patients with anterior subluxation. Most of the patients with anterior subluxations had minor and rapidly recovering neurological deficit and therefore were much more mobile than the majority of the patients with bilateral facet dislocations.

It is important to recognize that the literature documents stable healing of most cervical spine injuries with conservative care alone, regardless of the degree of ligamentous disruption. However, this conservative care may involve many weeks of bedrest and traction. In deciding how to manage an individual patient with a cervical spine injury these factors must be kept in mind.

Injury to the cervical spine often occurs as one part of multisystem trauma, particularly after high velocity motor vehicle accidents. Management of life-threatening injuries may preclude an immediate thorough evaluation of cervical spine stability. An algorithm for the evaluation and management of possible cervical spine instability is illustrated in Figure 4.

Thoracic Spine and Thoracolumbar Spine

Stability in the thoracic and thoracolumbar spine depends upon several anatomical factors that differ from those found in the cervical spine. The anterior and posterior longitudinal ligaments are more distinct and stronger structures here than in the cervical spine. The articulations between the ribs and spine, which are buttressed further by the costotransverse ligaments, provide additional internal support.[59] The ligamentum flavum, being thicker and better developed, is an important structure that resists hyperflexion of the spine. The orientation of the facet joints is also different. The joints are oriented in a sagittal plane that limits axial rotation and provides stability against horizontal translation.[60] As the orientation of the facet joints changes in the lower thoracic spine, they provide less resistance to horizontal translation. The capsular ligaments also differ from those present in the cervical spine. In the thoracic spine they are thinner and much less able to resist flexion forces than in the cervical spine.[61]

White and his colleagues have performed several biomechanical studies of the thoracic spine similar in concept to their experiments in the cervical spine that have been described above.[62,63,79] These studies have demonstrated that increased flexion, extension, and axial rotation follow removal of the posterior elements. However, motion segment failure does not occur until all the posterior ele-

Clinical Assessment

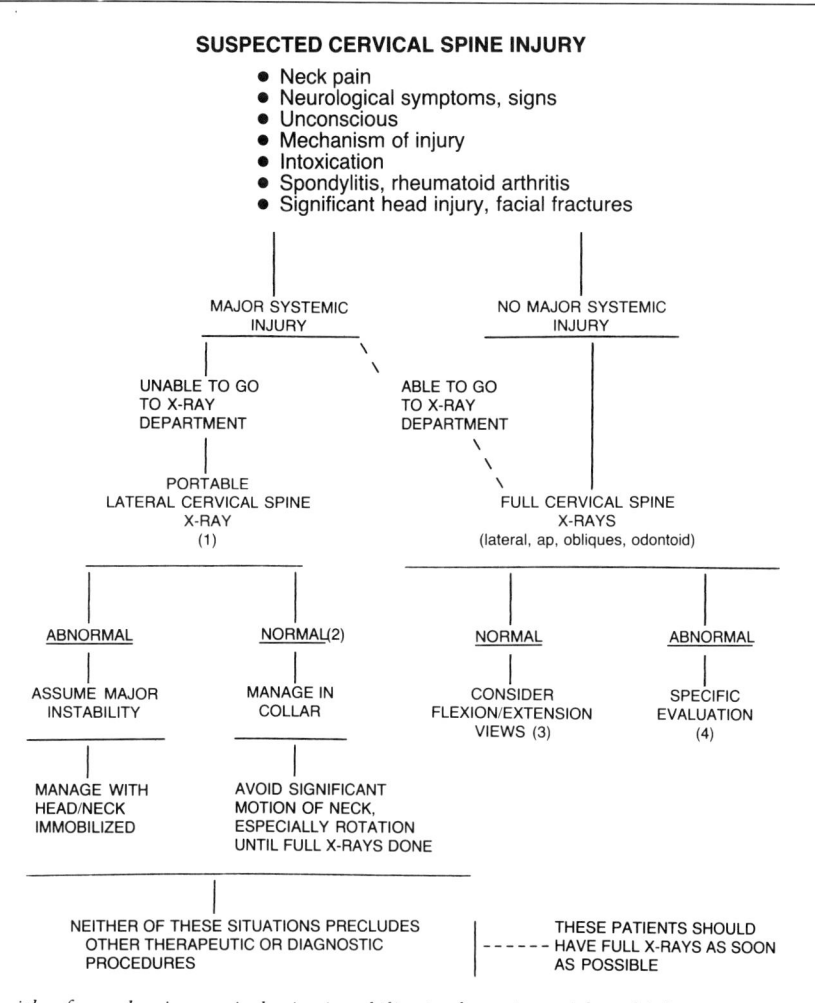

```
                    SUSPECTED CERVICAL SPINE INJURY
                    • Neck pain
                    • Neurological symptoms, signs
                    • Unconscious
                    • Mechanism of injury
                    • Intoxication
                    • Spondylitis, rheumatoid arthritis
                    • Significant head injury, facial fractures
```

Figure 4. Algorithm for evaluating cervical spine instability in the patient with multiple trauma:

1. The portable lateral cervical radiograph must visualize the entire cervical spine and include all of C7. A bilateral facet dislocation of C7 on T1 may be missed unless the top of T1 also is seen. Visualizing down to T1 may require a swimmer's view, pulling the shoulders down, or tomography.
2. To be considered normal, the lateral radiograph must be 100% normal. Any degree of translational or angulation effect is considered abnormal under these circumstances.
3. Flexion-extension radiographs are performed when there is concern about possible ligamentous instability. They should be performed cautiously with only the patient moving the neck. These studies may be falsely normal shortly after injury due to cervical paraspinal muscle spasm.
4. Abnormal radiographic findings evaluated with additional diagnostic techniques including computed tomography, conventional tomography, and magnetic resonance imaging.

ments plus the costovertebral articulation, or all the anterior elements plus at least one posterior component, are destroyed. Furthermore, stability in extension could be maintained with the anterior longitudinal ligament alone, while stability in flexion could be maintained with posterior longitudinal ligament and other anterior ligaments intact. Based on these studies, these investigators have concluded that a horizontal displacement of greater than 2.5 mm or an angulation greater than 5° between thoracic vertebral bodies as seen on a standard lateral radiograph may indicate an unstable spine.

Several clinical studies have attempted to define criteria to determine if fractures and fracture dislocations of this region are stable or unstable. Nicoll[64] studied 166 fractures of the dorsolumbar spine in 152 miners. He stated that anterior and lateral wedge fractures were stable, while fracture-dislocations were unstable. The most significant feature that determined instability was loss of support from the posterior ligamentous structures.

Other investigators have offered additional classification schemes for determining the presence of instability.[49,65-67] From the information available at present, it is possible to conclude that anterior wedge fractures, lateral wedge fractures, and bursting compression fractures are likely to be stable unless the posterior ligaments are destroyed. One clue that the posterior ligaments may not be intact is a loss of vertebral body height by 50%, although this observation alone cannot be considered positive proof of instability.[68] Dislocations and fracture-dislocations, particularly those with rotational deformities, should be considered to be unstable.[69]

White and Panjabi[63] have suggested a checklist system for assessing instability in the thoracic and thoracolumbar spine (Table 2). This system offers a useful framework within which to consider these fractures, although its precise details have yet to be validated in a large clinical series.

Determining that a thoracolumbar fracture is unstable does not necessarily mean that surgical intervention is required. Unstable fractures managed with long-term bedrest can heal in a stable manner.[49,64,70] However, conservative treatment will result in a longer hospital stay than surgical therapy.

Lumbar Spine

In contrast to the thoracic spine, the facet joints and their tough capsular ligaments play a major role in stability of the lumbar spine. Axial rotation of 30° or more between adjacent lumbar vertebrae results in facet dislocation or fracture and can be considered evidence of instability.[71] The anterior longitudinal ligament is also well developed in the lumbar spine as is the annulus fibrosus. However, the interspinous ligaments may be deficient in up to 21% of normal adults,[72] and are probably not of major importance in lumbar spine stability.

A biomechanical analysis of stability has been performed by Posner et al.[73] Using a method similar to that described previously they studied 18 motion segments from the lumbar spines of cadavers. During loading in flexion, all the motion segments failed when all the posterior components plus one anterior component were destroyed. With loading in extension all the motion segments failed when all the anterior components plus two posterior components were destroyed.

TABLE 2
Diagnosis of Instability in the Thoracic and Thoracolumbar Spine

Criteria	Point Value
Anterior Elements Not Functional	2
Posterior Elements Not Functional	2
Relative Sagittal Plane Translation > 2.5 mm	2
Relative Sagittal Plane Angulation > 5°	2
Injury to Spinal Cord or Cauda Equina	2
Disruptions of Costovertebral Articulations	1
Dangerous Loading Anticipated	2
Clinical Instability If > 5	

Adapted from Reference 63.

The anterior components generally failed at the disc with the annulus fibers and cartilaginous end-plate pulling away from the vertebral body. The posterior components failed at the attachment of ligaments to bone. These authors used this information to propose a checklist for lumbar (Table 3) and lumbosacral instability (Table 4).

Kaufer and Hayes[74] collected 21 cases of lumbar fracture-dislocation in a retrospective analysis of 525 spine fractures seen at the University of Michigan Medical Center between 1956 and 1963. All of these were unstable injuries. However, some bias was evident here since patients had to have subluxation or dislocation of either or both articular processes or of the vertebral bodies to be included in this review.

It is apparent from the reviews of Nicoll[64] and Holdsworth,[49] which also included many patients with lumbar spine injuries, that not all of these injuries are unstable. It seems safe to conclude from these reviews that anterior wedge and lateral wedge fractures are stable injuries if the posterior ligamentous structures remain intact. Isolated neural arch fractures are also stable injuries. Fracture-dislocations as defined above should be considered unstable. Rotational deformities of 30° or greater and loss of vertebral body height of more than 50% should be considered unstable. Lumbar spine injuries are described in depth in Chapter 9.

Sacrum

Stability of sacral fractures has been reviewed in detail by Schmidek et al.[75] They emphasize the importance of considering not only the type of sacral fracture itself, but also

TABLE 3
Diagnosis of Instability in the Lumbar Spine

Criteria	Point Value
Cauda Equina Injury	3
Relative Flexion Sagittal Plane Translation > 8% or Relative Extension Sagittal Plane Translation > 9%	2
Relative Flexion Sagittal Plane Rotation < 9°	2
Anterior Elements Not Functional	2
Posterior Elements Not Functional	2
Dangerous Loading Anticipated	1
Clinical Instability If > 5	

Adapted from Reference 73.

TABLE 4
Diagnosis of Instability in the Lumbosacral Spine

Criteria	Point Value
Cauda Equina Injury	3
Relative Flexion Sagittal Plane Translation > 6% or Relative Extension Sagittal Plane Translation > 9%	2
Anterior Elements Not Functional	2
Posterior Elements Not Functional	2
Dangerous Loading Anticipated	1
Clinical Instability If > 5	

Adapted from Reference 73.

the integrity of the pelvic ring in determining stability in sacral fractures. Thus a cleaving fracture of the sacrum is inherently unstable and likely to be associated with a pelvic ring disruption, while a lateral mass fracture may be stable in the face of lateral compression of the pelvic ring. The addition of a sacroiliac joint disruption, however, would render the lateral mass fracture unstable. Since these fractures involve osseous disruptions, which usually heal, late instability is uncommon. A full discussion of these fractures is the subject of Chapter 10.

References

1. Fielding JW, Burstein AH, Frankel VH. The nuchal ligament. *Spine.* 1976;1:3-14.
2. Hohl M. Normal motions in the upper portion of the cervical spine. *J Bone Joint Surg Am.* 1964;46A:1777-1779.
3. Jofe MH, White AA, Panjabi MM. Kinematics. In: Research Society editorial subcommittee, ed. *The Cervical Spine.* Philadelphia, Pa: JB Lippincott Co; 1983:23-25.
4. Werne S. Studies in spontaneous atlas dislocation. *Acta Orthop Scand.* 1957;23(suppl):1-50.
5. Bucholz RW, Burkhead WZ. The pathological anatomy of fatal atlanto-occipital dislocations. *J Bone Joint Surg Am.* 1979;61A:248-250.
6. Eismont FJ, Bohlman HH. Posterior atlanto-occipital dislocation with fractures of the atlas and odontoid process. *J Bone Joint Surg Am.* 1978;60A:397-399.
7. Evarts CM. Traumatic occipito-atlantal dislocation: report of a case with survival. *J Bone Joint Surg Am.* 1970;52A:1653-1660.
8. Farthing JW. Atlantocranial dislocation with survival: a case report. *N Carolina Med J.* 1948;9:34-36.
9. Fruin AH, Pirotte TP. Traumatic atlantooccipital dislocation. *J Neurosurg.* 1977;46:663-666.
10. Gabrielson TO, Maxwell JA. Traumatic atlanto-occipital dislocation: with case report of a patient who survived. *AJR.* 1966;97:624-629.
11. Page CP, Story JL, Wissinger JP, Branch CL. Traumatic atlantooccipital dislocation. *J Neurosurg.* 1973;39:394-397.
12. Pang D, Wilberger JE Jr. Traumatic atlanto-occipital dislocation with survival: case report and review. *Neurosurgery.* 1980;7:503-508.
13. Powers B, Miller MD, Kramer RS, Martinez S, Gehweiler JA. Traumatic anterior atlanto-occipital dislocation. *Neurosurgery.* 1979;4:12-17.
14. Wholey MH, Bruwer AJ, Baker HL Jr. The lateral roentgenogram of the neck. *Radiology.* 1958;71:350-356.
15. Dublin AB, Marks WM, Weinstock D, Newton TH. Traumatic dislocation of the atlanto-occipital articulation (AOA) with short term survival. *J Neurosurg.* 1980;52:541-546.
16. Wood-Jones F. The ideal lesion produced by judicial hanging. *Lancet.* 1913;1:53-55.
17. Fielding JW, Cochran GVB, Lawsing JF III, Hohl M. Tears of the transverse ligament of the atlas: a clinical and biomechanical study. *J Bone Joint Surg Am.* 1974;56A:1683-1691.
18. Steele HH. Anatomical and mechanical considerations of the atlanto-axial articulations. In: Proceedings of the American Orthopaedic Association. *J Bone Joint Surg Am.* 1968;50A:1481-1482.
19. Jefferson G. Fracture of the atlas vertebra: review of four cases, and a review of those previously recorded. *Br J Surg.* 1920;7:407-422.
20. Sherk HH, Nicholson JT. Fractures of the atlas. *J Bone Joint Surg Am.* 1970;52A:1017-1024.
21. Spence KF Jr, Decker S, Sell RW. Bursting atlantal fracture associated with rupture of the transverse ligament. *J Bone Joint Surg Am.* 1970;52A:543-549.
22. Levine AM, Edwards CC. Treatment of injuries in the C1-C2 complex. *Orthop Clin North Am.* 1986;17:31-44.
23. Anderson LD, D'Alonzo RT. Fractures of the odontoid process of the axis. *J Bone Joint Surg Am.* 1974;56A:1663-1674.
24. Fielding JW, Hawkins RJ. Atlanto-axial rotatory fixation. *J Bone Joint Surg Am.* 1977;59A:37-44.
25. Fielding JW, Hawkins RJ, Hensinger RN, Francis WR. Atlantoaxial rotary deformities. *Orthop Clin North Am.* 1978;9:955-967.
26. Greenberg AD. Atlanto-axial dislocations. *Brain.* 1968;91:655-684.
27. Coutts MB. Atlanto-epistropheal subluxations. *Arch Surg.* 1934;29:297-311.
28. Brashear HR, Venters GC, Preston ET. Fractures of the neural arch of the axis. *J Bone Joint Surg Am.* 1975;57A:879-887.
29. DeLorme TL. Axis pedicle fractures. *J Bone Joint Surg Am.* 1967;49A:1471-1474.
30. Schneider RC, Livingston KE, Cave AJE, Hamilton G. Hangman's fracture of the cervical spine. *J Neurosurg.* 1965;22:141-154.
31. Williams TG. Hangman's fracture. *J Bone Joint Surg Br.* 1975;57B:82-88.
32. Effendi B, Roy D, Cornish B, Dussault RG, Laurin CA. Fractures of the ring of the axis: a classification based on the analysis of 131 cases. *J Bone Joint Surg Br.* 1981;63B:319-327.
33. Seljeskog EL, Chou SN. Spectrum of the hangman's fracture. *J Neurosurg.* 1976;45:3-8.
34. Francis WR, Fielding JW, Hawkins RJ, Pepin J, Hensinger R. Traumatic spondylolisthesis of the axis. *J Bone Joint Surg Br.* 1981;63B:313-318.
35. Grady MS, Howard MA, Jane JA, Persing JA. Use of the Philadelphia collar as an alternative to the halo vest in patients with C-2, C-3 fractures. *Neurosurgery.* 1986;18:151-156.
36. Bedrock GM. Are cervical spine fractures ever unstable? *J West Pac Orthop Assoc.* 1969;6:7-29.
37. Bailey RW. Fractures and dislocations of the cervical spine: orthopedic and neurosurgical aspects. *Postgrad Med.* 1964;35:588-599.
38. Bailey RW. Observations of cervical intervertebral-disc lesions in fractures and dislocations. *J Bone Joint Surg Am.* 1963;45A:461-470.
39. Roaf R. A study of the mechanics of spinal injuries. *J Bone Joint Surg Br.* 1960;42B:810-823.
40. Munro D. The factors that govern the stability of the spine. *Paraplegia.* 1965;3:219-228.

41. Holdsworth FW. Fractures, dislocations, and fracture-dislocations of the spine. *J Bone Joint Surg Br.* 1963;45B:6-20.
42. Halliday DR, Sullivan CR, Hollinshead WH, Bahn RC. Torn cervical ligaments: necropsy examination of the normal cervical region of the spinal column. *J Trauma.* 1964;4:219-232.
43. Johnson RM, Crelin ES, White AA III, Panjabi MM, Southwick WO. Some new observations on the functional anatomy of the lower cervical spine. *Clin Orthop.* 1975;111:192-200.
44. Panjabi MM, White AA III, Johnson RM. Cervical spine mechanics as a function of transection of components. *J Biomech.* 1975;8:327-336.
45. White AA III, Johnson RM, Panjabi MM, Southwick WO. Biomechanical analysis of clinical stability in the cervical spine. *Clin Orthop.* 1975;109:85-96.
46. White AA, Southwick WO, Panjabi MM. Clinical instability in the lower cervical spine. *Spine.* 1976;1:15-27.
47. White AA III, Panjabi MM, Saha S, Southwick WO. Biomechanics of the axially loaded cervical spine: development of a clinical test for ruptured ligaments. In: Proceedings of The Orthopaedic Research Society. *J Bone Joint Surg Am.* 1975;57A:582.
48. Beatson TR. Fractures and dislocations of the cervical spine. *J Bone Joint Surg Br.* 1963;45B:21-35.
49. Holdsworth F. Fractures, dislocations, and fracture-dislocations of the spine. *J Bone Joint Surg Am.* 1970;52A:1534-1551.
50. Whitehill R, Moran DJ, Fechner RE, Ruch WW, Drucker S, Hooper WE, et al. Cervical ligamentous instability in a canine in vivo model. *Spine.* 1987;12:959-963.
51. Cheshire DJE. The stability of the cervical spine following the conservative treatment of fractures and fracture-dislocations. *Paraplegia.* 1969;7:193-203.
52. Braakman R, Vinken PF. Unilateral facet interlocking in the lower cervical spine. *J Bone Joint Surg Br.* 1967;40B:249-257.
53. Rorabeck CH, Rock MG, Hawkins RJ, Bourne RB. Unilateral facet dislocation of the cervical spine. *Spine.* 1987;12:23-27.
54. O'Brien PJ, Schweigel JF, Thompson WJ. Dislocations of the lower cervical spine. *J Trauma.* 1982;22:710-714.
55. Sonntag VKH. Management of bilateral locked facets of the cervical spine. *Neurosurgery.* 1981;8:150-152.
56. Maiman DJ, Barolat G, Larson SJ. Management of bilateral locked facets of the cervical spine. *Neurosurgery.* 1986;18:542-547.
57. Webb JK, Broughton RBK, McSweeney T, Park WM. Hidden flexion injury of the cervical spine. *J Bone Joint Surg Br.* 1976;58B:322-327.
58. Mazur JM, Stauffer ES. Unrecognized spinal instability associated with seemingly "simple" cervical compression fractures. *Spine.* 1983;8:687-692.
59. Andriacchi TP, Schultz AB, Belytschko TB, Galante J. A model for studies of mechanical interactions between the human spine and rib cage. *J Biomech.* 1974;7:497-507.
60. White AA III, Panjabi MM. The basic kinematics of the human spine: a review of past and current knowledge. *Spine.* 1978;3:12-20.
61. Markolf KL. Deformation of the thoracolumbar intervertebral joints in response to external loads. *J Bone Joint Surg Am.* 1972;54A:511-533.
62. White AA III, Hirsch C. The significance of the vertebral posterior elements in the mechanics of the thoracic spine. *Clin Orthop.* 1971;81:2-14.
63. White AA, Panjabi MM. *Clinical Biomechanics of the Spine.* Philadelphia, Pa: JB Lippincott Co; 1978:236-251.
64. Nicoll EA. Fractures of the dorso-lumbar spine. *J Bone Joint Surg Br.* 1949;31B:376-394.
65. Denis F. The three column spine and its significance in the classification of acute thoracolumbar spinal injuries. *Spine.* 1983;8:817-831.
66. Riggins RS, Kraus JF. The risk of neurologic damage with fractures of the vertebrae. *J Trauma.* 1977;17:126-133.
67. Kelly RP, Whitesides TE Jr. Treatment of lumbodorsal fracture-dislocations. *Ann Surg.* 1968;167:705-717.
68. Larson SJ. The thoracolumbar junction. In: Dunsker SB, Schmidek HH, Frymoyer J, Kahn A III, eds. *The Unstable Spine.* Orlando, Fla: Grune & Stratton Inc; 1986:127-152.
69. Whitesides TE Jr. Traumatic kyphosis of the thoracolumbar spine. *Clin Orthop.* 1977;128:78-92.
70. Davies WE, Morris JH, Hill V. An analysis of conservative (non-surgical) management of thoracolumbar fractures and fracture-dislocations with neural damage. *J Bone Joint Surg Am.* 1980;62A:1324-1328.
71. Sullivan JD, Farfan HF. The crumpled neural arch. *Orthop Clin North Am.* 1975;6:199-214.
72. Rissanen PM. The surgical anatomy and pathology of the supraspinous and interspinous ligaments of the lumbar spine with special reference to ligament ruptures. *Acta Orthop Scand.* 1960;46(suppl):1-20.
73. Posner I, White AA III, Edwards WT, Hayes WC. A biomechanical analysis of the clinical stability of the lumbar and lumbosacral spine. *Spine.* 1982;7:374-389.
74. Kaufer H, Hayes JT. Lumbar fracture-dislocation. *J Bone Joint Surg Am.* 1966;48A:712-730.
75. Schmidek HH, Smith DA, Kristiansen TK. Sacral fractures: issues of neural injury, spinal stability, and surgical management. In: Dunsker SB, Schmidek HH, Frymoyer J, Kahn A III, eds. *The Unstable Spine.* Orlando, Fla: Grune & Stratton, Inc; 1986:191-220.
76. Dvorak J, Panjabi MM. Functional anatomy of the alar ligaments. *Spine.* 1987;12:183-189.
77. Maiman DJ, Sances A Jr, Myklebust JB, Larson SJ, Houterman C, Chilbert M, et al. Compression injuries of the cervical spine: a biomechanical analysis. *Neurosurgery.* 1983;13:254-260.
78. Monu J, Bohrer SP, Howard G. Some upper cervical spine norms. *Spine.* 1987;12:515-519.
79. Panjabi MM, Hausfeld JN, White AA III. A biomechanical study of the ligamentous stability of the thoracic spine in man. *Acta Orthop Scand.* 1981;52:315-326.

CHAPTER 4

Spinal Orthoses

Mark N. Hadley, MD

A number of spinal orthotic devices have been used to limit motion, correct deformities, and reduce pain in patients with vertebral column disorders. Depending on the abnormality, a spinal orthosis may be applied for comfort and a reminder, or may be used in an attempt to immobilize an injured vertebral segment.

Because all spinal orthotic devices are applied externally, the degree of immobilization is dependent on the design of the orthotic device, the tightness with which it is worn, points of fixation with the body, the vertebral segment to be immobilized, and the movement and shape of the patient's body.[1,2] These features will be discussed in the following review of the practical application of spinal orthoses.

Clinical Application

The goal in using a spinal orthotic device is control of the position of the spine. Usually this is directed to a specific vertebral column segment. Control of the position of the spine and the reduction or elimination of motion at an unstable vertebral segment may be required to reduce pain, allow healing of bony and ligamentous injuries, correct a deformity, and/or protect adjacent associated neurological structures. The latter principle of spinal immobilization is of greatest concern to neurological surgeons, whether in the early phase of evaluation of an acute traumatic injury or in the postinjury or postoperative management phase of a patient's treatment course. Longer, contiguous vertebral column segments (thoraco-lumbar and sacral segments) can be braced or immobilized as required in the treatment and correction of progressive spinal deformities, such as scoliosis and kyphosis.[3,4] The management of patients with these disorders, however, rarely falls to the neurological surgeon alone.

A spinal orthosis controls positions of the spine by the application of external forces. The applied external forces alter and limit the preexisting motion and deformation of the vertebral column.[2,5,6] When used in the treatment of spinal instability with subluxation of any cause, spinal injuries, or as a postoperative immobilization device, the orthosis must perform functions which would normally be accomplished by the spinal column and its associated supporting structures. The more rigid forms of spinal orthoses must serve their purpose until healing has occurred and structural competence has returned to the injured vertebral segments.

A less rigid orthosis may be used for lesser degrees of injury such as a sprain, or for patients with musculoskeletal pain of spinal origin. In these situations, the orthotic device is not responsible for the structural integrity of the vertebral column, but is used to assist the spinal column and axial musculature during the treatment period.[1] Devices of this type (collars, corsets) have addi-

---

The views of the author are his own and are not to be construed as official or reflecting the position of the Department of the Air Force or the Department of Defense.

tional benefit as a reminder to patients to limit their activities.

Biomechanics of Spinal Bracing

The spine may be considered as a series of semirigid bodies (the vertebrae) separated by viscoelastic linkages (the discs).[2] This biomechanical model of the spine explains both the rigid and plastic qualities of the spine and is the basis of spinal kinematics: the study of the motion of the spinal column without consideration of associated muscular and ligamentous structures. The semirigid, mobile spinal column is encased within the body muscle, the thoracic rib cage, abdominal viscera, and surrounded by the pelvis. Each of these structures is semirigid with variable degrees of compression, distortion, and viscoelasticity.

Spinal orthoses limit motion of the vertebral column by indirect means. They exert no direct force upon the spine, but instead, rely upon device designs and points of fixation with the body to effect vertebral column immobilization.[1,2,5,7] From the perspective of spinal orthotics, the spine is contained within a cylinder or series of cylinders of varying diameters and varying degrees of stiffness. The orthotic device must exert its influence and transmit forces through these cylinders (the neck, the torso, the abdomen, the pelvis) to the vertebral column to achieve its desired effect.[1,2]

Several major mechanical factors limit the application of force to the vertebral column and hinder effective spinal immobilization. First, the orthotic device must transmit force through low-stiffness, viscoelastic transmitters, each of which is different from another. The skull, the thoracic cage, and the pelvis are relatively rigid transmitters while muscle, fat, and the abdominal viscera are not. Second, within the various cylinders of the body lie structures which do not tolerate direct pressure or compression. These include major vascular structures, the larynx, trachea, and lower abdominal-perineal organs. An orthotic device must have specific points of fixation with relatively rigid body parts (skull, thoracic rib cage, pelvis) yet avoid compression and the transmission of force through the structures least tolerant of pressure and most easily compromised. Finally, the sensitivity and durability of the skin and subcutaneous structures must be considered in the application of spinal orthoses. Broad-based pressure is preferred over focal compression to avoid skin erosion, pain, and ulceration.

Spinal Motion

White and Panjabi have outlined six degrees of freedom intrinsic to each vertebral unit.[2] The complex motions of the cervical spine in space, for example, may be described by the determination of 42 independent displacements: seven vertebrae each with six degrees of freedom. Kinematic analysis reveals the cervical spine to be the most mobile of spinal segments.[2,5-12] Axial rotation is maximal at C1-C2, sagittal plane motion is greatest at C5-C6 and C6-C7, and lateral bending is maximal at C4-C5.

The thoracic spine is the least mobile of the three spinal regions, but still allows a significant amount of flexion and extension and a lesser degree of lateral bending, particularly at the distal thoracic spine and the thoracolumbar junction. The lumbosacral spinal segment is limited with respect to lateral bending and axial rotation, but demonstrates a remarkable degree of flexion and extension from the L1 level increasing through the lumbosacral junction.[2,6] Distal sacral segments are firmly joined to the pelvis and have little independent mobility. Pelvic motion translates directly to the lumbosacral spinal segment.[1,2,6]

In general, axial rotation is greatest at the superior aspect of the spinal column and decreases with lower vertebral segments. Lateral bending and sagittal plane motion are significant in the cervical spinal segment, decrease at the cervicothoracic junction, and then increase distally from the thoracolumbar junction through the lumbar vertebrae.

Spinal Bracing

Spinal orthoses must control the movement of a single spinal column motion segment, each with a variable number of vertebra, and must also limit the effects of motion of the adjacent spinal segments. To limit motion at the thoracolumbar junction, for example, the orthosis must limit the influence of motion of both the thoracic and lumbosacral spinal segments. To achieve immobilization, the orthotic device will typically span beyond the segment to be immobilized to limit the influences of contiguous spinal segments on the area of injury or instability. Effective motion control is one of the primary goals of spinal bracing. Other beneficial objectives of spinal bracing include spinal realignment, trunk support, weight transfer, and irritative reminder.[1,7] To accomplish these objectives, several biomechanical principles have been incorporated into the design and utilization of spinal orthoses. They include the following:

1. balancing of forces via mechanical three-point fixation (including skeletal fixation)
2. distraction
3. fluid compression and the sleeve principle (the construction of a cage around the patient)
4. irritative restraint[1,2,7]

Three-point fixation is essential to achieve motion control of a spinal column segment. Skeletal fixation appears to be the most effective method of three-point fixation if rigid spinal immobilization is desired. Spinal realignment with or without distraction cannot be accomplished without using three-point fixation. It is an essential component of any orthotic device used in the treatment of kyphotic, scoliotic, or rotational spinal deformities.

Distraction is accomplished by weight transfer, most effectively and consistently with three-point fixation/skeletal fixation devices. Distraction forces may be required to facilitate spinal column realignment and are the rationale behind the use of cranial tongs in the early management of cervical spinal segment fracture-dislocations. Once realignment has been achieved, lesser degrees of distraction will usually be required to maintain alignment during healing. Rigid immobilization devices using three-point fixation are typically used for this purpose.

Fluid compression plays a role when attempting to immobilize the thoracic or lumbosacral spinal segments. Compression of the viscoelastic abdominal cavity and viscera elevates intraabdominal pressure and permits transfer of force to the desired spinal segment(s). The sleeve principle is used to create a sleeve or cast around the thoracic or abdominal cavities to convert them into semirigid cylinders through which force may be exerted on the spinal column. Orthotic devices that use these principles provide weight transfer and trunk support.

Lastly, a spinal orthosis may be useful in providing an irritative reminder to the patient. Irritative restraints provide stimuli for corrective muscle activity in response to uncomfortable pressure points and serve as reminders to patients to limit their exertion and curb their activities.

Cervical Orthoses

The support and immobilization provided by orthotic devices varies widely and depends on the biomechanical principles used in their construction and application. The clinician must decide which type of device is best suited to achieve the specific treatment goals for an individual patient (Table 1). Cervical spinal segment orthoses have been categorized into four distinct types: collars, poster-type orthoses, cervicothoracic devices, and halo orthoses.[1,8]

Collars

Collars provide little support for the cervical spine and are ineffective as cervical spinal immobilization devices.[3,9,11-16] Three main types are the soft collar, the hard collar,

TABLE 1
Cervical Orthoses

Device	Disorder	Comments
All collars	Acute trauma	Do not immobilize
Tape-sandbags	Acute trauma	Best motion control
Tape-rolled blankets	Acute trauma	Excellent alternative
Soft collars	Muscle spasm Mild strain Postop ACD without fusion	Irritative reminder
Philadelphia collar	Stable spine Postop ACD with fusion Nondisplaced Cl Fractures Minimal body or spinous process fractures	Some limitations of flexion and extension
Four poster brace	Stable spine	Alternative to Philadelphia collar
SOMI brace	Nondisplaced Cl fractures Some C2 fractures, not odontoid type II	More motion control, particularly at C1-C3
Halo vest	Spinal instability	Most effective motion control device
	Displaced atlas fractures Type II odontoid fractures Combination Cl-C2 fractures Postop immobilization	
	Other significant fractures	Thermoplastic Minerva Jacket is alternative

and the Philadelphia collar (Figure 1). Compared to healthy patients without collars, the soft collar provides little limitation of axial rotation, flexion, extension or lateral bending of the cervical spinal segment. The hard collar, such as the Thomas collar, is little better. The Philadelphia collar provides significantly more limitation of cervical motion than the soft collar, particularly with respect to flexion and extension, but is ineffective in limiting axial rotation and lateral bending.[9,11,12,15] Collars in general do not provide motion control, spinal realignment, or weight transfer and serve primarily as irritative reminder-restraints.

Poster-Type Orthoses

A more rigid orthosis, the poster-type brace, uses the principles of three-point fixation with fixation at the mandible, occiput and shoulder or upper thorax. Three major poster-type orthoses are commonly used: the four-poster brace, the two-poster Guilford orthosis, and the SOMI (sterno-occipito-mandibular immobilization) brace (Figure 2). Three-point fixation with these devices allows for some degree of weight transfer for spinal realignment and/or distraction and provides increased cervical segment immobilization compared to cervical collars. The

Spinal Orthoses

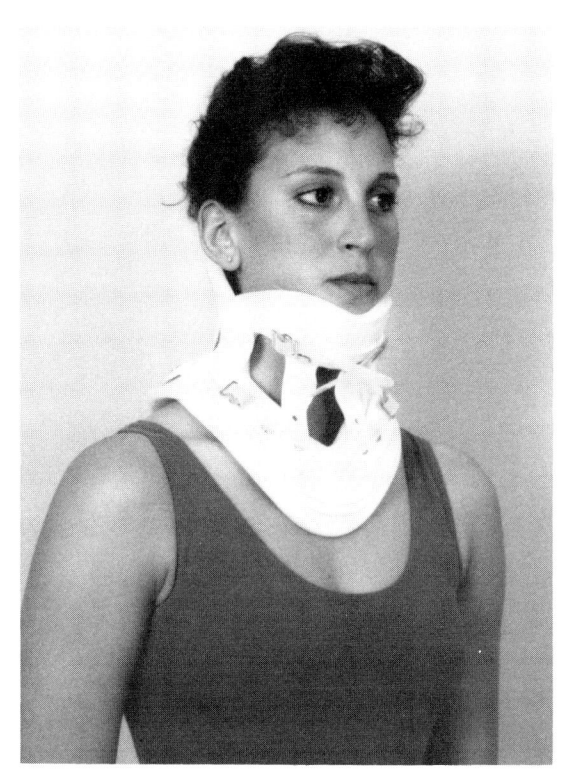

Figure 1. The Malibu Collar, a hard collar similar in design to the Philadelphia Collar. The height and circumference may be adjusted for a tighter fit (Manufactured by Johnson Orthopedic Appliances, Inc.).

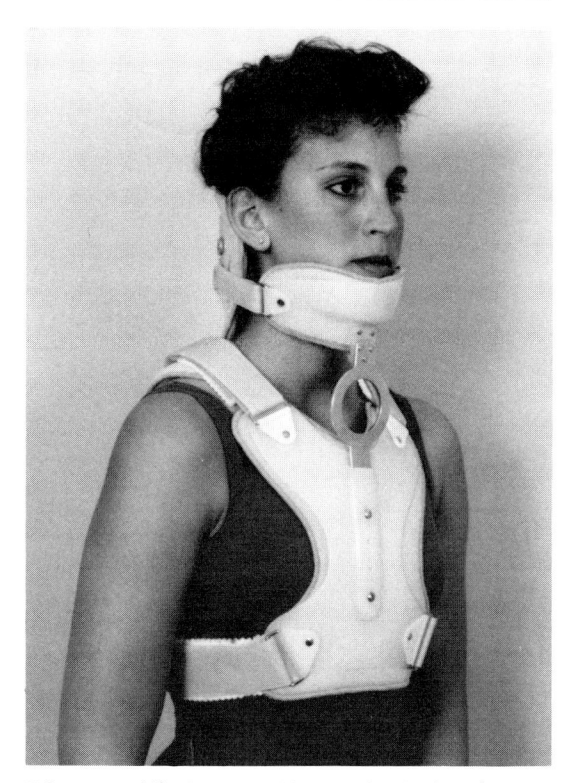

Figure 2. The Lerman Minerva Cervical Orthosis, a poster type brace of Polyethylene and aluminum with a velour lining (Made by the United States Manufacturing Corp.).

four-poster brace provides significantly more motion control of the cervical spine than the Philadelphia collar but does not restrict axial rotation and lateral bending.[1,8,11,12] While the thoracic attachments of the four-poster brace limit flexion and extension to a greater extent than the Philadelphia collar, significant sagittal plane motion is still allowed.

The Guilford brace has a firm circumferential chest attachment and is therefore more effective than the four-poster brace in motion control of the cervical spinal segment.[1,9,11,17] The Guilford orthosis limits flexion and extension, particularly of the lower and mid-cervical spine. However, it does not control flexion and extension at the superior cervical spine, nor does it limit axial rotation or lateral bending. The SOMI brace has three rigid post attachments to the chest: one supports the mandible anteriorly and the other two support the occiput posteriorly. The chin plate and occipital supports are strapped together and the brace is firmly secured around the upper thoracic cage. When applied properly the SOMI is quite effective in limiting sagittal plane motion at the superior cervical spine. It is not as effective as the other poster-type orthoses in limiting lateral bending and rotational movement.[1,9,11,17]

Cervicothoracic Orthoses

Cervicothoracic braces are a more rigid extension of the Philadelphia collar and poster type devices (Figure 3). They provide greater degrees of cervical spinal segment motion control by improved three-point fixation and increased contact with the skull, mandible, and thoracic chest wall. The Yale orthosis is a commonly used cervicothoracic brace consisting of a Philadelphia collar with rigid, molded extensions down over the anterior

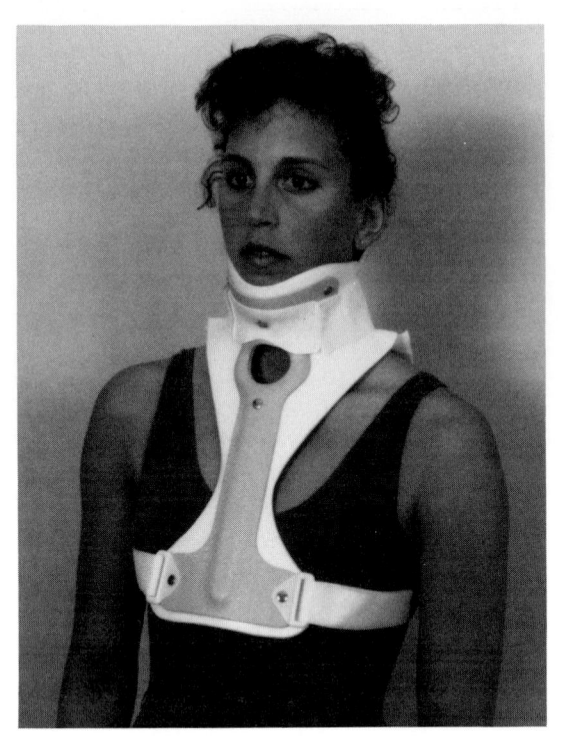

Figure 3. Cervicothoracic orthosis made of heat molded polyethylene (Manufactured by Camp International).

and posterior chest walls secured by a circumferential strap.[18] These devices limit cervical spine flexion, extension, and axial rotation by about 90% and restrict lateral bending by 50%.[1,9,11,17,18] The Minerva jacket is very effective in limiting motion of the cervical spine but it is a heavy, uncomfortable plaster body cast. The thermoplastic Minerva body jacket is a modification of the old plaster jacket constructed of rigid but light thermoplastic materials.[19,20] This new device rivals the halo vest with its ability to immobilize the head and neck in relation to the torso and appears to limit cervical spine "snaking" better than the halo orthoses.[19,20]

Halo Orthoses

The halo cast and halo vest are the standard orthoses for cervical immobilization by which other orthoses are compared.[8,9,11,16,17,19-26] The halo vest is used far more frequently than the cast and may be employed for cervical spine motion control in patients three years of age and older.[16,27,28] Because the halo is a metallic ring affixed by four or more pins to the outer table of the skull, it uses skeletal fixation to restrict the motion of the head and neck with respect to the torso. The halo ring is attached to a form-fitting, lined rigid jacket by four metal posts. The jacket or vest is fitted securely around the thoracic rib cage and extends in a circumferential fashion around the thoracic cavity to the level of the umbilicus. Wang et al evaluated the effect of halo-vest length on motion control of the cervical spine and found no significant control differences between vest length to the xiphoid process, the umbilicus, and superior iliac crest levels.[26]

The halo orthoses represent the most reliable and secure devices designed to control motion of the cervical spinal segment.[8,9,11,16,17] Their greatest contribution is their ability to limit axial rotation, lateral bending, flexion, and extension of the upper cervical spine (C1-C4), planes of motion, and spinal levels poorly immobilized by other devices. The halo orthoses cannot eliminate all motion of the cervical spine, but they represent the best external immobilization devices available for the cervical spine. Immobilization of the head and neck in relation to the torso can be maximized in the halo device if the cervical spine is placed into a position of slight distraction.[1] The devices are easily applied and may be used in the acute setting. New, nonmagnetic, rigid materials are used in the construction of contemporary halo devices to allow magnetic resonance imaging of the patient's head and/or spine while wearing the halo orthosis.

Recommended Use of Cervical Orthoses

The soft cervical collar has no significant utility in neurosurgical practice other than for mild neck strain or muscle spasms without radiographic evidence of vertebral injury or instability. The Philadelphia collar has been advocated in the treatment of nondisplaced or minimally displaced atlas and axis fractures. It is an adequate form of immobilization for minimally displaced atlas fractures uncomplicated by another vertebral segment injury, but it should be used with caution for all but the most benign axis fractures.[16,23,24,29,30-33]

Only the halo vest significantly limits motion of the cervical spinal segment from the occiput through C3.[8,9,11,17] Odontoid fractures, particularly Type II fractures and displaced hangman's fractures, are notorious for poor healing and chronic nonunion.[16,23,24,31,32] Because these fracture-dislocation injuries occur at the superior cervical spine at levels where the greatest degrees of motion occur in virtually all planes, the halo vest should be used for markedly displaced atlas fractures, combination C1-C2 fracture injuries, and virtually all complicated axis fractures.[16,23,24,28,29,30-34]

Patients with mid-cervical vertebral injuries may be treated with a Guilford or SOMI brace, a cervicothoracic brace, or the halo device, depending on the severity of injury and the need for distraction. The cervicothoracic braces and thermoplastic Minerva jackets are adequate alternatives to the halo orthosis for mid and lower cervical spinal injuries.[1,16,18-20]

Thoracic Orthoses

Immobilization of the thoracic spine cannot be accomplished without motion control of the closest adjacent spinal column segment. Proximal thoracic vertebral injuries require immobilization of the adjacent cervical spinal segments in addition to the proximal thoracic spine. This is best accomplished with a cervicothoracic orthosis, a thermoplastic Minerva body jacket, or a halo orthosis.[1,8,9,11,16-19,25,35]

The treatment of injuries or instability of the lower thoracic spinal segment, including the thoracolumbar junction, requires motion control of both the thoracic and lumbosacral spinal segments. A number of orthotic devices are available to provide immobilization and support or to correct progressive spinal deformities of the lower thoracic and upper lumbar spine. These include thoracic corsets, a variety of thoracolumbar braces including hyperextension braces, the Milwaukee brace, and molded body jackets.

Thoracic Corsets

Even when applied properly these devices provide little motion control of the thoracic or lumbosacral spinal segments.[1] They, like cervical collars, appear to serve as an irritative reminder to limit a patient's physical exertion. Because they do elevate intraabdominal pressure some force is exerted on the spine, providing a variable degree of weight transfer and unloading of trunk structures.

Thoracolumbar Braces

A variety of thoracolumbar braces are available to treat thoracolumbar spinal disorders (Figure 4). These are similar in forming contact with the thoracic chest wall, compressing of the abdominal cavity and viscera, and fitting on the pelvis and symphysis pubis. The chairback brace and other dorsolumbar orthoses, including the Taylor brace, rely in part on the principle of three-point fixation and in part on the sleeve principle (indirect force transmitted to the spine by way of compression of the abdomen). These devices limit flexion and extension to variable degrees but do not significantly reduce rotational and lateral bending motions.[2,7,36]

The hyperextension braces such as the Jewett brace rely on three-point fixation to maintain hyperextension for the treatment of thoracolumbar vertebral body collapse and/or kyphotic deformities. These devices maintain hyperextension by force applied to the anterior and lateral aspects of the chest wall and abdomen. They do not significantly limit further extension, lateral bending, or rotational movement of the thoracic or lum-

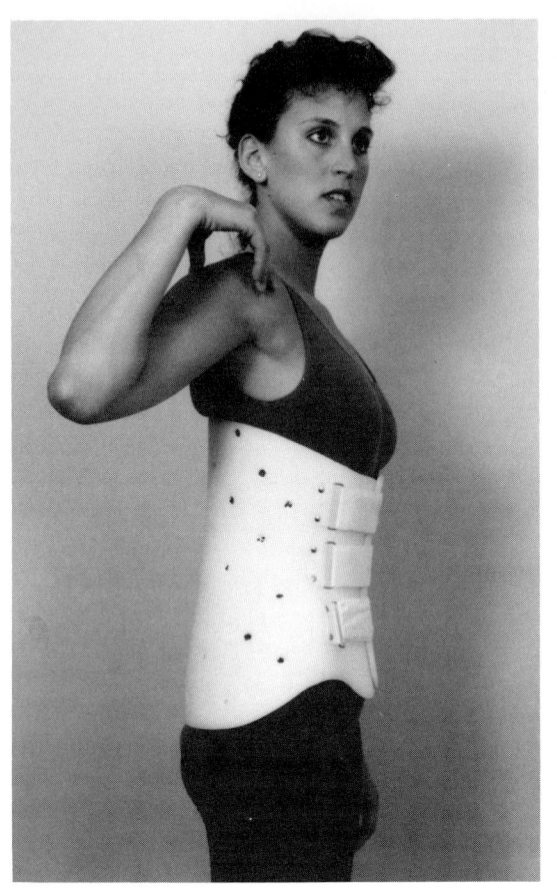

Figure 4. A custom-made thoracolumbar brace of polyethylene (Arimed Orthopedics, New York, NY).

bosacral spinal segments. Despite their ability to maintain hyperextension of the thoracolumbar spine they do not prevent further collapse of severe compression fractures or burst fractures of the thoracolumbar junction.[1,2,5,35]

The Milwaukee Brace with Molded Body Jackets

These orthoses are often used in the treatment of progressive kyphosis, scoliosis, and lordosis. They are multisegmental spinal corrective devices which span the thoracic and lumbosacral spinal segments. The Milwaukee brace, the Wilmington jacket, and other dynamic orthoses use three-point fixation and the sleeve principle to restrict the progression of the deformity, and to redirect spinal growth by stimulating corrective trunk muscle development.[1,3,4] In effect, they unload specific forces from one portion of the spine and redirect them toward another. Neurological surgeons rarely use these types of devices in the treatment of nontraumatic progressive scoliotic or kyphotic spinal deformities. Molded body jackets are used by neurological surgeons in the treatment of some types of traumatic thoracolumbar junction injuries, neoplastic or infectious spinal instability, and in the postoperative period after spinal decompression and instrumentation.

Biomechanical studies reveal that the plastic, molded thoraco-lumbosacral orthosis (TLSO), while not perfect in its ability to control motion of the thoracic and lumbosacral spinal segments, is a far better immobilization device than the thoracic or lumbar corset and the chairback brace type of thoracic orthoses. Recommendations regarding the use of thoracic spinal[1,4,36] segment orthotic devices in neurosurgical practice are listed in Table 2.

Lumbosacral Orthoses

Lumbosacral orthoses are used as a vertebral column support or immobilization device following lumbosacral spine fusion or trauma and as a therapeutic adjunct in the treatment of low back pain.[1,37] There is little evidence of their merit in the treatment of chronic musculoskeletal low back pain, yet many patients report at least temporary symptomatic relief with their use. Some clinicians rationalize their application as a diagnostic trial for the evaluation of candidates for lumbosacral spinal fusion. Many devices are employed for immobilization of the lumbosacral spinal segment. From the least restrictive to the most restrictive they include: corsets, braces and jackets, and lumbosacral spicas.

TABLE 2
Thoracic Orthoses

Device	Disorder	Comments
Long spine board, Tape and body straps	Acute trauma	Immobilize one segment above and one level below suspected injury
Halo vest or Thermoplastic Minerva	Proximal thoracic fracture/instability	High thoracic levels only
Corsets	None Muscle spasm	Irritative reminder
Thoracolumbar braces	Thoracic fractures without instability	Some motion control, especially flexion
Molded body jackets	Thoracic fracture Thoracic instability Postoperative fusion	Best available thoracic motion control device

Lumbosacral Corsets

These devices, the least restrictive of the lumbosacral orthoses, are frequently used in the treatment of chronic low back pain.[1,37] Made of canvas with several metallic support struts, the corset is snugly worn around the abdomen from the lower aspect of the thoracic rib cage, over the sacrum to the level of the buttocks posteriorly and the symphysis pubis anteriorly. There is little motion control or weight transfer with the lumbosacral corset.[38] It serves primarily as an irritative restraint.

Lumbosacral Braces

The length of lumbosacral braces and jackets and their effectiveness as motion control devices vary widely. Several have been discussed in the review of thoracolumbar braces. The majority of lumbosacral braces and jackets use three-point fixation across the thoracic rib cage and throughout the pelvis, in conjunction with the sleeve principle of abdominal cavity compression, to elevate intraabdominal pressure. Through these mechanisms a modest degree of weight transfer and motion control is achieved, with the primary motion restriction in sagittal plane flexion and extension, rather than in lateral bending or axial rotation.[2,7,36,38,39] A key principle for all lumbosacral orthoses is secure fixation to the pelvis to achieve motion control of the lower lumbar segments.

Lumbosacral Spicas

Spicas, lumbosacral jackets with a thigh extension, are the most restrictive of lumbosacral orthoses (Figures 5a,b).[1,38,39] They use three-point fixation and the sleeve principle, but because they include thigh immobilization they also limit the motion of the pelvis and eliminate its influence on movement of the lumbosacral spine.[1,38,39] These are form fitted, light cast or polyform jackets with an extension that encases the thigh, usually on the most symptomatic side. They are worn whenever the patient is weight-bearing and are easily removed when resting for skin care or for comfort.

In comparison with other types of lumbosacral spinal orthoses, the lumbosacral spica provides the greatest degree of lumbosacral spinal segment motion control, particularly at the L4 through S1 motion segments, which are typically the most difficult to immobilize.[1,38,39] Lumbosacral spica orthoses are recommended for use as immobilization devices in patients with lumbosacral spinal segment instability, in postoperative patients after lumbosacral spinal stabilization procedures, or as a diag-

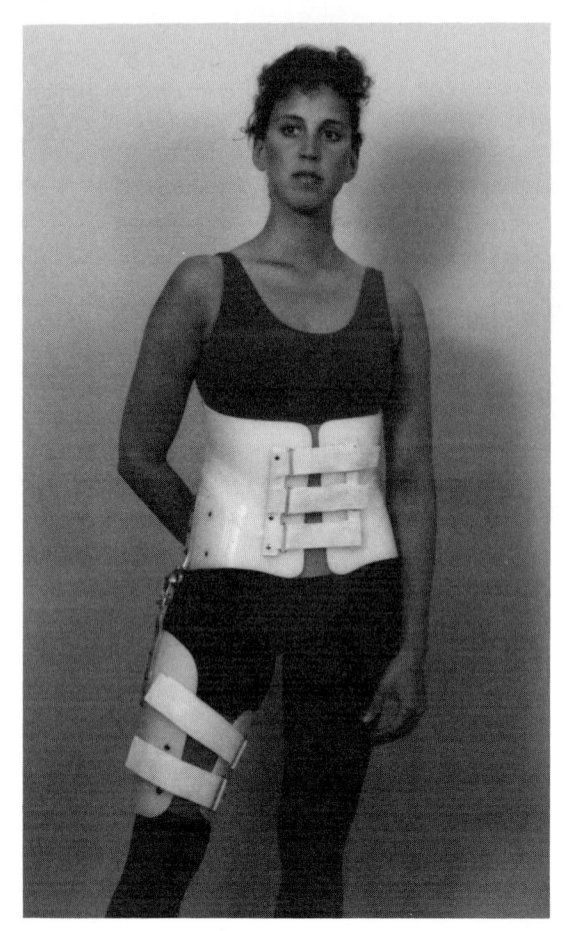

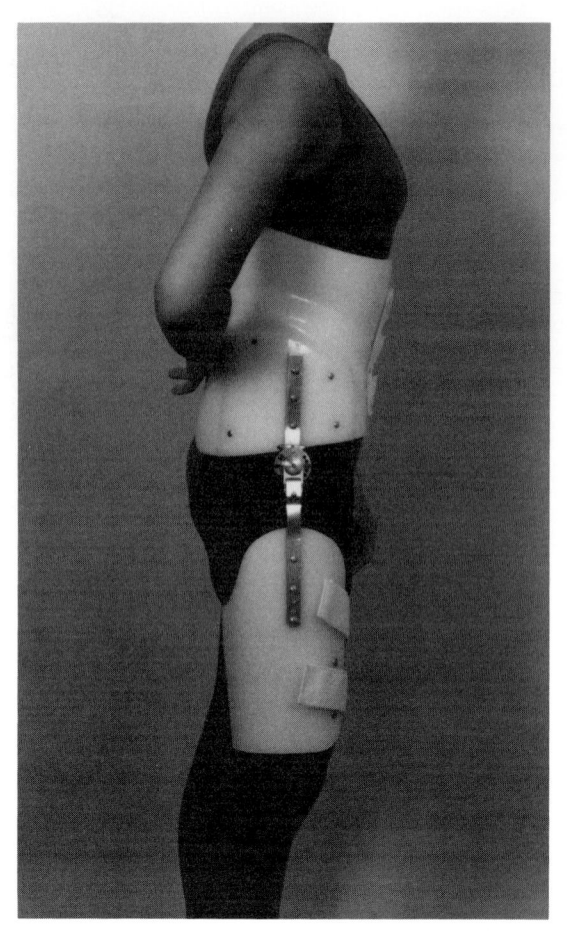

Figure 5. (*a*) *Lumbosacral orthosis with a hip spica to limit pelvic movement custom made from a cast.* (*b*) *Lateral view (Arimed Orthopedics, New York, NY).*

nostic adjunct in the preoperative assessment of lumbosacral spine fusion candidates (Table 3).

Complications of Spinal Orthoses

The most serious complication of a spinal orthotic device is failure to fulfill the objectives for which it was intended. Typically, this is manifested by a lack of adequate spinal segment immobilization with spinal instability, exacerbation of neurological injury, worsening of pain, loss of vertebral column alignment, and/or breakdown or nonunion of a stabilization-fusion mass. The primary causes of orthosis failure are inappropriate selection and/or improper application of the device.

The onus is on the physician to carefully select and appropriately apply spinal orthoses with knowledge of their clinical usefulness and awareness of device limitations. The assistance of a skilled, experienced orthotist is essential for proper fitting and adjustment of most immobilization devices. The recommended usage of orthoses in the treatment of disorders of each of the three spinal motion segments is outlined in Tables 1-3.

Complications of spinal orthosis use other than inadequate immobilization include pain, skin erosion, reduced pulmonary function, and infection.[1,21,25,29,40,41] Skin erosion, pressure sores, and friction burns occur with the loose application of immobilization

TABLE 3
Lumbosacral Orthoses

Device	Disorder	Comments
Long spine board, Tape and body straps	Acute trauma	Immobilize one segment above and one segment below injury. Immobilize legs.
Lumbosacral corsets	None Muscle spasm Musculoskeletal pain without instability	Irritative reminder
Lumbosacral braces	Lumbar fracture without instability	See Table 2, Thoracolumbar braces
Spicas	Lumbar fracture Lumbosacral instability Postoperative fusion or stabilization	Best motion control device for lumbosacral spine Incorporates one thigh to limit pelvic motion

orthoses which rely on three-point fixation and/or the sleeve principle. Corsets and collars are easily removed and cause few skin problems. A skilled orthotist must snugly fit the thermoplastic Minerva jacket, halo vest body jacket, TLSO or lumbosacral spica to avoid irritative and erosive motion over the skin surface. These devices are designed to be removed at periodic intervals for skin cleansing and airing.

Devices that restrict the thoracic or abdominal cavities reduce pulmonary compliance and vital capacity.[5,41] In most patients these reductions in pulmonary function amount to only a 10% compromise over baseline function. No significant differences in the degree of pulmonary compromise from an immobilization orthosis have been identified when comparing neurologically intact and neurologically impaired patients.[41]

The halo orthoses, considered by many to be the best available orthotic devices for rigid cervical spinal segment immobilization, have been criticized because of the number of complications associated with their use.[1,19,21,22,25,40,41] Because the halo ring must be fixed to the skull with four or more torque-tightened pins, the potential exists for skull fracture, perforation, CSF leak, and cranial nerve palsies. All have been reported. The device is usually worn between six and 16 weeks and pin site infection can become a major problem. Serious infections, including cranial vault osteomyelitis and brain abscess have been described. Close attention to pin site care and daily (three times) cleaning with saline–hydrogen peroxide solution will reduce the incidence of infection.[40] Rotation or changing pin sites during the course of therapy will reduce the likelihood of serious pin site complications if long-term immobilization is required. A halo immobilization brace care treatment protocol has been published which has proven to be efficacious in the management of patients requiring halo immobilization.[40]

Summary

A wide variety of spinal orthoses exist to assist the neurosurgeon in the management of patients with spinal disorders. The orthoses are designed utilizing one or two of several biomechanical principles and functions, on one extreme as irritative reminders and on the other as spinal segment motion control devices. It is the decision of the clinician to select and apply the appropriate orthosis for a given patient's pathological condition, with full awareness of the functions and liabilities of the device chosen. The most serious complication resulting from use of an immobilization orthosis is failure to achieve motion control of the desired spinal segment. Persistent instability may lead to further patient morbidity. Knowledge of the use of spinal orthoses, insight into their practical application, appropriate fitting, and compulsive follow-up including patient education will optimize their effectiveness.

References

1. Sypert GW. External spinal orthotics. *Neurosurgery.* 1987;20:642-649.
2. White AA III, Panjabi MM. *Clinical Biomechanics of the Spine.* Philadelphia, Pa: Lippincott; 1978.
3. Bassett GS, Bunnell WP. Influence of the Wilmington brace on spinal decompensation in adolescent idiopathic scoliosis. *Clin Ortho.* 1987;223:164-169.
4. Hanks GA, Zimmer B, Nogi J. TLSO treatment of idiopathic scoliosis: an analysis of the Wilmington jacket. *Spine.* 1988;13:626-629.
5. Morris JM. Spinal bracing. In: Wilkins RH, Rengachary SS, eds. *Neurosurgery.* New York, NY: McGraw-Hill; 1985:2300-2305.
6. Panjabi MM, Thibodeau LL, Crisco JJ, White AA III. What constitutes spinal instability? *Clinical Neurosurg.* 1986;34:313-339.
7. Morris JM, Lucas DB. Biomechanics of spinal bracing. *Ariz Med.* 1964;21:170-176.
8. Wolf JW Jr, Johnson RM. Cervical orthoses. In: The Cervical Spine Society, ed. *The Cervical Spine.* Philadelphia, Pa: JB Lippincott; 1983:54-61.
9. Hartman JT, Palumbo F, Hill BJ. Cineradiography of the braced normal cervical spine: a comparative study of five commonly used cervical orthoses. *Clin Orthop.* 1975;109:97-102.
10. Heiden JS, Weiss MH, Rosenberg AW, Apuzzo MLJ, Kurze T. Management of cervical spinal cord trauma in Southern California. *J Neurosurg.* 1975;43:732-736.
11. Johnson RM, Hart DL, Simmons EF, Ramsby GR, Southwick WO. Cervical orthoses: a study comparing their effectiveness in restricting cervical motion in normal subjects. *J Bone Joint Surg Am.* 1977;59A:332-339.
12. Johnson RM, Owen JR, Hart DL, Callahan RA. Cervical orthoses: a guide to their selection and use. *Clin Orthop.* 1981;154:34-45.
13. Jones MD. Cineradiographic studies of the collar-immobilized cervical spine. *J Neurosurg.* 1960;17:633-636.
14. Colachis SC Jr, Strohm BR, Ganter EL. Cervical spine motion in normal women: radiographic study of effect of cervical collars. *Arch Phys Med Rehabil.* 1973;54:161-169.
15. Podolsky S, Baraff LJ, Simon RR, Hoffman JR, Lamon B, Ablon W. Efficacy of cervical spine immobilization methods. *J Trauma.* 1983;23:461-465.
16. Sonntag VKH, Hadley MN. Nonoperative management of cervical spine injuries. *Clin Neurosurg.* 1988;31:630-649.
17. Wolf JW, Jones HC. Comparison of cervical immobilization of the cervical spine by halo casts versus halo plastic jackets. *Orthop Trans.* 1981;5:118.
18. Zeleznik R, Chapin W, Hart D, Smith H, Southwick WO, Zito M. Yale cervical orthosis: fabrication. *Phys Ther.* 1978;58:861-864.
19. Benzel EC, Hadden TA, Saulsbery CM. A comparison of the Minerva and halo jackets for stabilization of the cervical spine. *J Neurosurg.* 1989;70:411-414.
20. Millington PJ, Ellingsen JM, Hauswirth BE, Fabian PJ. Thermoplastic Minerva body jacket—a practical alternative to current methods of cervical spine stabilization: a clinical report. *Phys Ther.* 1987;67:223-225.
21. Chan RC, Schweigel JF, Thompson GB. Halo-thoracic brace immobilization in 188 patients with acute cervical spine injuries. *J Neurosurg.* 1983;58:508-515.
22. Glaser JA, Whitehill R, Stamp WG, Jane JA. Complications associated with the halo-vest: a review of 245 cases. *J Neurosurg.* 1986;65:762-769.
23. Hadley MN, Browner C, Sonntag VKH. Axis fractures: a comprehensive review of management and treatment in 107 cases. *Neurosurgery.* 1985;17:281-290.
24. Hadley MN, Sonntag VKH. Acute axis fractures. *Contemp Neurosurg.* 1987;9:1-6.
25. Lind B, Sihlbom H, Nordwall A. Halo-vest treatment of unstable traumatic cervical spine injuries. *Spine.* 1988;13:425-432.
26. Wang GJ, Moskal JT, Albert T, Pritts C, Schuch CM, Stamp WG. The effect of halo-vest length on stability of the cervical spine. *J Bone Joint Surg Am.* 1988;70A:357-360.
27. Hadley MN, Sonntag VKH, Rekate HL. Pediatric vertebral column and spinal cord injuries. *Contemp Neurosurg.* 1988;10:1-4.
28. Hadley MN, Zabramski JM, Browner CM, Rekate H, Sonntag VKH. Pediatric spinal trauma: a review of 122 cases of spinal cord and vertebral column injuries. *J Neurosurg.* 1988;68:18-24.
29. Dickman CA, Hadley MN, Browner C, Sonntag VKH. Neurosurgical management of acute atlas-axis combination fractures: a review of 25 cases. *J Neurosurg.* 1989;70:45-49.
30. Hadley MN, Browner C, Sonntag VKH. Miscellaneous fractures of the second cervical vertebra. *BNI Quarterly.* 1985;1:34-39.
31. Hadley MN, Browner CM, Liu SS, Sonntag VKH. New subtype of acute odontoid fractures (Type IIA). *Neurosurgery.* 1988;22:67-71.
32. Hadley MN, Dickman CA, Browner CM, et al: Acute axis fractures: a review of 229 cases. *J Neurosurg.* 1989. In press.
33. Hadley MN, Dickman CA, Browner CM, Sonntag VKH. Acute traumatic atlas fractures: management and long-term outcome. *Neurosurgery.* 1988;23:31-35.
34. Reiss SJ, Raque GH Jr, Shields CB, Garretson HD. Cervical spine fractures with major associatd trauma. *Neurosurgery.* 1986;18:327-330.
35. Hadley MN, Browner CM, Dickman CA, Sonntag VKH. Compression fractures of the thoracolumbar junction: a treatment algorithm based on 110 cases. *BNI Quarterly.* 1989;5. In press.
36. Lantz SA, Schultz AB. Lumbar spine orthosis wearing, I: restriction of gross body motions. *Spine.* 1986;11:834-837.

37. Ahlgren SA, Hansen T. The use of lumbosacral corsets prescribed for low back pain. *Prosthet Orthot Int.* 1978;2:101-104.
38. Fidler MW, Plasmans CMT. The effect of four types of support on the segmental mobility of the lumbosacral spine. *J Bone Joint Surg Am.* 1983;65A:943-947.
39. Norton PL, Brown T. The immobilizing efficiency of back braces: their effect on the posture and motion of the lumbosacral spine. *J Bone Joint Surg Am.* 1957;39A:111-139.
40. Browner CM, Hadley MN, Sonntag VKH, Mattingly LG. Halo immobilization brace care: an innovative approach. *J Neurosci Nurs.* 1987;19:24-29.
41. Lind B, Bake B, Lundqvist C, Nordwall A. Influence of halo vest treatment on vital capacity. *Spine.* 1987;12:449-452.

CHAPTER 5

Management of Occipito-Cervical Instability

Arnold H. Menezes, MD, and Michael Muhonen, MD

The occipito-atlanto-axial complex is a transition zone between vertebral joint structures and the skull.[1] It is unique in that it allows extensive motion and yet its vertebrae are interlocked to form an amazingly stable three-dimensional structure.[2] The complex interaction between the occipital bone, its opening the foramen magnum, and the atlas and atlas vertebrae and their associated ligaments, strongly suggests that experimentally as well as in vivo, this complex acts as one unit.[2-4] The atlas serves as a washer or bearing between the occipital condyles and the axis vertebra. In order to understand, diagnose and treat traumatic disorders of this area, it is pertinent to review the osseous anatomy, ligamentous structures and their functional properties, together with the joint kinematics.[5]

Normal Anatomy

Osseous

The paired occipital condyles on either side of the foramen magnum are oval and convex with partially everted surfaces. The condyles articulate with the paired superior articular facets of the atlas, which are oval-shaped in the transverse plane and concave in the frontal section. Each facet functions as a cup for the corresponding condyle of the occipital bone. Such an arrangement permits flexion-extension and minimal lateral bending while allowing little axial rotation.[4,6-9]

In contrast, the atlanto-axial articulations consist of two lateral zygo-apophyseal and two median odontoid joints. The first joints, located laterally on either side, are between the inferior articular surfaces of the atlas and the corresponding superior articular surfaces of the axis. The articulating surfaces of the axis are round and slightly convex and those of the atlas are relatively flat. The joint capsule is wide and redundant. The second articulation is provided by another set of synovial cavities: one between the dens of the axis and the anterior arch of the atlas, and the other between the dens and the transverse ligament. The complex arrangement permits a very large amount of axial rotation, some flexion-extension, but very little lateral bending.

Rotation of the atlas occurs around the odontoid process like a wheel around an axle. Because the atlanto-axial-lateral facet articulations are convex, as rotation progresses there is a telescoping effect of the axis on the atlas with a decrease in the circumference of the cervical canal. The average rostral caudal movement of this joint with rotation is about 1.5 mm.[10]

Ligamentous Anatomy

The organization of the ligamentous tissue limits the range of motion of the craniovertebral joint, yet allows for its diverse motion.[1,11] The articular capsule ligaments, the anterior and posterior atlanto-occipital membrane, and the lateral atlanto-occipital ligaments unite the atlas to the cranium. The cruciate ligament contributes some strength to this articulation, especially in the transverse ligament complex. However, it is the paired alar ligaments, the broad tectorial membrane, and the secondary apical dens ligament that provide major structural support for the craniovertebral junction.[10]

Muscular Action

In vitro studies of the craniovertebral junction have shown that application of very small loads to the craniovertebral complex results in significant rotation, flexion, and extension in comparison to the lower cervical spine.[2,3] However, in vivo observations show that this is not the case. Thus, the principal muscular action has to be held responsible for holding the head firmly to the neck and preventing abnormal excursions.[2,12,13] When the protective muscles are relaxed or inadequately developed, as in the young child, the craniovertebral junction becomes inherently less stable than that of adults.[9] In children, this may also be due in part to small occipital condyles and an almost horizontal plane of the articulation between the cranium and the atlas. The full development of the occipital condyles produces more vertical orientation of this joint plane with advancing age. As muscular development occurs there also is less tendency for instability at the craniovertebral junction.

Biomechanics of the Occipito-Atlanto-Axial Complex

Both the occipito-atlantal and atlanto-axial articulations are involved in flexion and extension. The average range of this motion at the occipito-atlantal joint is 13-15°. An additional 10° of motion occurs at the atlanto-axial articulation.[4,6,8,10,14] Flexion is limited by the tectorial membrane and by contact between the dens and the occipital basion.[1,8,10] Extension is restricted by the stretching of the tectorial membrane and by bony contact between the opisthion and the posterior arch of the atlas.

The normal excursion between the anterior arch of the atlas and the dens is 3 mm in an adult and up to 4-5 mm in a child.[1,9,15,16] When the transverse component of the cruciate ligament has ruptured but the alar ligaments are still intact, up to 5 mm of displacement may occur at the atlanto-dental junction.[10,17,18] When both the transverse and the alar ligaments are incompetent, there is more than 5 mm separation between the odontoid process and the anterior atlas arch. Studies by Werne demonstrated that sectioning of the alar ligaments and the tectorial membrane produces instability of the occipito-atlantal joints, permitting luxation of these articulations.[10]

In contrast to the duality of the flexion-extension motion, rotation occurs only at the atlanto-axial joint.[1,4] The osseous geometry of the lateral atlanto-axial articular surfaces, together with the cartilaginous cover to the opposing surfaces make them convex with horizontal orientation, providing an optimal design to permit rotation. Maximal rotation of the atlanto-axial joints is 45°.[6] When rotation exceeds this, an interlocking of the lateral inferior facet of the atlas over the superior articular facet of the axis vertebra occurs. Should the transverse ligament be deficient, the anterior atlas arch will sublux forwards, producing a unilateral dislocation, and the facet will interlock at a rotation of less than 45°. However, should the transverse ligament remain intact, there is no subluxation between the odontoid process and the anterior atlas arch up to a higher degree of rotation.[6,9]

Rotation at the atlanto-axial joint of more than 30° produces an angulation of the contralateral vertebral artery.[19] With greater rotation, there is stretching of the vertebral artery, and at 45° the ipsilateral artery may demonstrate angulation and occlusion. This phenomenon may explain the neurological deficit from cervical traction, football and wrestling injuries, chiropractic manipulations and sudden head rotations with general anesthesia.[20,21,22]

Although the lateral rotation of the neck is 90°, only one-half of this movement occurs at the atlanto-axial joint.[2,4] The remainder of the lateral rotation occurs in the subaxial vertebra. This in vivo phenomenon is due to the muscular contraction and tone producing a compressive force across the cervical motion segments.[2,12] The initial axial twist produces a threshold value that overcomes the "interlocking-stiffening" of the subaxial segments, allowing for the completion of the rotation to 90°.

Translation and rotation occurring simultaneously is called coupling.[4] Coupling occurs at the atlanto-axial joint, due primarily to the geometry of the regional facet articulations. With axial rotation of the atlas around the axis, there is an associated upward and transverse movement of the dens in relation to the atlas. Thus, in rotatory luxations of the atlas beyond 35-40°, there is excessive translation of the axis-odontoid process with a relative "descent of the cervicomedullary junction."[1,9,11] This finding has led to a misdiagnosis of the Arnold Chiari Type I malformation and cerebellar tumors on magnetic resonance imaging (MRI) of these patients.[9]

The atlas-axis complex is not involved with lateral bending of the head. The normal distance from the basion to the odontoid process is about 5 mm (4-11 mm).[23] The normal translation between the clivus and the anterior arch of the atlas is no more than 1 mm. Any motion greater than this is considered to be pathological.

Occipito-Atlantal Instability/Dislocation

The literature concerning traumatic occipito-atlantal dislocation is limited, with the majority of reports being in the last decade.[9,24-32] The condition is not uncommon and appears to be associated with an extremely high mortality at the scene of the accident. Hence, this is presumed to be a rare occurrence.[24,25,32-43] The actual incidence of occipito-atlantal dislocation is obscured by the devastating nature of the injury itself.[32,36,44] In a review of 112 trauma victims who succumbed at the scene of the accident, Bucholz discovered that 26 had a cervical spine injury.[45] Of the 26 patients, nine had a traumatic occipito-atlantal dislocation and five had an odontoid fracture.

In a similar review, Alker et al found a 19% incidence of occipito-atlantal dislocation.[32] Woodring et al reviewed the literature in 1981 and found 15 survivors.[46] However, the number of survivors has increased dramatically due to improved on-scene resuscitation and transportation by emergency units.[44]

Our neurosurgical experience encompasses 12 patients with traumatic occipito-atlantal dislocation and four with lesser forms of ligamentous occipito-atlantal injury. Five patients succumbed to their injury. Of the 16 patients, 10 were children.

Several mechanisms have been implicated as the cause of occipito-atlantal dislocation.[26,27,29,30,39,43-45,47,48,49] We feel that the most frequent mechanism of injury is excessive hyperflexion of the skull in relation to the upper cervical spine, with distraction. The resulting separation of the posterior elements of the atlas and the axis is quite well visualized with MRI (Figures 1a-c). Other authors have implicated lateral flexion as the major etiology.

Some others believe that the primary mechanism is extreme hyperextension leading to disruption of the tectorial membrane. Ligamentous rupture of the anterior occipito-atlantal ligament, the tectorial membrane, the alar ligaments of the occipito-atlanto-axial joints and the posterior elements of the occipito-atlanto-axial complex produce forward dislocation of the cranium on the atlas. Although anterior occipito-atlantal dislocation is the most common injury, lateral occipito-atlantal dislocation as well as a posterior cranial dislocation have been reported.[43,47]

Based upon a review of the literature and our own series of patients, occipito-atlantal dislocation can be classified as follows: (1) anterior displacement of the cranium with respect to the atlas, (2) posterior displacement of the cranium on the atlas, and (3) a longitudinal distraction with separation of the skull from the cervical spine.

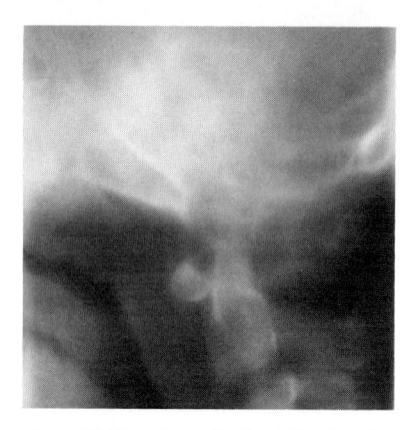

Figure 1a. Midline lateral pleuridirectional tomogram of the craniovertebral junction (CVJ). This eight-year-old boy was initially unconscious after a motor vehicle accident. He had excruciating headache and neck pain with arm weakness. Note increased predental space, mild shift of dens dorsally, and increased atlanto-axial interspinous distance.

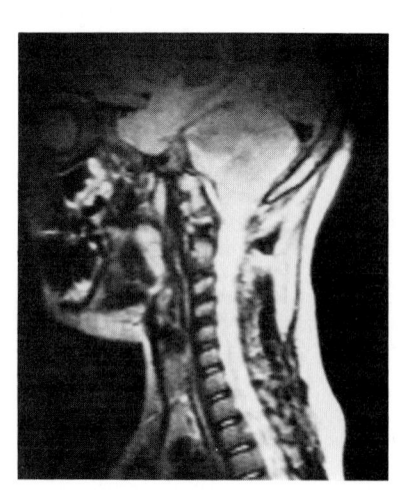

Figure 1b. Midsagittal T2 weighted MRI of CVJ of Figure 1a. Ligamentous injury to the interspinous tissue is seen dorsally between occiput, C1 and C2. The signal intensity of the tectorial membrane is increased.

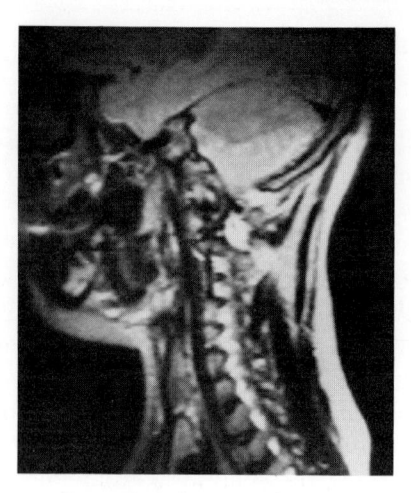

Figure 1c. Parasagittal T2 weighted MRI of CVJ of Figure 1a illustrating ligamentous injury of the interspinous, dorsal occipitoatlantal and capsular tissue. The flow void in the vertebrobasilar system indicates patency.

Presentation

The diagnosis of occipito-atlantal instability should be considered for any victim of a motor vehicle accident, especially if the patient has a submental laceration, mandibular fracture, or has had a cardiorespiratory arrest. The clinical presentation varies widely.

Neurological involvement can range from mild to catastrophic. In those survivors with neurological deficits, the most vulnerable neural structures are the caudal paired cranial and upper cervical nerves, the brain stem, and the rostral cervical spinal cord. Avulsion of the lower cranial nerves usually ends in permanent impairment. Quadriparesis, hemiparesis, and paraparesis have been recorded in survivors. Less severe brain stem insults may cause cardiopulmonary instability leading to bradycardia, irregular respirations, or apnea. Usually, the patient is comatose with hemiparesis or quadriparesis and has diaphragmatic breathing or is respirator dependent. Occlusion or stenosis of the anterior spinal artery has been reported.[39,43,47] Loss of autonomic function manifested by systemic hypotension can suggest blood loss and lead to unnecessary and negative abdominal or thoracic explorations.

Radiology of Atlanto-Occipital Dislocation

In our review of the literature and in our own experience, we found several radiographic findings that were helpful in establishing the diagnosis of occipito-atlantal dislocation. Retropharyngeal hematoma is commonly associated with this entity. Separation of the atlas from the occipital condyles is usually obvious. The "bare" or "naked" appearance of the occipital condyles and condylar fossa is caused by longitudinal distraction pulling the skull away from the cervical spine and exposing the condyles and fossae (Figure 2). It becomes more obvious with distraction. Significant anterior or posterior displacement of the odontoid from beneath the basion is highly suggestive of occipito-atlantal dislocation (Figure 3). This is analogous to bilateral facet interlock.

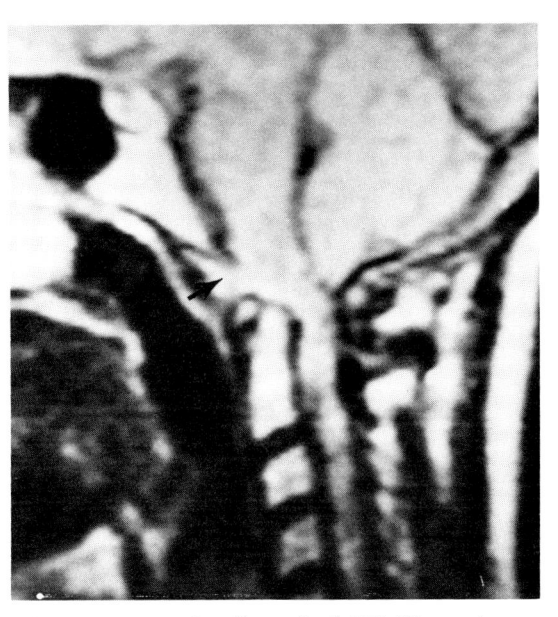

Figure 3. Lateral radiograph of CVJ illustrating an anterior occipito-atlantal dislocation.

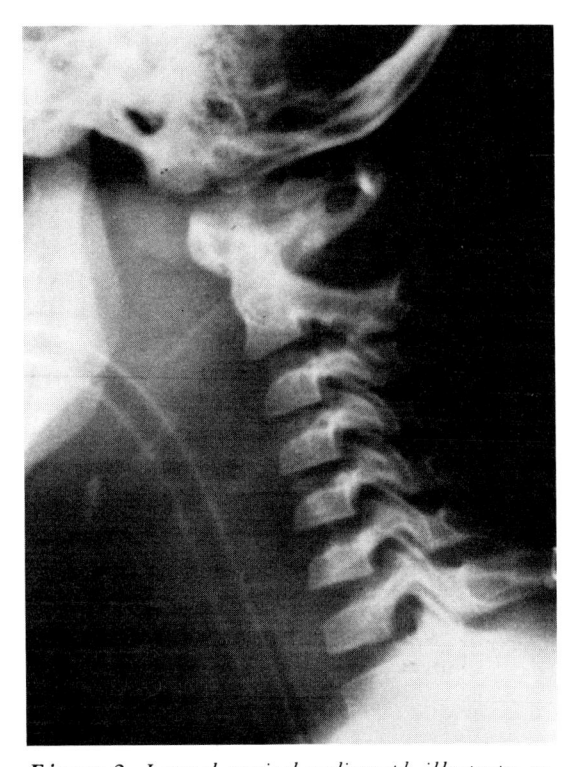

Figure 2. Lateral cervical radiograph illustrates occipitoatlantal dislocation. The occipital condyles and atlantal condylar fossae are separated and "bare." The retropharyngeal hematoma extends from the clivus to the mediastinum. Note the increased distance between the posterior arches of the atlas and axis.

The basion and opisthion indirectly reflect the location of the occipital condyles. The anterior C1 arch, dens, C1 and C2 spinal laminar line, and ramus of the mandible indirectly reflect the location of the atlas condylar fossa. Several radiographic criteria for the diagnosis of occipito-atlantal dislocation have been proposed to aid in the early diagnosis with lateral cervical radiographs. Powers et al described the relationship for diagnosis of anterior occipito-atlantal dislocation.[39] In the intact craniovertebral junction, the ratio of the distance between the basion and the posterior arch of the atlas and the distance between the opisthion and the anterior arch of the atlas should normally be 0.77. Any value greater than 1 is considered to be indicative of anterior occipito-atlantal dislocation. The measurement is unreliable in patients with congenital anomalies of the foramen magnum or fractures of the atlantal arch, or in patients with posterior displacement.

Dublin et al stated that the distance between the posterior mandibular cortex and the anterior arch of the atlas in a true lateral radiograph should normally measure between 2-5 mm.[47] The distance between the anterior dens and the posterior mandible has a mean value of 10 mm with extremes between 2-17 mm in the normal patient. Lee et al evaluated traumatic atlanto-occipital dislocation with cross table lateral radiographs in 12 cases and found that a combination of these methods was the most significant, correctly diagnosing the lesion in 75%.[50]

In cases of longitudinal distraction, Kaufman et al proposed measuring the actual distance between the occipital condyle and the superior facet of the atlas.[51] In children the normal distance is less than 5 mm. Other radiographic abnormalities include air in the soft tissue secondary to pharyngeal laceration.

We have found that thin-section computerized tomography (CT) with reconstruction and pleuridirectional polytomography are helpful in better defining the bony pathology.[9,43] In our last four patients, MRI has been used to visualize the dislocation and to identify the ligamentous disruption as well as to identify spinal cord and brain stem contusion. Vertebral angiography may demonstrate occlusion or stenosis, especially in cases of sudden neurological deterioration.

Treatment

The therapeutic objective is realignment and skeletal fixation. Initial management should be directed toward maintenance of adequate ventilation with immobilization of the cervical spine in a neutral position. Nasotracheal intubation may be unsuccessful to protect the airway and a tracheostomy may be necessary. Neurological structures may be further injured with traction, and in those individuals with longitudinal distraction cervical traction should be avoided. Immobilization in a neutral position and early occipito-cervical fixation is essential in this situation. However, with anterior or posterior displacement, alignment usually follows cervical traction, which should not exceed 4-5 lbs. The patient is maintained in this position until occipito-atlanto-axial fixation with wire and autogenous bone graft is achieved.

Ligamentous disruption is easily identified by MRI. In those individuals without true dislocation, halo immobilization for 10-12 weeks may allow ligamentous and possibly bony reconstruction. However, should instability persist, an occipito-cervical fixation is mandatory.

The majority of patients with occipito-cervical instability require skeletal traction with realignment of the craniovertebral junction. The small number of individuals who have longitudinal distraction and separation of the occiput from the atlas can be realigned by head positioning alone. However, skeletal traction with 3-4 lbs is essential in this situation. This is best achieved with halo skull traction using a minimum of four-point fixation. With atlanto-occipital dislocation, 3-4 lbs of skeletal traction is all that is required. However, with associated atlanto-axial instability, traction should be increased to 6-7 lbs.

If a tracheostomy has not been performed prior to surgery, the induction of anesthesia is accomplished as skeletal traction is maintained. An awake oral or nasal endotracheal fiberoptic intubation is performed.[52] Following this, the patient is placed on the operating table in the prone position while the traction is maintained and the head secured by the ring resting on a horseshoe headrest. The chest is elevated on laminectomy rolls or by using a Wilson frame. During the entire period of induction and positioning, median nerve somatosensory evoked potentials are monitored. After positioning, a lateral radiograph is performed to document alignment.

After the lateral radiograph is performed and adjustments in position made, the patient's neurological status is reassessed. Only then is general endotracheal and intravenous anesthesia induced.

We and others have previously described the technique of posterior occipito-cervical fusion.[53,54,55] Cephalothin sodium, 1 gm every six hours, is administered intravenously 12 hours prior to the start of the procedure and maintained for 48 hours postoperatively. The posterior scalp and cervical region are prepared, as is the donor site from the iliac crest or posterior rib cage. Our own preference is rib taken as close as possible to the posterior contour toward the vertebral transverse process, so it can conform to the curvature of the occiput and the upper cervical spine.[52,53] A midline incision is made from the inion to the spinous process of the fourth cervical vertebra and carried down to the deep cervical fascia. Sharp dissection must be used to achieve a subperiosteal exposure of the squamous occipital bone and the posterior arches of the upper cervical vertebrae. Blunt dissection is dangerous and should be avoided. As soon as the posterior arches of the atlas and axis are exposed, a towel clip is passed through the spinous process of C2 to stabilize it until fixation can be accomplished. Further stabilization of the operative site is obtained with self-retaining retractors placed at 90° angles to each other. This has the effect of both stretching the muscle and fixing the muscle-bone relationship to prevent motion at the occipito-cervical and atlanto-axial joints.

The posterior rim of the foramen magnum is excised using a high speed drill initially and is completed with fine rongeurs. This facilitates extradural passage of wires from two trephines which are made in the squamous occipital bone 2½ cm to either side of the midline and 2 cm above the rim of the foramen magnum. Braided #22 wire is passed beneath the laminae of the atlas as well as the axis on either side of the midline. The occipital trephines allow purchase of the occipital bone by wire that is passed epidurally from the trephine to the midline and then brought upwards. The bone graft is harvested from the rib or ilium. Careful decortication of the exposed laminae, spinous processes, and occipital bone is performed. The bone grafts are secured to the squamous occipital bone, as well as to the laminae of the atlas and axis in a vertical manner by passing the wire through the grafts. The wires are then approximated to each other to provide additional stability. Matchstick-sized slivers of harvested bone are packed into the remaining crevices and against the occipital bone.

In severe instability and in patients who are extremely disabled or debilitated, management in a halo vest becomes nearly impossible. In this situation, the bone fusion should be supplemented with acrylic and wire.[52] With this procedure there is a diminished requirement for external support, thus allowing the use of a sterno-occipital mandibular immobilizer or similar orthosis. We have used a contoured wire loop in only two individuals, with the loop fixating the occiput to the posterior arches of the first three cervical vertebrae.[54] A bone fusion must also be performed since metallic implants provide only temporary fixation until solid bony fusion occurs.

Postoperatively, occipito-cervical immobilization should be maintained for a minimum of four to six months. Ideally this is provided by a halo vest, but the type of orthosis may vary depending on the patient's neurological status, age, and medical condition.

Atlanto-Axial Instability— Rotatory Luxation

Atlanto-axial luxations are divided into anterior, posterior, and rotational types. The anterior and the rare posterior atlanto-axial luxations are a common finding in acute as well as chronic nonunited fractures of the odontoid process. This section will address only luxations not associated with fracture, and in particular, rotary luxations.

Fielding and Hawkins, in a biomechanical study of the strength of the atlanto-axial ligament complex, showed that the force required to fracture the odontoid process was much less than the force required to cause failure of all the ligaments in the same specimen.[17] In anterior-posterior atlanto-axial luxation, suboccipital and paracervical pain is a presenting symptom.[9,16,56,57] Delayed myelopathy is another finding. Conditions which predispose to traumatic or nontraumatic anterior-posterior atlanto-axial dislocation include basilar invagination, occipitalization of the atlas, os odontoideum, aplasia or dysplasia of the dens, Down's syndrome, rheumatoid arthritis, ankylosing spondylitis, and infections of the pharynx and upper neck.[5,9]

When the distance between the anterior arch of the atlas and the odontoid process exceeds 5 mm, the transverse ligament, as well as the alar ligaments, are presumed to be incompetent. In patients in whom the anterior predental space (distance between the anterior arch of the atlas and the dens) is more than 5 mm, realignment is accomplished quite easily with skeletal traction of about 7 pounds. If the luxation is acute and less than 5 mm, fixation for three months is usually sufficient to allow for ligamentous reconstitution. However, if the luxation is more than 6 mm, or if it is chronic, a posterior arthrodesis is necessary.

Atlanto-Axial Rotatory Luxation

Rotatory dislocation of the atlanto-axial segment was first noted by Corner in 1907.[58] Greeley, in 1930, reported the case of a boy with bilateral "90° rotatory dislocation of the atlas upon the axis" and included radiographs and illustrated the possible mechanism of the injury.[38] Atlanto-axial rotatory luxation was first described by Wortzman and Dewar in 1966,[59] and was further clarified by Fielding and Hawkins in 1977.[6] However, the majority of the patients were not examined during the acute stage since symptoms were mild and consequently did not warrant immediate reduction.[58]

The etiology of rotatory dislocation at the atlanto-axial level is not clear, but age may be a factor as described earlier. In our series of 22 patients with rotatory luxation beyond 35-40°, 18 were adolescents and trauma was the causative factor in all.[9] The luxation was caused by a football spearing injury in eight of the 18, by a motor vehicle accident in six, and by a wrestling injury in three others. A 10-year-old girl sustained her injury in a fall on the ice. In four patients, an associated occipito-atlantal rotatory luxation was also present, leading to a characteristic "cock robin" appearance of the head.[1]

Rotatory luxation of the atlanto-axial segment has been reported following surgical repair of cleft lip and cleft palate, as well as after removal of orthodontic devices and a body cast.[9] It may go unrecognized if the symptoms are minor or may be diagnosed when associated with brain stem dysfunction or cervical myelopathy. Children with this lesion have been erroneously diagnosed as having brain stem vascular insult, cerebellar tumor, Chiari malformation, syringomyelia, vertebral-basilar migraine, and ocular muscle palsies. Most of these patients present with a torticollis and diminished range of motion of the neck.

Symptoms of neural compression occur when the atlas is separated from the odontoid process by more than 5 mm, as a result of destruction of the transverse ligament.[6,9,58] This allows a rotational displacement of the atlas on the axis, causing spinal canal compromise.

Atlanto-axial rotatory dislocation may be difficult to diagnose due to radiographic problems in visualizing the complex anatomical structures in the area. Diagnostic procedures should include an anterior-posterior open-mouth view of the craniovertebral complex, as well as an attempt to obtain a true lateral cervical radiograph.

Overriding of the atlas in relationship to the axis and abnormal position of the odontoid process are possible clues to the diagnosis. On the open-mouth frontal roentgenogram, the odontoid is asymmetrical in relation to the atlas lateral masses manifested by asymmetry of the lateral atlanto-axial facet articulations (Figure 4a). On the lateral radiograph of the skull and upper cervical spine, there should normally be an alignment of the facet joints. Rotation of the atlas is usually seen in relation to the axis, with a forward projection of the lateral atlantal mass anterior to the odontoid process. This is represented by a large bulk of bone in front of the odontoid process (Figure 4b).

In addition, if the skull and C1 are in a

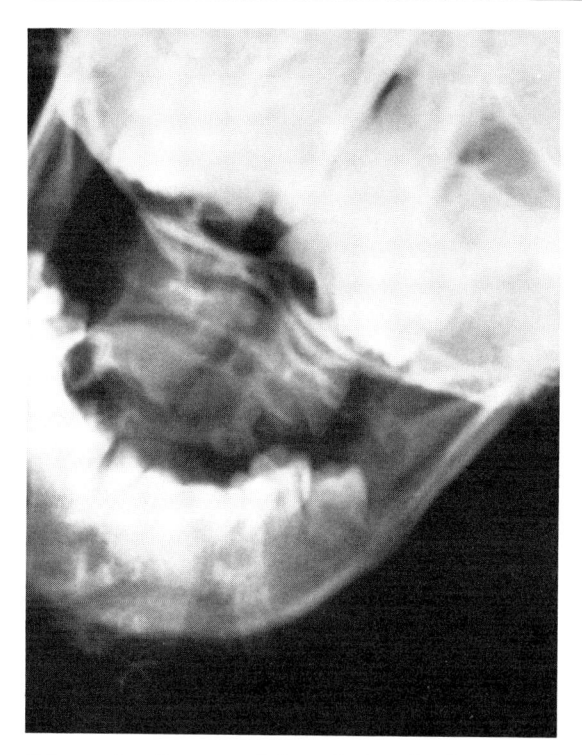

Figure 4a. Open-mouth frontal view of atlanto-axial articulation in a 12-year-old male who suffered trauma in a motor vehicle accident. The head was abnormally "cocked" to one side and fixed. Neck pain, arm paresthesias, and vertigo were prominent symptoms. There is marked lateral atlantal displacement in relation to the odontoid process.

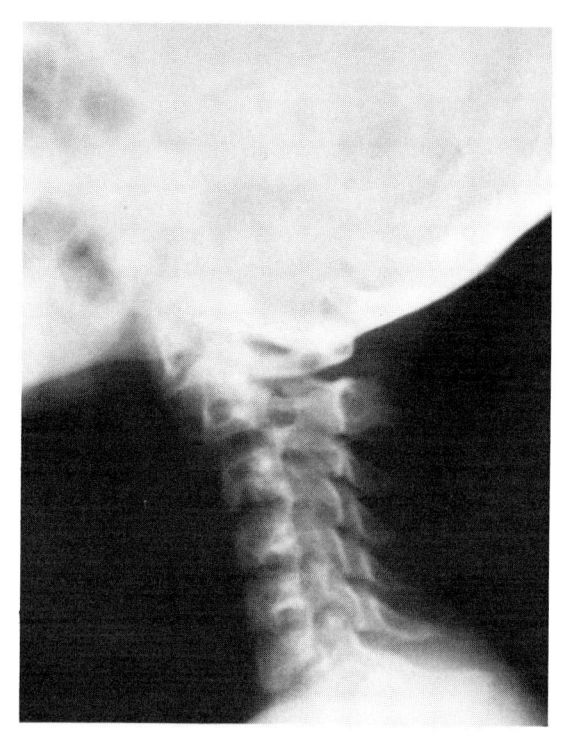

Figure 4b. Lateral skull and cervical roentgenogram of patient in Figure 4a. The atlas and skull are rotated 50° in relation to the axis. Note the lateral atlantal mass located in front of the dens.

true lateral position, the cervical spine then shows a prominence of the facet joints rather than a true lateral picture in the subaxial location. There is a persistent asymmetry in the atlanto-axial relationship that is not corrected by rotation unless it is reduced. This is easily seen on cine-roentgenography that shows the subluxed axis and atlas to move as a unit during neck rotation.

Multidirectional tomography should be obtained from facet to facet. This defines the abnormal bone articulation. It also distinguishes a unilateral from a bilateral facet luxation. A better conceptualization of the abnormality and definition of the interlocking of the facets is provided by illustrating the pathological state in a third dimension such as CT and MRI. A functional or dynamic CT study should be obtained through the craniovertebral junction.[9,60,61,62] The patients are initially scanned as they present with their heads fixed in lateral rotation (Figure 4c). Subsequent scans are obtained with the head turned to the contralateral side with maximum rotation. In patients with atlanto-axial rotatory fixation, there is no motion at the C1-C2 articulation during this maneuver,

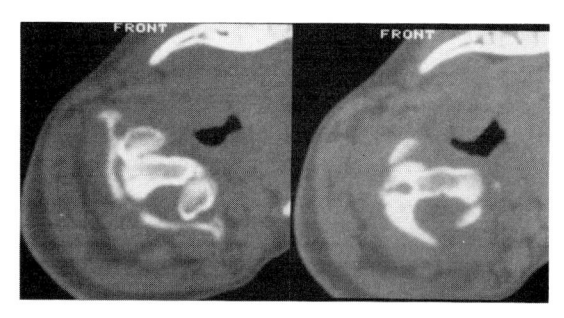

Figure 4c. Axial CT scans through the atlas and axis with head to the right as on presentation. There is bilateral facet interlock of C1 on C2 with rotational luxation. This did not change with head rotated to the left.

while with patients with transient torticollis, a reduction or reversal of the rotation of C1 on C2 occurs.[60] Dynamic MRI in the axial, sagittal, and coronal planes defines the bony pathology as well as any neural compromise.[9] It also provides indirect information regarding the patency of the vertebral-basilar vascular complex. Three-dimensional CT of the craniovertebral junction may clarify any doubts of the abnormality (Figure 5).

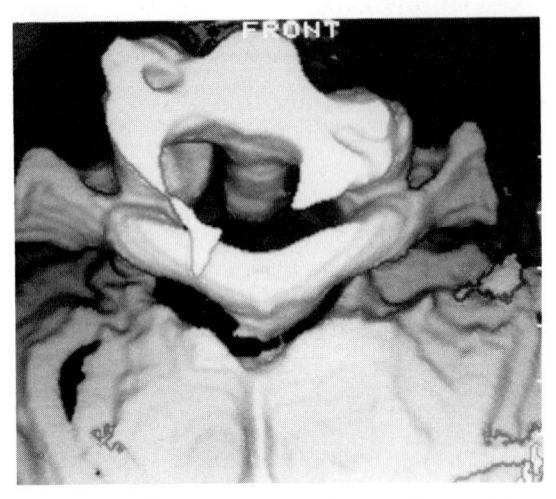

Figure 5. Three-dimensional CT of CVJ viewed from below C2 vertebra. Note the unilateral atlanto-axial rotational luxation. The left superior facet of the axis is displaced forward. Capsular interposition and subaxial fractures necessitated surgical reduction.

Fielding and Hawkins classified the atlanto-axial rotatory fixation-luxation into four types.[6] This was dependent upon the integrity of the transverse ligament and the secondary support ligament complex. If the transverse ligament is intact, and the dens acts as a pivot, the rotation is within 35° and is correctable with traction and realignment (Figure 6). It is seen in minor trauma and infections and is associated with inflammatory conditions of the craniovertebral junction. It is the most common of pediatric rotatory atlanto-axial luxations. However, when the transverse ligament ruptures, the atlas arch is displaced forward causing compromise of the spinal canal diameter. In this situation, rotation may exceed 40° with the atlas displaced

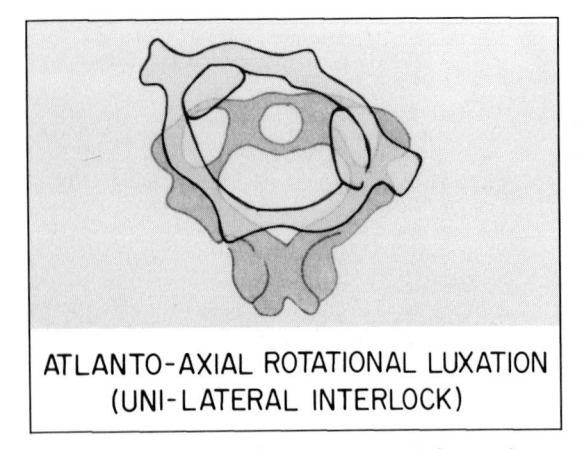

Figure 6. Drawing of unilateral interlock in atlanto-axial rotational luxation.

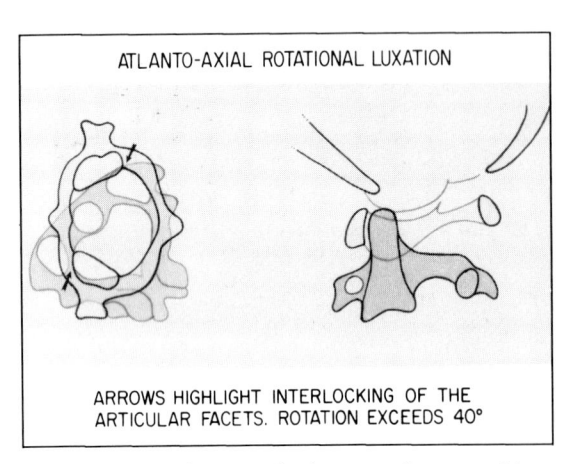

Figure 7. Line drawing of atlanto-axial rotational luxation with bilateral interlock. The axial view (left) and lateral view (right) are presented.

forward indicating rupture of both the transverse ligament complex as well as alar and accessory ligaments. This requires reduction and derotation. Internal fixation, bone fusion, and immobilization are essential (Figure 7).

References

1. Penning L. Normal movements of the cervical spine. *AJR.* 1978;130:317-326.
2. Goel VK, Clark CR, Gallaes K, Liu YK. Moment-rotation relationships of the ligamentous occipito-atlanto-axial complex. *J Biomechanics.* 1988; 21:673-680.
3. Panjabi MM, Summers DJ, Pelker RR, Videman T, Friedlander GE, Southwick WO. Three-dimensional load-displacement curves due to forces on the cervical spine. *J Orthop Res.* 1986;4:152-161.

4. White AA III, Panjabi MM. The clinical biomechanics of the occipitoatlantoaxial complex. *Ortho Clin North Am.* 1978;9:867-878.
5. Menezes AH, VanGilder JC, Graf CJ, McDonnell DE. Craniocervical abnormalities: a comprehensive surgical approach. *J Neurosurg.* 1980;53:444-455.
6. Fielding JW, Hawkins RJ. Atlanto-axial rotatory fixation. *J Bone Joint Surg Am.* 1977;59A:37-44.
7. Jirout J. Changes in the atlas-axis relations on lateral flexion of the head and neck. *Neuroradiology.* 1973;6:215-218.
8. Jones MD. Cineradiographic studies of the normal cervical spine. *Calif Med.* 1960;93:293-296.
9. Menezes AH. Traumatic lesions of the craniovertebral junction. In: VanGilder JC, Menezes AH, Dolan K, eds. *Textbook of Craniovertebral Junction Abnormalities.* Mt Kisco, NY: Futura Publishing Co; 1987.
10. Werne S. Studies in spontaneous atlas dislocation, I: the craniovertebral joints. *Acta Orthop Scand.* 1957;23(suppl):11-83.
11. Braakman R, Penning L. Atlanto-occipital and atlantoaxial luxations. In: Braakman R, Penning L, eds. *Injuries of the Cervical Spine.* Excerpta Medica. Royal Van Gorcum, Assen, Netherlands; 1971:125-131.
12. Fielding JW, Stillwell WT, Chynn KY, Spyropoulos EC. Use of computed tomography for the diagnosis of atlanto-axial rotatory fixation: a case report. *J Bone Joint Surg Am.* 1978;60A:1102-1104.
13. Jirout J. The rotational component in the dynamics of the C2-3 spinal segment. *Neuroradiology.* 1979;17:177-181.
14. Hohl M, Baker HR. The atlantoaxial joint. *J Bone Joint Surg Am.* 1964;46A:1739-1752.
15. Gehweiler JA, Osborne RL Jr, Becker RF. Atlantoaxial rotary fixation. *The Radiology of Vertebral Trauma.* Philadelphia, Pa: WB Saunders Co; 1980:145-147.
16. Maiman DJ, Cusick JF. Traumatic atlantoaxial dislocation. *Surg Neurol.* 1982;18:388-392.
17. Fielding JW, Cochran GB, Lawsing JF III, Hohl M. Tears of the transverse ligament of the atlas: a clinical and biomechanical study. *J Bone Joint Surg Am.* 1974;56A:1683-1691.
18. Jackson RH. Simple uncomplicated rotary dislocation of the atlas. *Surg Gynecol Obstet.* 1927;45:156-164.
19. Selecki BR. The effects of rotation of the atlas on the axis: experimental work. *Med J Aust.* 1969;1:1012-1015.
20. Barton JW, Margolis MT. Rotational obstruction of the vertebral artery at the atlantoaxial joint. *Neuroradiology.* 1975;9:117-120.
21. Okawara S, Nibbelink D. Vertebral artery occlusion following hyperextension and rotation of the head. *Stroke.* 1974;5:640-642.
22. Schneider RC, Schemm GW. Vertebral artery insufficiency in acute and chronic spinal trauma with special reference to the syndrome of acute central cervical spinal cord injury. *J Neurosurg.* 1961;18:348-360.
23. Wiesel SW, Rothman RH. Occipitoatlantal hypermobility. *Spine.* 1979;4:187-191.
24. Banna M, Stevenson GW, Tumiel A. Unilateral atlanto-occipital dislocation complicating an anomaly of the atlas. *J Bone Joint Surg Am.* 1983;65A:685-687.
25. Bools JC, Rose BS. Traumatic atlantooccipital dislocation: two cases with survival. *AJNR.* 1986;7:901-904.
26. Eismont FJ, Bohlman HH. Posterior atlantooccipital dislocation with fractures of the atlas and odontoid process: report of a case with survival. *J Bone Joint Surg Am.* 1978;60A:397-399.
27. Evarts CM. Traumatic occipito-atlantal dislocation: report of a case with survival. *J Bone Joint Surg Am.* 1970;52A:1653-1660.
28. Farthing JW. Atlantocranial dislocation with survival: a case report. *N Carolina Med J.* 1948;9:34-36.
29. Gabrielsen TO, Maxwell JA. Traumatic atlantooccipital dislocation with case report of a patient who survived. *AJR.* 1966;97:624-629.
30. Georgopoulos G, Pizzutillo PD, Lee MS. Occipitoatlantal instability in children. *J Bone Joint Surg Am.* 1987;69(A):429-436.
31. Grobovschek M, Scheibelbrandner W. Atlantooccipital dislocation. *Neuroradiology.* 1983;25:173-174.
32. Alker AJ, Oh YS, Leslie EV. High cervical spine and craniocervical junction injuries in fatal traffic accidents: a radiological study. *Orthop Clin North Am.* 1978;9:1003-1010.
33. Blackwood NJ. Atlas-occipital dislocation. *Ann Surg.* 1908;47:654-658.
34. Bohlman, HH. Acute fractures and dislocations of the cervical spine: an analysis of three hundred hospitalized patients and review of the literature. *J Bone Joint Surg Am.* 1979;61A:1119-1142.
35. Collalto PM, DeMuth WW, Schwentker EP, Boal DK. Traumatic atlanto-occipital dislocation: case report. *J Bone Joint Surg Am.* 1986;68(A):1106-1109.
36. Davis D, Bohlman H, Walker AE, Fisher R, Robinson R. The pathological findings in fatal craniospinal injuries. *J Neurosurg.* 1971;34:603-613.
37. Englander O. Non-traumatic occipito-atlanto-axial dislocation: a contribution to the radiology of the atlas. *Br J Radiol.* 1942;15:341-345.
38. Greeley PW. Bilateral (ninety degrees) rotary dislocation of the atlas upon the axis. *J Bone Joint Surg.* 1930;12:958-962.
39. Page CP, Story JL, Wissinger JP, Branch CL. Traumatic atlanto-occipital dislocation: case report. *J Neurosurg.* 1973;39:394-397.
40. Powers B, Miller MD, Kramer RS, Martinez S, Gehweiler JA Jr. Traumatic anterior atlantooccipital dislocation. *Neurosurgery.* 1979;4:12-17.
41. Rockswold GL, Seljeskog EL. Traumatic atlantocranial dislocation with survival. *Minn Med.* 1979;62:151-152.
42. VanDenBout AH, Dommisse GF. Traumatic atlanto-occipital dislocation. *Spine.* 1986;11:174-176.
43. Watridge CB, Orrison WW, Hendrick A, Woods GA. Lateral atlanto-occipital dislocation: case report. *Neurosurgery.* 1985;17:345-347.
44. Traynelis VC, Marano GD, Dunker RO, Kaufman HH. Traumatic atlanto-occipital dislocation: case report. *J Neurosurg.* 1986;65:863-870.
45. Bucholz RW, Burkhead WF. The pathological anatomy of fatal atlanto-occipital dislocations. *J Bone Joint Surg Am.* 1979;61A:248-250.
46. Woodring JH, Selke AC Jr, Duff DE. Traumatic atlantooccipital dislocation with survival. *AJR.* 1981;2:251-254.
47. Dublin AB, Marks WM, Weinstock D, Newton

TH. Traumatic dislocation of the atlanto-occipital articulation (AOA) with short-term survival: with a radiographic method of measuring the AOA. *J Neurosurg.* 1980;52:541-546.
48. Finney HL, Roberts TS. Atlantooccipital instability: case report. *J Neurosurg.* 1978;48:636-638.
49. Fruin AH, Pirotte TP. Traumatic atlantooccipital dislocation: case report. *J Neurosurg.* 1977; 46:663-666.
50. Lee C, Woodring JH, Goldstein SJ, Daniel TL, Young BA, Tibbs PA. Evaluation of traumatic atlantooccipital dislocations. *AJNR.* 1987;8:19-26.
51. Kaufman RA, Dunbar JS, Botsford JA, McLaurin RL. Traumatic longitudinal atlanto-occipital distraction injuries in children. *AJNR.* 1982; 3:415-419.
52. Menezes AH. "Cranial settling" in rheumatoid arthritis. *Contemp Neurosurg.* 1984;6(16):1-8.
53. Menezes AH, VanGilder JC. Abnormalities of the craniovertebral junction. In: Youmans J, ed. *Neurological Surgery*, 3rd ed. Philadelphia, Pa: WB Saunders Co: chap 45. In press.
54. Ransford AO, Crockard HA, Pozo JL, Thomas NP, Nelson IW. Craniocervical instability treated by contoured loop fixation. *J Bone Joint Surg Br.* 1976;68B:173-177.
55. VanGilder JC, Menezes AH. Craniovertebral abnormalities and their treatment. In: Schmidek HH, Sweet WH, eds. *Operative Neurosurgical Techniques*, 2nd edition. Orlando, Fla: Grune & Stratton Inc; 1988:1281-1293.
56. DeBeer JV, Thomas M, Walters J, Anderson P. Traumatic atlanto-axial subluxation. *J Bone Joint Surg Br.* 1988;70(B):652-655.
57. Spence KF Jr, Decker S, Sell KW. Bursting atlantal fracture associated with rupture of the transverse ligament. *J Bone Joint Surg Am.* 1970;52A:543-549.
58. El-Khoury GY, Clark CR, Gravett AW. Acute traumatic rotatory atlanto-axial dislocation in children. *J Bone Joint Surg Am.* 1984;66(A):774-777.
59. Wortzman G, Dewar FP. Rotary fixation of the atlantoaxial joint: rotational atlantoaxial subluxation. *Radiology.* 1968;90:479-487.
60. Kowalski HM, Cohen WA, Cooper P, Wisoff JH. Pitfalls in the CT diagnosis of atlantoaxial rotary subluxation. *AJNR.* 1987;8:697-702.
61. Ono K, Yonenobu K, Fuji T, Okada K. Atlantoaxial rotatory fixation: radiographic study of its mechanism. *Spine.* 1985;10:602-608.
62. Rinaldi I, Mullins WJ Jr, Delaney WF, Fitzer PM, Tornberg DN. Computerized tomographic demonstration of rotational atlanto-axial fixation: case report. *J Neurosurg.* 1979;50:115-119.

CHAPTER 6

The Evaluation and Management of Trauma to the Odontoid Process

Craig T. Clark, MD, and Michael L. J. Apuzzo, MD

Fractures of the odontoid process have been the subject of considerable debate in both the neurosurgical and orthopedic literature for the past 80 years. Recent advances in the radiologic evaluation of odontoid fractures have led to an improved diagnosis, yet there continues to be argument over the management of this lesion. This chapter will review the etiology, diagnosis, and management of odontoid fractures.

The first reported case of odontoid fracture is unclear. Sir Charles Bell in 1824 described the sudden death of a young man following a fall. An autopsy revealed an atlanto-axial subluxation with transection of the cord.[1] Other early accounts of death from atlanto-axial trauma with associated odontoid fractures were reported by Lambotte in 1894, Bernstein in 1903, and Cortes in 1907.[2-4] In 1928 Osgood and Lund reviewed the literature related to fractures of the odontoid and found a total of 55 cases.[5]

Embryology

The second cervical vertebra develops from four primary ossification centers at birth. At eight weeks of fetal life, chondrification of the axis is complete. Both the odontoid process and the axis are present as a single cartilaginous mass. By the fourth or fifth gestational month the odontoid process develops separately from right and left ossification centers, which normally fuse in the midline by the seventh gestational month. If fusion fails to take place by birth, a vertical line can sometimes be seen between the right and left ossification centers and can be misinterpreted as a fracture. At birth the odontoid is joined to the body of the axis by a cartilaginous plate which may occasionally resemble a fracture.

The apical portion of the dens is derived from the fourth occipital sclerotome which is unossified at birth and is sometimes referred to as the summit ossification center. Between two and five years of age ossification begins in the apical segment, and fusion with the remainder of the odontoid normally occurs by age 12. If this apical segment does not form, the odontoid process is called hypoplastic. In contrast, when this apical segment is present but does not unite with the main portion of the odontoid, the term *ossiculum terminale* is used. If the odontoid process develops but does not unite with the main body of the axis, the lesion is called *os odontoideum*. Failure of development of the entire dens is known as odontoid agenesis or aplasia.

The odontoid fuses with the body of the axis between the ages of three and six years. By seven years of age all synchondroses of the axis should be united, although the bony coalescence of dens and axis proper may be delayed until adolescence.[6-9]

Anatomy

The anatomy of the atlanto-axial junction is unique. The atlas is a bony ring and does not have a body or a spinous process. The articular surfaces of the atlanto-axial junction are slightly oval and are oriented in a nearly horizontal plane, in contradistinction to the rest of the spine where the joints lay in an oblique orientation. This difference in anatomy is easily understandable when one considers that the primary function of the atlanto-axial junction is rotation rather than flexion and extension. As a result of these anatomic and functional differences of the atlanto-axial junction, injuries at this level result in different patterns of fractures and dislocations compared to the rest of the cervical spine.

At the atlanto-axial joint movement occurs as flexion, extension, and rotation. The majority of rotation of the head and cervical spine occurs at this joint and usually accounts for 40 to 50° of rotatory motion. Rotation at the facet joints of the rest of the cervical spine contributes to the remainder of rotational movement; the full rotary motion of the head can be as much as 90°.[10]

When the transverse ligament is intact, the atlanto-axial articulation pivots on the eccentrically placed odontoid and complete dislocation of both articular processes can occur at approximately 65 to 70° of rotation if the remainder of the cervical spine does not rotate. When this occurs, there is a narrowing of the diameter of the average-sized canal at the level of the atlas to approximately 7 mm, at which point spinal cord injury can occur.[11,12]

Ligaments

The transverse or cruciate ligament is composed of transverse and vertical bands and is the primary stabilizer of the atlanto-occipital junction.[13-16] The paired alar ligaments function as secondary stabilizers preventing anterior subluxations. They also prevent excessive rotation of the atlas on the axis. The right alar ligament limits left rotation and the left alar prevents right rotation. The alar ligaments alternatively relax on one side and tighten on the other during rotation. Laxness or absence of these ligaments will allow excessive rotation to take place.[17]

The most common dislocation of the atlanto-axial junction is an anterior subluxation of the atlas on the axis usually associated with fracture of the odontoid process during trauma. However, a pure ligamentous injury involving the transverse ligament can also result in anterior or posterior subluxation. While trauma accounts for a large percentaage of atlanto-axial instability, other conditions that can result in subluxation include infections, rheumatoid arthritis, ankylosing spondylitis, congenital anomalies including partial and complete absence of the odontoid, Klippel-Feil syndrome, Morquio syndrome, and Down's syndrome.[12,18-23]

The ligaments associated with the atlanto-axial articulation in children differ from those of adults in that they are extremely lax until the patient reaches the age of six years. The neonate's neck is therefore at increased risk of injury during birth and shortly after.

Blood Supply

Paired anterior and posterior arterial branches arise from each vertebral artery at the C3 level and run cephalad to supply the base of the odontoid process by way of the accessory ligaments. Branches then run along the periphery to supply the tip of the odontoid process. Here the arteries anastomose freely with each other and with the transverse, superior, and inferior arteries that originate from the internal carotid arteries to form the apical arcade.[24-27]

Using a canine model, Schatzker and associates studied the canine odontoid, which has a rich blood supply similar to that of humans. In their model, they created osteotomies of the odontoid above and below the insertion of the accessory ligaments. The animals were sacrificed at eight weeks, and microangiographic studies showed an extensive vascular network in the proximal fragment.

Some investigators interpreted the data to mean that poor blood supply is not a significant factor in the etiology of nonunion of odontoid fractures.[26] However, others maintained that significant displacement of the odontoid may disrupt the arterial arcade and compromise the vascularization of the bony elements of the region, thus predisposing to nonunion.[27-29] Hensinger et al pointed out that the dens is surrounded by four synovial joints and this may play a role in the diminished bony revascularization after a fracture.[29] Although there has been intensive investigation of the role of devascularization in odontoid fractures, the reason for a high rate of nonunion remains unclear.

Pathology and Epidemiology

Mechanism of Injuries

The mechanism of injury of odontoid fractures cited in older literature was mostly severe falls or blows to the head.[5] Road traffic accidents now account for a majority of the cases.[30] Sorenson and Husby in 1974 published a series in which motor vehicle accidents accounted for over 80% of the odontoid fractures.[31] In Hadley's series of axis fractures, motor vehicle accidents were associated with five cases and miscellaneous accidents accounted for eight cases.[32]

Some authors report that in children less severe trauma can result in odontoid fractures. Falls from heights as low as 60 cm and 90 cm have been reported to result in odontoid fractures in otherwise healthy children.[33] The youngest reported patient with an axis fracture was a two-month-old with a hangman's fracture.[32] In a Japanese series fractures of the atlas or axis comprised 16% of adult cervical spine fractures, but 70% of cervical spine injuries in children.[34] Hubbard reported a series of 42 children with spinal injuries in which nearly 50% involved the atlas or axis, or both.[35]

Fractures of the odontoid with atlanto-axial dislocations and fractures of the neural arch are the most common spinal injuries seen in children. This is thought to be due to the increased laxity of ligaments in this region, along with the incomplete ossification of the dens in younger patients.[36,37]

The biomechanics involved in odontoid fractures is complex and not fully understood. In flexion injuries, the odontoid is fractured when the transverse ligament is pushed forward, resulting in anterior subluxation. With extension the anterior arch of the atlas is forced backward against the odontoid, which is held stationary by the transverse ligament, producing posterior subluxation.[38] In the presence of intact atlanto-axial ligaments the normal joint space between the odontoid process and anterior arch of the atlas does not exceed 3 mm in adults or 4 mm in children, and is usually unchanged during flexion and extension. When these ligaments are injured the distance between the arch of the atlas and the odontoid process increases. Menezes has shown that sectioning of the transverse ligament will allow up to 4 mm of displacement of the dens. Any further dorsal displacement is prevented by the alar ligaments.[39]

Classification of Odontoid Fractures

Various classification schemes for odontoid fractures have been proposed. Anderson and D'Alonzo in 1974 proposed a system for classification that has been widely accepted.[40-44] In a series of 60 patients with odontoid fractures they were able to distinguish three distinct types based on the anatomical location of the fracture line as seen in roentgenograms: Type I fractures have an oblique fracture line through the upper one-third of the odontoid process. This probably represents an avulsion fracture where the alar ligament attaches.

A Type II fracture occurs at the lower third of the odontoid at the junction of the odontoid process and the vertebral body of C2.

Type III fractures extend down into the cancellous bone of the body of the axis and the fracture line usually extends into the superior articular facets of C2 (Figure 1).

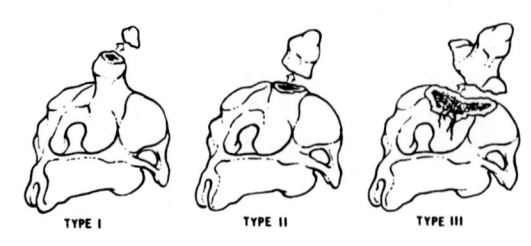

Figure 1. The Anderson and D'Alonzo scheme classifies the type of odontoid fracture according to the location of the fracture on the dens. A Type I fracture involves the distal tip of the dens. A Type II fracture involves the base of the dens. A Type III fracture extends into the body of the axis.

Congenital Conditions Related to C1-C2 Instability

Congenital anomalies of the odontoid are usually discovered incidentally during radiologic examination following trauma to the neck. The trauma may also initiate symptoms by causing atlanto-axial instability or aggravate conditions caused by an already compromised spinal canal. Odontoid anomalies can be divided into three main categories: (1) aplasia or complete absence of the dens, (2) hypoplasia or partial formation of the dens, (3) os odontoideum, the most common, in which the base of the dens fails to unite with the axis.

Aplasia is rare while hypoplasia is only slightly more common. The hypoplastic odontoid arises from the base of the axis as a short peg projecting only a short distance above the plane of the C1-C2 facet articulation. This can often be difficult to distinguish from the more common os odontoideum which is usually seen as an oval or round ossicle, usually approximately half the normal size of the odontoid, with a smooth cortical border of the body of the axis. The ossicle is variable in size and location and most often is located in the position of the normal odontoid tip (orthotopic). Occasionally it is located near the foramen magnum and may fuse with the clivus (dystopic). There is a jointlike articulation between the os odontoideum and the body of the axis. Os odontoideum can be difficult to distinguish from an old odontoid fracture on radiographs.

In adults the diagnosis of os odontoideum is suggested when a radiolucent defect is seen between the odontoid and the body of the axis. The gap between the axis and dens usually extends above the level of the superior facets and the margins are smooth. The odontoid may be up to 50% smaller than normal and is rounded or oval in shape with smooth cortical margins along the entire circumference. In a traumatic nonunion of the odontoid the gap is usually narrow and extends below the level of the superior facets often into the body of the axis. The margins are irregular and the two surfaces can appear to match. A cortical margin is not seen at the level of the fracture line. Anteroposterior and lateral tomograms are useful to supplement the plain film examination. The extent to which atlanto-axial instability is present is determined by lateral tomograms obtained in various degrees of flexion and extension.

The incidence of the three types of anomalies is unclear since they often remain occult unless trauma results in atlanto-axial instability. Attempting to distinguish between the three types of lesions is of little practical significance. The most important point is that they all can predispose to atlanto-axial instability after minor trauma.

Epidemiology of Odontoid Fractures

Odontoid fractures are thought to comprise more than 11% of all cervical fractures.[45] The number of cases of odontoid fractures has steadily increased over the past 50 years, probably as a result of an increase in spine trauma due to traffic accidents and improved radiologic imaging. Acute axis fractures represent approximately 7% to 17%

of all cervical spine fractures in most recent large series.[32,45-49]

In Hadley's series of 625 cervical fractures, 17% involved the axis. Forty percent of the axis fractures were associated with head injuries and 18% were associated with other cervical spine injuries.[32] In most series the average age of patients with odontoid fractures is approximately 40 years and males outnumber females 3:1.[25,28,40,50]

Morbidity and Mortality of Odontoid Fractures

Odontoid fractures are potentially lethal lesions and if improperly treated or unrecognized they may be a cause of significant neurological injury.[51-58] The mortality associated with acute odontoid fractures is less than the 50% described by Osgood and Lund and is probably closer to the 8% figure quoted by Amyes and Anderson.[5,30] The true incidence is difficult to ascertain because a high percentage of patients who die of odontoid fractures probably do so at the scene of trauma as a result of respiratory arrest and are never hospitalized.

Initial Diagnosis and Assessment

Fractures of the odontoid can present with a wide variety of symptoms, many of which are nonspecific. Suboccipital pain, headaches, and neck stiffness are among the most common complaints. Compression of the greater occipital nerve can produce an occipital neuralgia associated with painful paresthesias of the scalp. Hematoma formation often occurs in the retropharyngeal space.

The patient with atlanto-axial instability from an odontoid fracture can present with clinical signs of a myelopathy immediately after the injury, or can remain neurologically intact for many years. There are reports of clinically silent odontoid fractures that presented with the first signs of a myelopathy up to 25 years after initial injury.[52,59]

Nearly 50% of patients with cervical spine trauma will not sustain neurological injury.[46,60-63] In Hadley's series of 150 axis fractures, 91 patients presented with pain, 11 had paresthesias, 8 complained of specific motor weakness, and 14 had some form of paralysis at the time of presentation. On physical examination 104 patients were neurologically intact with respect to their axis fractures. Two patients had signs of a central cord syndrome and one was quadriplegic as a result of a C2 injury. Twenty-two had significant deficits from an associated head or cervical spine injury unrelated to the C2 fracture.[32] These data emphasize the role of maintaining proper cervical spine immobilization and performing careful serial neurological evaluations. In some series 10% of the patients developed signs of cervical spinal cord compression during evaluation in the emergency room or shortly after hospitalization.[63,64]

A high level of suspicion of spinal injury must be maintained until a cervical fracture or instability can be ruled out. Maintaining the head and cervical spine in a neutral, anatomic position with respect to the torso is the mainstay of treatment that begins with paramedics in the field and continues when the patient arrives in the emergency room. During transport and while in the emergency room the patient should be kept in a cervical collar with the head taped to a spine board with a sandbag on each side of the head.[28,46,49,60-65]

Associated Injuries

In some series as many as 60% of the patients with cervical fractures have other major organ system trauma. This fact underscores the importance of basic life support and resuscitation in the field and in the emergency room. Some of the frequently encountered problems include hypoxia, hypovolemia, and hypotension that may exacerbate the damage to the spinal cord.[28,61,63]

In Apuzzo's series, injuries associated with odontoid fractures included: 14 scalp lacerations, 8 cerebral concussions, 8 mandibular fractures, 5 limb fractures, 4 skull fractures, 4 facial bone fractures, 1 lung contusion, 1 hemothorax, 1 splenic rupture, 1 colonic tear, and 1 rib fracture.[28]

Radiographic Evaluation

The initial radiographic evaluation of the patient with a suspected spine injury has been discussed in detail in Chapter 2, but the specific details of the radiologic examination as it pertains to patients with odontoid fractures will be reviewed here.

Open-mouth views of the odontoid are essential and often provide definitive information (Figure 2). If the patient is uncooperative, intubated, or if it is technically impossible to obtain an open-mouth view of the odontoid, tomograms or high resolution computerized tomography (CT) scans should be obtained through the areas of suspected pathology. While CT scanning is the most popular additional radiologic exam after plain films, CT scans are less helpful than standard biplanar tomography to evaluate the odontoid if the fracture is located transversely, parallel to the plane of the axial CT scan. When there is suspicion of an odontoid fracture and CT scans fail to demonstrate a fracture, standard tomograms should be obtained (Figures 3 and 4).

The choice of additional diagnostic tests depends on several factors: (1) rapidly progressive and otherwise unanticipated neurologic deterioration; (2) significant neurological injury in the setting of normal radiographs; (3) abrupt plateauing of neurological deficit after progressive neurological improvement; (4) suspicion of anterior pannus at the odontoid in rheumatoid patients or those with fibrous tissue as a result of chronic subluxations.[66] Until recently the most popular imaging study used to evaluate compression of the spinal cord was a CT scan after intrathecal contrast injection. At this time MRI scanning, if available, is used in place of CT/myelography.

If the CT/myelogram scan is normal in appearance but clinically the suspicion of spinal instability remains, careful flexion and extension plain films of the lateral cervical spine can be obtained if the patient is awake and cooperative. A physician should be present at all times and the patient's neurological status monitored closely. The patient is asked to flex his or her neck until there is any degree of discomfort. Only 20° of flexion or extension is needed to rule out subluxations (Figure 5).

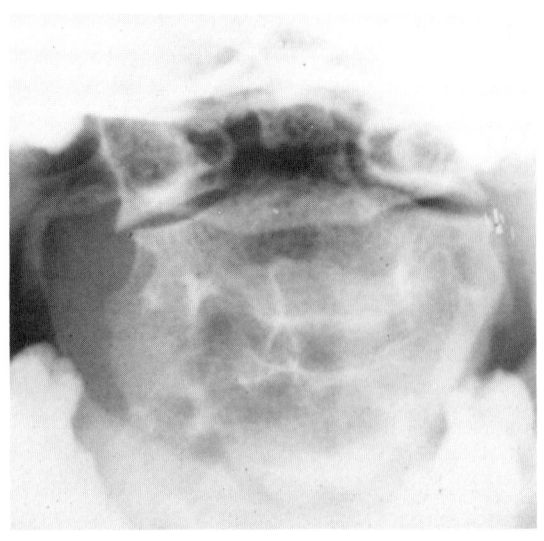

Figure 2. A Type III fracture as seen on an AP open-mouth view utilizing routine tomography.

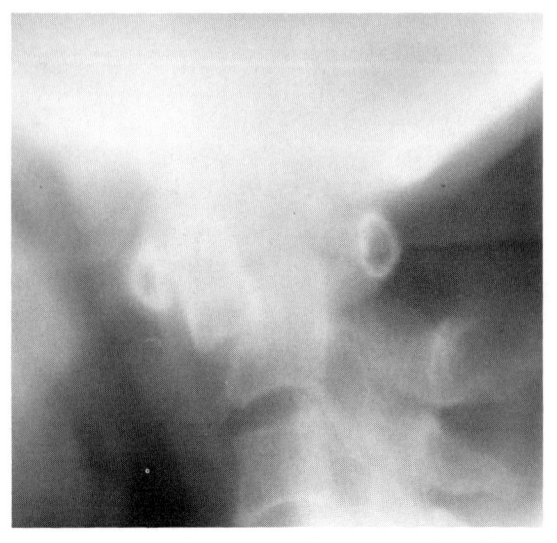

Figure 3. Lateral tomogram of a Type II odontoid fracture with anterior displacement.

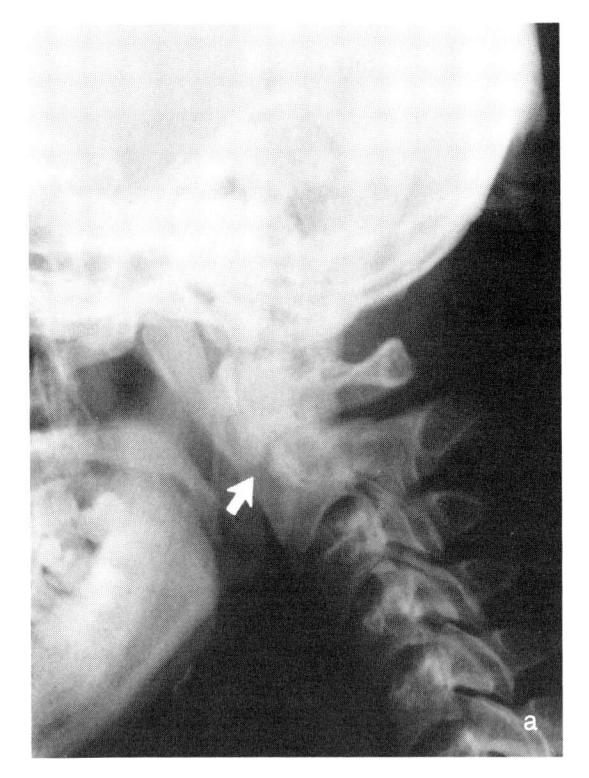

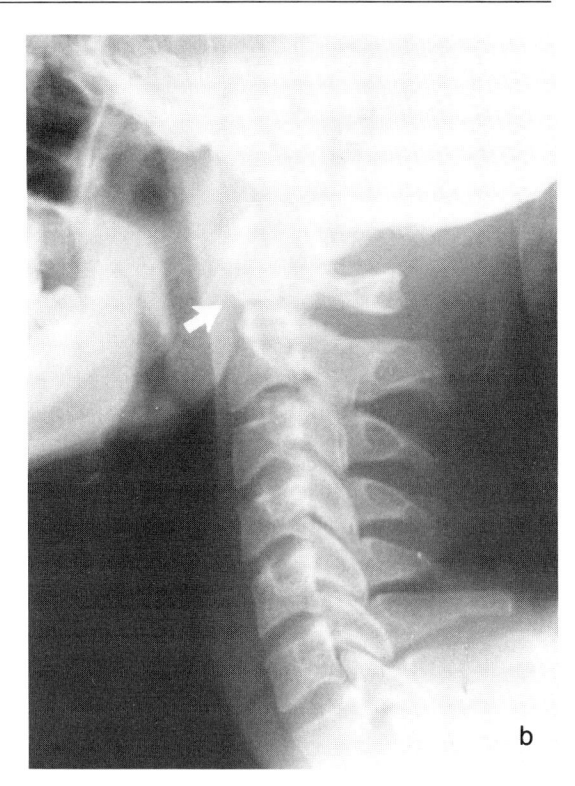

Figure 4. Flexion (a) and extension (b) films of a Type II odontoid fracture demonstrating motion of the odontoid. Note the relationship of the posterior elements of C1 and C2 during flexion and extension.

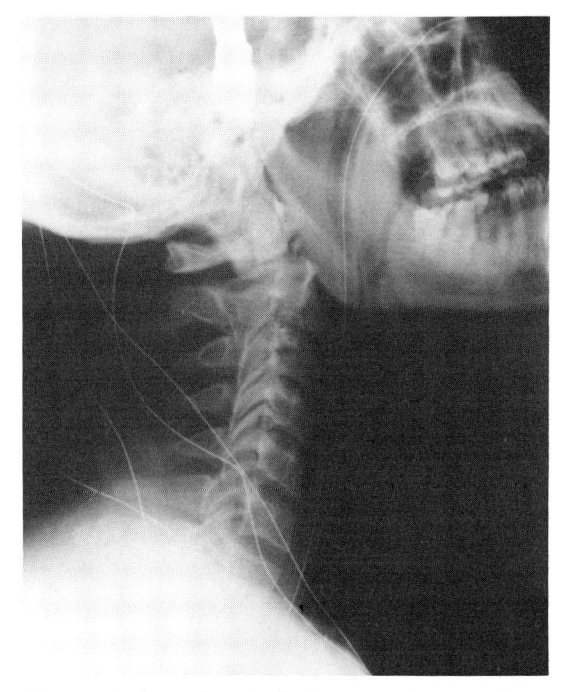

Figure 5. Lateral cervical spine x-ray demonstrating a Type II odontoid fracture with posterior displacement.

In Apuzzo's series of odontoid fractures, the initial radiographs demonstrated fractures at the base of the odontoid in 80% of the cases. Fractures involving the base and body of the axis were seen in the remaining 20% of cases. Fractures of the apical portion of the odontoid rostral to the accessory ligaments were not observed. Displacement of the dens (defined as loss of cortical alignment in lateral views taken in neutral position) was seen in 17 patients. Anterior displacement of the dens greater than 4 mm was seen in eight cases. Anterior displacement less than 4 mm was found in seven patients. Posterior displacement was seen in only two patients, in both instances less than 4 mm.[28]

In Dickman's report of 25 patients presenting to the emergency room with combination C1-C2 fractures, the patients were evaluated with plain cervical radiographs and standard biplanar tomography or computerized tomography. Ninety-two percent of the C2 fractures and 76% of the C1 fractures in patients with combined C1-C2 fractures were identified on plain cervical spine series (anteroposterior, lateral, and open-mouth odontoid views). When either tomography or CT scans were used both the C1 and C2 fractures were identified in 100% of the cases. When there is a suspicion of combination fractures of C1-C2 a thin section CT scan through the C1-C2 region can be useful.[32,66,67]

In viewing plain radiographs the distance between the posterior arch of C1 and the anterior surface of the dens (atlas-dens interval) should be no greater than 3 mm in adults and 4 mm in children. If this interval is increased the transverse ligament is usually injured.

Management Options and Guidelines

Initial Stabilization of Odontoid Fractures

Patients with unstable odontoid fractures are admitted to the intensive care unit. Skeletal traction is applied to achieve reduction and maintain alignment. A variety of devices may be used and include: Gardner-Wells tongs, Trippe-Wells tongs, Vinke tongs, Crutchfield tongs, or a halo ring.

At our institution we prefer Gardner-Wells tongs because of their ease of application. Reduction of the fracture is accomplished using no more than 5-10 lbs of skeletal traction under fluoroscopy or serial lateral radiographs with constant monitoring of the neurological status by the physician. Once reduction has been achieved, traction is reduced two to three pounds to prevent overdistraction. The patient is then placed in a halo vest for external immobilization. This is done whether the patient is to undergo early operative fusion or is to be treated with a trial of external immobilization.

Operative versus Nonoperative Treatment

Controversy over management of odontoid fractures centers around the indications for operative versus nonoperative treatment. The debate regarding operative management concerns the type of operative procedure, the timing of surgery, the type of postoperative immobilization, and the length of immobilization.

Nonoperative management issues include the duration of traction, the type of external immobilization device, and the total length of time for immobilization. The most controversial issue is the appropriateness of nonoperative treatment for Type II fractures. Some authorities recommend early operation for stabilization of nearly all odontoid fractures. Others advocate initial conservative management with a trial of external immobilization. Although considerable scrutiny has been devoted to these issues, the controversies are unresolved (Table 1).[32,44,45,61,68-70]

Factors in Decision Making

Review of the literature reveals several radiologic and clinical factors that have been used to predict the likelihood of fusion without operation. These include the following: (1) age of the patient, (2) location of the fracture on the odontoid, (3) displacement, (4) degree, (5) age of the fracture, (6) combined C1-C2 fractures, and (7) preexisting pathology.

Age of the Patient

In general, the younger the patient the more likely it is that healing will take place without an operation. Apuzzo's data show that if the patient is more than 40 years old, displaced odontoid fractures carry nearly an 80% rate of nonunion. This is twice the nonunion rate for displaced odontoid fractures in patients under 40 years of age.[28]

TABLE 1
Nonunion Rate

Study	# of Cases	Rate (%)
Amyes et al., 1956 [30]	3/48	6
Anderson et al., 1974 [40]	9/37	24
Apuzzo et al., 1978 [28]	13/45	29
Baker et al., 1966 [93]	22/35	63
Blockey et al., 1956 [38]	22/35	63
Bohler, 1965 [82]	2/36	6
Dickman et al., 1989 [67]	1/10	10
Dunn et al., 1986 [68]	19/74	26
Ekong et al., 1981 [71]	7/17	41
Griswold et al., 1978 [94]	7/15	47
Hadley et al., 1985 [32]	8/51	16
Hentzer et al., 1971 [95]	4/7	57
Horlyck et al., 1974 [96]	2/11	18
Husby et al., 1974 [73]	3/21	14
Landells et al., 1988 [97]	1/34	3
Maiman et al., 1982 [69]	15/17	88
Mouragues et al., 1972 [98]	12/52	23
Nachemson, 1960 [99]	7/21	33
Paradis et al., 1973 [50]	2/13	15
Pepin et al., 1985 [74]	9/26	35
Pringle, 1974 [100]	21/62	34
Raimadier et al., 1977 [101]	12/26	46
Roberts et al., 1973 [102]	8/40	20
Rogers, 1957 [64]	4/9	44
Schatzker et al., 1971 [25]	14/22	63
Seljeskog, 1978 [103]	2/27	7

Average nonunion rate = 30%

The data of Dunn and Seljeskog show that nonunion in Type II fractures increases from 22% in patients less than 50 years of age to 60% in patients over 50 years old.[68] A possible explanation for the high rate of nonunion in this group of patients is alteration in blood supply to the fractured dens.[25,27]

Location of the Fracture on the Odontoid

In Anderson's series it was felt that Type I fractures are very rare and are considered stable injuries with a good prognosis. Type II fractures were the most common and were considered unstable and often had a high rate of nonunion when treated with conservative methods. Because of the large cancellous surface, Type III fractures have a higher rate of union when treated conservatively (Table 2).[40]

Displacement

In his series of 37 patients in 1971, Schatzker reported an overall nonunion rate of 63%. If the fracture was displaced there was a higher incidence of nonunion compared to fractures that were not displaced. In nondisplaced fractures the rate of nonunion was 42%. If the fractures were displaced the nonunion rate doubled.[25]

Apuzzo and others reported that when Type II fractures were anteriorly subluxed a distance of 4 mm or more, they had a high incidence of nonunion and should be treated with an operation.[28,71] In Hadley's review, if the dens displacement was 6 mm or greater the nonunion rate was 67%, regardless of the age of the patient or direction of dislocation. In this circumstance early operation was recommended (Table 3).

The ratio of anterior to posterior subluxation is approximately 6:1.[28,50,72,73] Schatzker found that when the fractures were anteriorly displaced the rate of nonunion was 63% and in posteriorly displaced fractures the rate was 93%.[25] Dunn and Seljeskog could not find a relationship between the amount of anterior subluxation and the incidence of nonunion. On the other hand a posterior subluxation of greater than 2-3 mm was associated with a very high incidence of nonunion, and they felt that these fractures should be fused primarily.[68,74]

Age of Fracture

Fractures that are months or years old with sclerosis around the fracture margins will not heal, even with extended immobilization, and should be treated with operative stabilization and fusion. In general, fractures older than two weeks have a high rate of nonunion and often require fusion.[66]

Combined C1-C2 Fractures

In 1988, Hadley and associates reviewed several large series of atlanto-axial fractures including 170 cases of acute C2 fractures from their institution.[47] They recommended that the decision to perform early operation (3-10 days postinjury) on combined C1-C2 fractures should be based on the type of axis fracture present.

In odontoid Type III fractures, hangman's fractures, and nearly all miscellaneous C2 fractures, conservative treatment with external immobilization alone for 8 to 14 weeks was suggested. They also found that 90% of odontoid Type II fractures with odontoid dislocations of less than 6 mm healed with external immobilization. If the odontoid dislocation was more than 6 mm the incidence of nonunion was 70% regardless of the type of immobilization, the age of the patient, the direction of dens dislocation, or the degree of neurological impairment. Therefore, early operative stabilization was recommended.[45,47,63,67,75] Pure ligamentous disruption between the odontoid process and C1 without a fracture of the dens can also result in instability of the C1-C2 complex. These injuries do not heal spontaneously and require fusion.

TABLE 2
Relationship of Fracture Type and Nonunion Rate

Study	Fracture	(%)	Nonunion Rate (%)
Pepin, 1985 [74]	Type I	0	0
	Type II	51	54
	Type III	49	15
Griswold, 1978 [94]	Type I	0	0
	Type II	81	44
	Type III	19	0
Apuzzo, 1978 [28]	Type I	0	0
	Type II	80	46
	Type III	20	54
Hadley, 1985 [32]	Type I	0	0
	Type II	68	26
	Type III	32	0
Dunn, 1986 [68]	Type I	0	0
	Type II	80	32
	Type III	20	0
Anderson, 1974 [40]	Type I	5	0
	Type II	59	36
	Type III	36	8
Ekong, 1981 [71]	Type I	0	0
	Type II	73	38
	Type III	27	17
Paradis, 1973 [50]	Type I	0	0
	Type II	100	15
	Type III	0	0
Maiman, 1982 [69]	Type I	0	0
	Type II	88	100
	Type III	22	0
Landells, 1988 [97]	Type I	46	6
	Type II	37	7
	Type III	17	0
Roberts, 1973 [102]	Type I	5	0
	Type II	59	32
	Type III	36	8
Schweigel, 1987 [104]	Type I	0	0
	Type II	60	17
	Type III	40	10

Preexisting Pathology

In the presence of preexisting pathology at the atlanto-axial junction, an odontoid fracture has an increased risk of nonunion and should be fused primarily. This includes patients with Down's syndrome, patients with rheumatoid involvement at the C1-C2 junction, patients with neoplastic involvement of the atlas or axis, and finally patients with any other condition that may predispose to a nonunion.

TABLE 3
Relationship of Amount of Displacement to Nonunion Rate

Study	Nonunion Rate (%)	Displacement
Hadley et al., 1985 [32]	6/23 (26%)	>4mm
	1/23 (4%)	<4mm
Pepin, 1985 [74]	19/26 (75%)	>4mm
	7/26 (25%)	<4mm
Apuzzo, 1978 #17 [28]	7/8 (88%)	>4mm
	2/7 (29%)	<4mm
Dunn, 1986 [68]	7/27 (26%)	>4mm
	2/27 (7%)	<4mm
Ekong, 1981 [71]	3/4 (75%)	>4mm
	3/8 (38%)	<4mm
Paradis, 1973 [50]	13/17 (76%)	>4mm
	2/17 (12%)	<4mm
Griswold, 1978 [94]	15/16 (94%)	>4mm
	1/16 (6%)	<4mm
Maiman, 1982 [69]	7/15 (47%)	>4mm
	8/15 (53%)	<4mm

Nonoperative versus Operative Treatment Summarized

Odontoid Type I fractures are rare and are usually stable. The nonunion rate for this type of fracture approaches 0 unless there is coexisting ligamentous injury, in which case a posterior fusion may be necessary if there is persistent instability after the trial of external immobilization. Similarly, odontoid Type III fractures have an excellent prognosis with conservative management and can be treated with external immobilization in most instances.

The majority of disagreement centers around the management of odontoid Type II fractures. While some authors advocate primary operative fusion for all cases, others advocate a trial of external immobilization in all cases. Some predictions can be made regarding the likelihood of nonunion. The older patient is at greater risk of nonunion with conservative therapy.

In most series the rate of nonunion is significantly increased when patients over 60 are compared with patients less than 40 years of age. If a patient with an odontoid fracture is over 60 years of age, the risk of nonunion should be weighed against the risk of early operation. In most instances a primary fusion should be considered. The rate of nonunion also is increased if the displacement of the dens is 6 mm or greater. In this instance a primary fusion should be considered regardless of the patient's age.

In combined C1-C2 fractures, management is determined by the type of axis fracture present. An odontoid fracture in a patient with a preexisting condition that can cause atlanto-axial instability will frequently require a fusion that incorporates the occiput. An example would be an odontoid fracture in a Down's syndrome patient, with increased laxity of the cruciate ligament. When a patient has a pathologic process that can result in soft tissue deposition anterior to the spinal cord—as occurs in patients with rheumatoid arthritis—the evaluation should include a magnetic resonance imaging (MRI) scan or CT/myelogram. An algorithm can be helpful in selecting optimum managment for pa-

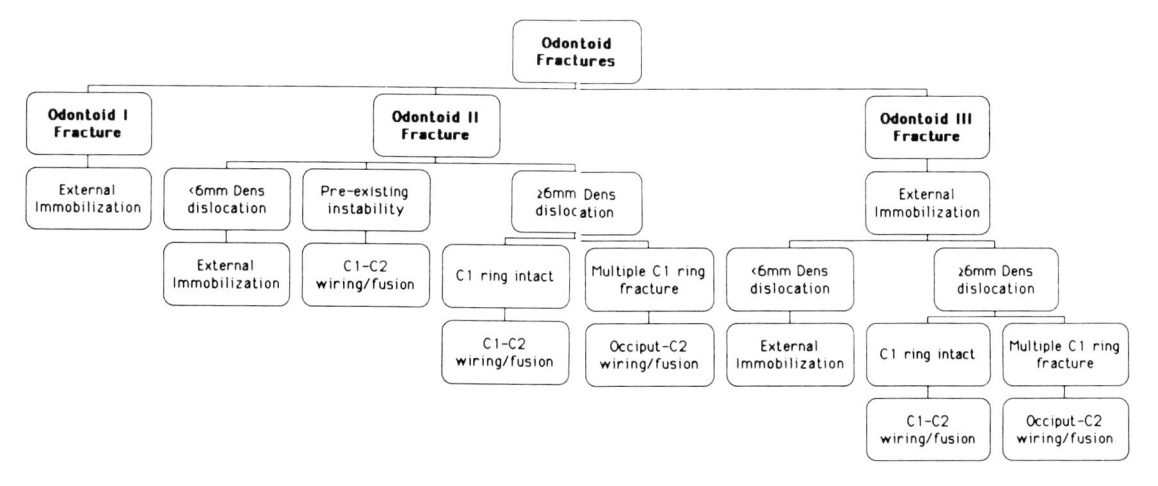

Figure 6. General guidelines for the management of odontoid fractures.

tients with C1-C2 instability from odontoid fractures or ligamentous instability (Figure 6).

Nonoperative Management

After selecting patients using the aforementioned criteria, external immobilization can be used as the initial definitive treatment. The recommended length of skeletal traction and immobilization varies. Some authors suggest skeletal traction for a period of one to five weeks, followed by external fixation with a device that allows ambulation. More commonly, skeletal traction is used mainly for reduction of the fracture. Once the fracture is reduced, external fixation with a halo or similar device will allow the patient to get out of bed or ambulate. The goal is to prevent the complications of deep venous thrombosis and pneumonia associated with prolonged bedrest. Using this approach in Apuzzo's series, patients were placed in external immobilization shortly after reduction of the fracture for a minimum of 14 weeks (range 14-20 weeks). Films were obtained at intervals to monitor alignment and maintenance of fracture reduction. These patients were assessed radiographically for nonunion at the conclusion of this period. If there was a nonunion with instability, the patients underwent operative stabilization.[28]

In 1985, Pepin reviewed a series of 39 patients with odontoid fractures comparing the morbidity associated with the management of fractures in elderly patients with that observed in younger patients. The fractures were grouped into Types I through III according to the Anderson and D'Alonzo classification scheme. Type II fractures were observed more frequently in the younger patients, while Type III fractures were the most common in the elderly group. In reviewing the results of their data they concluded that the use of the halo apparatus in elderly patients (more than 75 years of age) required extreme caution and close nursing supervision to avoid pneumonia. Younger, active patients tolerated the external immobilization well and did not experience pulmonary complications. In active, elderly patients with nonunion, posterior operative stabilization with bone or methylmethacrylate was advocated. In the sedentary, high-risk elderly patient with a nonunion, treatment with a collar for protection when ambulatory or while riding in a car was recommended when operation was deferred.[74]

Orthotic Devices

Several long-term external immobilization devices are available. These include: the halo vest, the Jason brace, the Minerva Plaster jacket, and the SOMI brace. The Jason brace is an excellent method for external immobilization of the upper cervical spine. It maintains cervical immobility by occipital-mandibular noninvasive fixation. We have used it in more than 50 patients and it has proven to be well tolerated and a reasonable alternative to halo fixation (Figure 7).

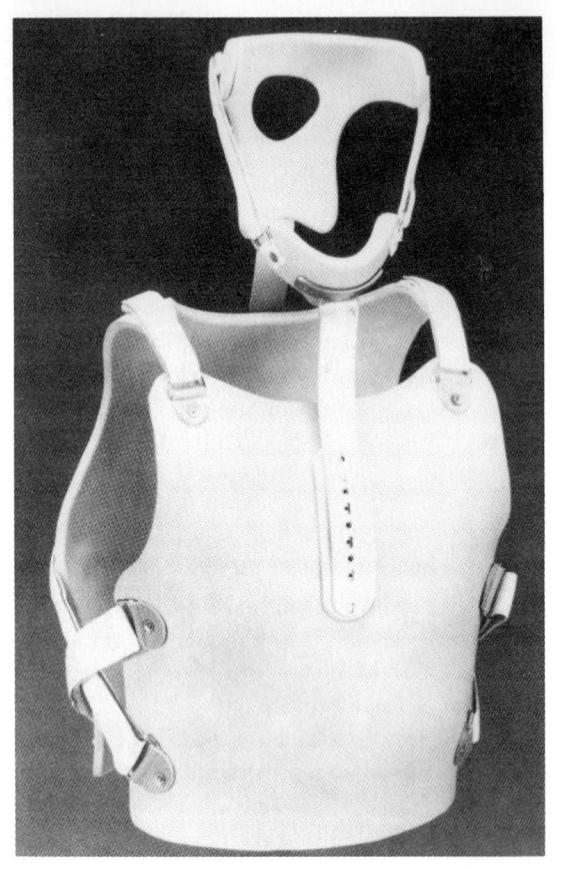

Figure 7. The Jason brace provides excellent external immobilization of the cervical spine.

Operative Management

Internal fixation using a posterior approach was initially described by Church and Eisendrath in 1892. The spinous processes and laminae were tied together with silk. Since that time numerous posterior and anterior techniques have been described for stabilization of the atlanto-axial junction.

The early techniques used a midline posterior approach.[76] In 1910, Mixter and Osgood described a technique using a loop of fascia around the posterior elements of the atlas and axis. In 1935, Gallie revised this technique using a combination of sublaminar wires and a corticocancellous bone graft. The wire provided short-term stabilization until the bone graft fused. Since that time numerous variations of Gallie's technique have been reported. Most variations involve modifications of the wiring technique or the shape of the bone graft. In 1957, Southwick and Robinson[77] described an anterolateral approach to the mid and lower cervical spine. Modifications were later made to allow exposure of the axis and atlas.

Timing of surgery

In general, fusion procedures are performed electively. However, in patients with either complete or partial neurological deficit and radiographic evidence of spinal cord compression, the timing of surgery is controversial. Some authors believe that the spinal cord compression must be relieved as soon as possible to increase the chance of neurological recovery. This situation is rare with isolated dens fractures as they are generally reduced without difficulty, although maintenance of reduction may pose a problem.

Methods of Fusion

Gallie Fusion

A posterior incision is made in the midline from the inion to the level of the third or fourth cervical vertebra, and the lamina of the first three vertebrae are exposed using electracautery and subperiosteal dissection. Two sublaminar wires are passed under posterior elements of C1 and C2. The cortical surfaces of C1 and C2 are abraded. The wires are tightened and a bone graft is then placed over the decorticated fusion site.[78] The patient is immobilized in a halo apparatus, a Philadelphia, or similar orthosis for 8-12 weeks postoperatively.

Apuzzo Modification of the Gallie Fusion

At our institution a modification of the Gallie fusion developed by Apuzzo is most frequently used. With this method, two wires are passed under the posterior arch of C1. Each wire is tightened around the posterior arch of C1. The free ends of each wire are passed around the spinous process of C2 and tightened (Figure 8). The posterior elements on each side of the spinous process of C2 and the posterior arch of C1 are roughened. Bicortical bone grafts and morselized bone obtained from the iliac crest are then placed over the denuded surfaces of the posterior elements of C1 and C2. The patient is maintained in external immobilization for 6-12 weeks postoperatively.

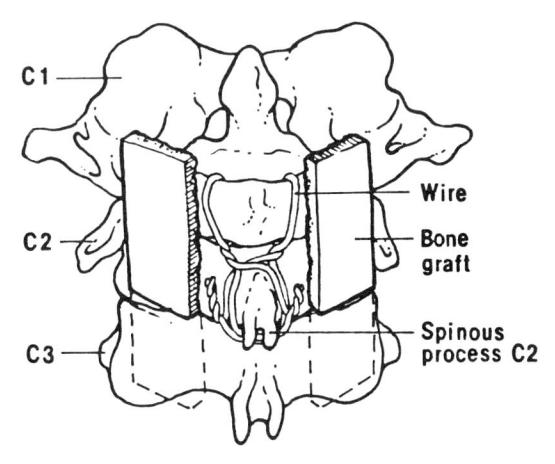

Figure 8. Apuzzo modification of the basic wiring technique for a C1-C2 fusion with bone graft.

Over a 15-year period, we have found this technique to be a safe, easy, and effective method to fuse C1 to C2. Successful fusion has been achieved in 95% of the 40 patients in whom it has been used. This method has the advantage of passing wires only under the posterior arch of C1. This has proven to be useful in cases where the operative exposure is limited or when there is concern over a narrow canal diameter at C2.

Brooks Modification of the Gallie Fusion

In this procedure one wire is passed under each side of the lamina of C1 and C2. Wedge-shaped bone grafts are then placed horizontally between the inferior ring of C1 and the superior surface of lamina of C2. The bone grafts act as struts to prevent collapse of the posterior elements of C1 and C2 when the wires are tightened. The grafts also prevent posterior subluxation of C1 on C2 (Figure 9).[79] The patient is maintained in external immobilization for 8-12 weeks postoperatively.

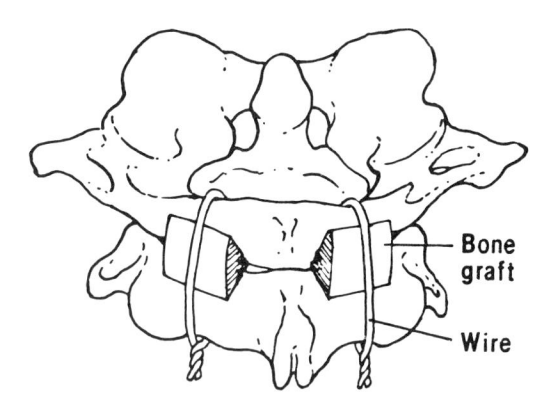

Figure 9. Brooks modification of Gallie fusion. Bone grafts act as struts to prevent collapse of the posterior elements of C1-C2.

Callahan Modification

Callahan described a modification of the Brooks fusion which differs in the positioning of the wires. To prevent possible spinal cord damage during the passing of the sublaminar wires, Callahan recommended drilling two perpendicular holes through the posterior arch of C1. The wires are then passed through these holes and tightened over the bone graft.[80] This procedure has the disadvantage of depending on an intact posterior arch of C1 that is weakened by the drill holes. As a result, even slight tension may result in pulling out of the wires and loss of reduction.

Occipital-C2 Fusions/C1-C3 Fusions

These techniques are used when there is severe instability of the atlanto-axial junction, usually secondary to an underlying pathological process, atlanto-occipital instability, or an incompetent C1 ring. The occiput is included in the fusion by creating two burr holes in the occipital bone and passing the wires through these holes to hold the bone graft in place. The external cortical surface of the inferior calvarium is abraded and incorporated into the bony fusion mass. Fusion of the occiput to C1 and C2 severely limits rotational movement between C1 and C2 and flexion and extension at the atlanto-occipital articulation.

Anterolateral Approach

The anterolateral approach to the atlanto-axial region has been described by several authors. DeAndrade and McNab[81] reported a technique that is a variation of an approach previously described by Southwick and Robinson.[77] The skin incision is made on either side of the neck along the anterior border of the sternocleidomastoid from the mastoid prominence to the level of the cricoid cartilage, and is carried through the platysma and the superficial and deep cervical fascial layers. The plane of dissection is continued posteriorly and the omohyoid is divided if necessary. The recurrent laryngeal nerve is identified and mobilized medially while the carotid sheath is mobilized laterally. The anterior aspect of the atlas and the body of the axis can be palpated. The posterior pharynx is retracted medially and the longus coli and capitus muscles are divided longitudinally and dissected medially and laterally. The bony surfaces of the atlas and axis are now exposed. A fusion can be accomplished by carefully creating a shallow trough between the superior margin of the body of the axis and the inferior margin of the atlas. A thin strip of corticocancellous bone is harvested from the iliac crest and placed in the trough. The longus coli muscles are reapproximated over the midline. The patient is maintained in a halo for three months postoperatively.

Anterior Wiring and Bony Fusion

Bohler described a technique that involves anterior wiring and fusion of the atlas and axis.[82] A transverse skin incision is made at the level of the cricoid cartilage and is continued along the anteromedial aspect of the neck. The carotid sheath is identified and gently retracted laterally and the plane of dissection is continued to the anterior aspect of the atlas and axis. Fluoroscopy or a plain radiograph can be obtained to confirm the level if necessary. Two holes are then placed through the antero-inferior body of C2 extending cephalad into the proximal tip of the dens. Two stabilizing wires are then passed under fluoroscopic guidance.

After the wires have been secured, a horizontal trough is created between the wires extending from the body of C2 into the dens. Corticocancellous bone graft dowels are then placed in the trough across the fracture site and the wound is closed in a standard fashion. The patient is maintained in a halo for six to eight weeks postoperatively.

Newer Methods for Stabilization of the Cervical Spine

Methylmethacrylate

The use of methylmethacrylate has been advocated by some authors for use in patients with C1-C2 instability secondary to malignancy. The methylmethacrylate is applied over the posterior wires for reinforcement and to eliminate the need for postoperative external immobilization.[83] The use of methylmethacrylate to stabilize nonpathological fractures is controversial and we limit its use to patients with malignancy.

Interlaminar Clamps

Interlaminar clamps are gaining popularity in some centers. The hooks of the clamp are seated under the lamina of adjacent vertebrae and a screw couples the hooks together and compresses the lamina together. The clamps are adjustable using a central screw, which joins two interlaminar hooks. These can be used in combination with bone grafting or methylmethacrylate.[84] Although attractive in principle, the clamps, and instruments designed to tighten them are awkward and difficult to use and are currently undergoing modification.

Plating

Roy-Camille and co-workers in France have developed a plate and screw combination that can be used between C1-C2 or the occiput-C2.[85]

Anterior Screw Fixation

Direct screw fixation with osteosynthesis of the odontoid process has recently been described. The technique uses a retropharyngeal approach and screws the fractured odontoid process to the body of the axis. The advantage of this technique over posterior wiring and C1-C2 fusion is maintenance of normal movement between C1 and C2.[86]

Transoral Exposure of the Atlanto-Axial Region

The transoral approach to the atlanto-axial region is useful in decompressing masses of various etiologies in the anterior portion of the upper spinal canal. The stabilization of the atlanto-axial junction by a fusion through a transoral approach was initially described in 1962 by Fang and Ong. Since their report a number of other investigators have refined the technique and reported its safe use in several large series of patients.[87-90]

Operative Technique

The midline of the soft palate is infiltrated with a solution of 1% lidocaine with epinephrine and is incised to the margin of the hard palate. A curvilinear incision that skirts the lateral margin of the uvula is made. This incision has provided optimal exposure for the basiclival odontoid procedure. In many patients exposure of the anterior arch of C1 or even the most inferior portion of the clivus can be obtained by lifting the soft palate with red rubber catheters placed through the nose and brought out through the mouth.

The incision in the posterior pharynx is centered at the level of the anterior tubercle and is extended approximately 2 cm superiorly and 2.5 cm inferiorly. The incision is extended through the posterior pharyngeal mucosa, the superior constrictor muscle of the pharynx and the anterior longitudinal ligamentary complex of the region. These tissues are dissected laterally to the level of the anterolateral joints. If instability is present at this level, there is usually considerable tissue reaction with thickening of the ligaments and granulation tissue at the junction of the body of C2 and the inferior margin of the atlas. These tissues are mobilized laterally and fixed with a Gelpi retractor. Upon complete mobilization of these soft tissues, visualization of the midline inferior clival region, the atlas, and the body of the axis is excellent.

A high-speed air drill is then employed to excise a window extending approximately 1 cm on either side of the midline. Excision is carried posteriorly until the transverse fibers of the transverse ligament are visualized. When the excision is considered to be complete, radiographs may be taken to assess and document the extent of bony excision.

An anterior fusion can be performed by creating a shallow trough in the inferior rim of the atlas and the superior aspect of the axis. A corticocancellous graft can then be placed in this trough. When this is completed, the posterior pharyngeal musculature is closed with a single layer of 3-0 chromic suture.[60,77,87-92]

Although this procedure has been described by a number of authors, in practice it is difficult to perform and provides little or no early stability. We would consider utilizing this procedure only if posterior fusion was not technically feasible. Most often, however, anterior decompression is followed by a posterior fusion.

Summary

The management of odontoid fractures remains a challenge for the clinician. The algorithms presented in this chapter summarize our decision making for the management of odontoid fractures. A brief summary follows:

1. The radiographic evaluation begins with plain films followed by a CT scan without contrast.
2. All displaced fractures are reduced initially with skeletal traction.
3. Routine tomograms in the frontal and lateral projection are performed if there is any question of the presence of an odontoid fracture on the plain films.
4. If a neurological deficit is present, an MRI or CT/myelogram is obtained to evaluate the presence of neural compression.
5. In cases where stability is uncertain, flexion-extension films are obtained.
6. Type I and Type III fractures are treated initially with external immobilization for three months, and if nonunion occurs a C1-C2 fusion is performed.
7. Type II fractures with more than 5 mm of displacement of those that occur in the presence of preexisting pathology are treated with operative stabilization as the primary treatment.
8. Type II fractures with less than 5 mm of displacement are treated with external immobilization initially for three months, and if nonunion occurs fusion is performed.
9. A posterior fusion is normally done unless there is anterior spinal cord compression, in which case a transoral or retropharyngeal approach is used for decompression and a posterior fusion is performed after anterior decompression.

References

1. Bell C. *The Nervous System of the Human Body*. London, England: Longman, Rees, Orme, Brown, and Green; 1830.
2. Bernstein R. Zur diagnnose und prognose der Ruckenmarksverletzungen. Ein Fall von Luxation mit Fradtur des Epistropheus. *Deutsche Zeitschrift fur Chirurgie*. 1903;70:175.
3. Cortes W. Unilateral rotatory dislocation of the atlas, with fracture of the odontoid process. *Ann Surg*. 1907;45:16.
4. Lambotte A. Un cas de fracture ancienne de l'apophyse odontöide avec luxation de l'atlas en avant. *Ann Sac Med*. 1894;56:131.
5. Osgood RB, Lund CC. Fractures of the odontoid process. *N Engl J Med*. 1928;198:61-71.
6. Anderson LD. Fractures of the odontoid process of the axis. In: Baily and Sherk, eds. *The Cervical Spine*. Philadelphia, Pa: JB Lippincott Co; 1983:206-223.
7. Greenberg AD. Atlanto-axial dislocations. *Brain*. 1968;91:655-684.
8. Lang J. Cranio-cervical region: osteology and articulations. *Neuroorthopaedics*. 1986;1:67-92.
9. Michaels M, Prevost MJ, Crang DF. Pathological changes in a case of os odontoideum (separate odontoid process). *J Bone Joint Surg Am*. 1969;51A:965-972.
10. Jacobson G, Adler DC. Evaluation of lateral atlanto-axial displacement in injuries of the cervical spine. *Radiology*. 1953;61:355-362.
11. Fielding JW, Hawkins RJ. Atlanto-axial rotatory fixation. *J Bone Joint Surg Am*. 1977;59A:37-44.
12. Wortzman G, Dewar FP. Rotatory fixation of the atlantoaxial joint: rotational atlantoaxial subluxation. *Radiology*. 1968;90:479-487.
13. Borden, AGB, Wohl MA. Roentgenographic demonstration of unilateral subluxation of the cervical spine. *J Albert Einstein Med Center*. 1962;10:26-30.
14. Dankmeijer J, Rethmeier BJ. The lateral movement in the atlanto-axial joints and its clinical significance. *Acta Radiol*. 1943;24:55-66.
15. Hohl M, Baker HR. The atlanto-axial joint: roentgenographic and anatomical study of normal and abnormal motion. *J Bone Joint Surg Am*. 1964;46A:1739-1752.
16. Werne S. Studies in spontaneous atlas dislocation. *Acta Orthop Scand*. 1957;23(suppl):1-150.
17. Crockard HA. Anterior approaches to lesions of the upper cervical spine. In: Little Jr, ed. *Clinical Neurosurgery: Proceedings of the Congress of Neurological Surgeons*. Baltimore, Md: Williams & Wilkins; 1986:389-416.
18. Lourie H, Stewart WA. Spontaneous atlantoaxial dislocation: a complication of Rheumatoid disease. *N Engl J Med*. 1961; 265:677-681.

19. Martel W. The occipital-atlanto-axial joints in rheumatoid arthritis and ankylosing spondylitis. *AJR*. 1961;86:223-240.
20. Pratt T. Spontaneous dislocation of the atlanto-axial articulation occurring in ankylosing spondylitis and rheumatoid arthritis. *J Fac Radiologists*. 1959;10:40-43.
21. Sharp J, Purser DW. Spontaneous atlanto-axial dislocation in ankylosing spondylitis and rheumatoid arthritis. *Ann Rheum Dis*. 1961;20:47-77.
22. Skok P, Kapp J, Troland CE. Spontaneous dislocation of the atlas: report of a case simulating syringomyelia with discussion of etiology and methods of treatment. *J Neurosurg*. 1964;21:219-222.
23. Spitzer R, Rabinowitch JY, Wybar KC. A study of the abnormalities of the skull, teeth and lenses in Mongolism. *Can Med Assoc J*. 1961;84:567-572.
24. Althoff B, Goldie IF. The arterial supply of the odontoid process of the axis. *Acta Orthop Scand*. 1977;48:622-629.
25. Schatzker J, Rorabeck CH, Waddell JP. Fractures of the dens (odontoid process): an analysis of thirty-seven cases. *J Bone Joint Surg Br*. 1971;53B:392-405.
26. Schatzker J, Rorabeck CH, Waddell JP. Nonunion of the odontoid process: an experimental investigation. *Clin Orthop*. 1975;108:127-137.
27. Schiff DCM, Parke WW. The arterial supply of the odontoid process. *J Bone Joint Surg Am*. 1973;55A:1450-1456.
28. Apuzzo MLJ, Heiden JS, Weiss MH, Ackerson TT, Harvey JP, Kurze T. Acute fractures of the odontoid process: an analysis of 45 cases. *J Neurosurg*. 1978;48:85-91.
29. Hensinger R, Fielding J, Hawkins R. Congenital anomalies of the odontoid process: an experimental investigation. *Clin Orthop*. 1978;9:901-912.
30. Amyes EW, Anderson FM. Fracture of the odontoid process: report of sixty-three cases. *Arch Surg*. 1956;72:377-393.
31. Husby J, Sorensen KH. Fracture of the odontoid process of the axis. *Acta Orthop Scand*. 1974;45:182-192.
32. Hadley MN, Browner C, Sonntag V. Axis fractures: a comprehensive review of management and treatment in 107 cases. *Neuorosurg*. 1985;17:281-290.
33. Seimon LP. Fracture of the odontoid process in young children. *J Bone Joint Surg Am*. 1977;59A:943-947.
34. Hasue M, Hoshino S, Omata S, Kuramochi E, Furukawa K, Nakamura T. Cervical spine injuries in children. *Fukushima J Med Sci*. 1974;20:115-123.
35. Hubbard DD. Injuries of the spine in children and adolescents. *Clin Orthop*. 1974;100:56-65.
36. Allen BL Jr, Ferguson RL. Cervical spine trauma in children. In: Bradford DS, Hensinger RM, eds. *The Pediatric Spine*. New York, NY: Thieme, Inc; 1985:89-104.
37. Sherk HH, Schut L, Lane JM. Fractures and dislocations of the cervical spine in children. *Ortho Clin North Am*. 1976;7:593-604.
38. Blockey NJ, Purser DW. Fractures of the odontoid process of the axis. *J Bone Joint Surg Br*. 1956;38B:794-817.
39. Menezes AH, Graf CJ, Hibri N. Abnormalities of the cranio-vertebral junction with cervico-medullary compression: a rational approach to surgical treatment in children. *Childs Brain*. 1980;7:15-30.
40. Anderson LD, D'Alonzo RT. Fractures of the odontoid process of the axis. *J Bone Joint Surg Am*. 1974;56A:1663-1674.
41. Donovan MM. Efficacy of rigid fixation of fractures of the odontoid process and retrospective analysis of fifty-four cases. *Orthop Trans*. 1979;3:309.
42. Fielding W, Hawkins RJ. Roentgenographic Diagnosis of the Injured Neck. American Association of Orthopaedic Surgeons: instructional course lectures. 1976;15:149-169.
43. Pierce DS, Barr JS. Use of the halo and cervical spine problems. *Orthop Trans*. 1979;3:125-126.
44. Southwick WO. Management of fractures of the dens (odontoid process). *J Bone Joint Surg Am*. 1980;62A:482-486.
45. Lipson SJ. Fractures of the atlas associated with fractures of the odontoid process and transverse ligament ruptures. *J Bone Joint Surg Am*. 1977;59A:940-943.
46. Bohlman HH. Acute fractures and dislocations of the cervical spine: an analysis of three hundred hospitalized patients and a review of the literature. *J. Bone Joint Surg Am*. 1979;61A:1119-1142.
47. Hadley MN, Dickman CA, Browner CM, Sonntag VKH. Acute traumatic atlas fractures: management and long term outcome. *Neurosurg*. 1988;23:31-35.
48. Pierce DS, Barr JS Jr. Fractures and dislocations at the base of the skull and upper cervical spine. In: Society, ed. *The Cervical Spine*. Philadelphia, Pa: JB Lippincott Co; 1983:196-206.
49. Weiss M. Mid- and lower cervical spine injuries. In: Wilkins RH, Rengachary SS, eds. *Neurosurgery*. New York: McGraw-Hill; 1985:1708-1716.
50. Paradis GR, Janes JJ. Posttraumatic atlantoaxial instability: the fate of the odontoid process fracture in 46 cases. *J Trauma*. 1973;13:359-367.
51. Askenasy HM, Braham J, Kosary IZ. Delayed spinal myelopathy following atlanto-axial fracture dislocation. *J Neurosurg*. 1960;17:1100-1104.
52. Bachs A, Barraquer-Bordas L, Barraquer-Ferre L, Canadell JM, Modolell A. Delayed myelopathy following atlanto-axial dislocation by separated odontoid process. *Brain*. 1955;78:537-553.
53. Craig WM. Fracture dislocation of the cervical vertebrae with injury to the spinal cord. *Surg Clin North Am*. 1931;11:841-852.
54. Dastur DK, Wadia NH, Desai AN, Sinh G. Medullospinal compression due to atlanto-axial dislocation and sudden haematomyelia during decompression. *Brain*. 1965;88:897-924.
55. Kahn EA, Yglesias L. Progressive atlanto-axial dislocation. *JAMA*. 1935;105:348-352.
56. Kamman GR. Recurring atlanto-axial dislocation with repeated involvement of the cord and recovery. *JAMA*. 1939;112:2018-2020.
57. Rana NA, Hancock DO, Taylor AR, Hill AGS. Atlanto-axial subluxation in rheumatoid arthritis. *J Bone Joint Surg Br*. 1973;55B:458-470.
58. Schwarz GA, Wigton RS. Fracture-dislocations in the region of the atlas and axis, with consideration of delayed neurological manifestations and some roentgenographic features. *Radiology*. 1937;28:601-607.
59. Stratford J. Myelopathy caused by atlanto-axial dislocation. *J Neurosurg*. 1957;14:97-104.

60. Apuzzo M, Weiss M, Heiden J. Transoral exposure of the atlantoaxial region. *Neurosurgery*. 1978;3:201-207.
61. Heiden JS, Weiss MH, Rosenberg AW, Apuzzo MLJ, Kurze T. Management of cervical spinal cord trauma in Southern California. *J Neurosurg*. 1975;43:732-736.
62. Reiss SJ, Raque GH Jr, Sheilds CB, Garretson HD. Cervical spine fractures with major associated trauma. *Neurosurgery*. 1986;18:327-330.
63. Sonntag VKH, Hadley MN. Nonoperative management of cervical spine injuries. *Clin Neurosurg*. 1986;34:630-649.
64. Rogers WA. Fractures and dislocations of the cervical spine: an end-result study. *J Bone Joint Surg Am*. 1957;39A:341-376.
65. Sonntag VKH. The early management of cervical spine injuries. *Ariz Med*. 1982;39:644-647.
66. Cooper PR. Operative management of cervical spine injuries. *Clin Neurosurg*. 1986;34:650-674.
67. Dickman CA, Hadley MN, Browner C, Sonntag VKH. Neurosurgical management of acute atlas-axis combination fractures. *J Neurosurg*. 1989;70:45-49.
68. Dunn ME, Seljeskog EL. Experience in the management of odontoid process injuries: an analysis of 128 cases. *Neurosurgery*. 1986;18:306-310.
69. Maiman DJ, Larson SJ. Management of odontoid fractures. *Neurosurgery*. 1982;11:471-476.
70. Schiess RJ, DeSaussure RL, Robertson JT. Choice of treatment of odontoid fractures. *J Neurosurg*. 1982;57:496-499.
71. Ekong CEU, Schwartz ML, Tator CH, Rowed DW, Edmonds VE. Odontoid fracture: management with early mobilization using the halo device. *Neurosurgery*. 1981;9:631-637.
72. Blockey NJ, Purser DW. Fractures of the odontoid process of the axis. *J Bone Joint Surg Am*. 1978;60A:279-284.
73. Husby J, Sorensen KH. Fracture of the odontoid process of the axis. *Acta Orthop Scand*. 1974;45:182-192.
74. Pepin JW, Bourne RB, Hawkins RJ. Odontoid fractures, with special reference to the elderly patient. *Clin Orthop*. 1985;193:178-183.
75. Hadley M, Sonntag V. Acute axis fractures. *Contemp Neurosurg*. 1986;9:1-6.
76. Church A, Eisendrath DW. A contribution to spinal-cord surgery. *Am J Med Sci*. 1892;103:395-412.
77. Southwick WO, Robinson RA. Surgical approaches to the vertebral bodies in the cervical and lumbar regions. *J Bone Joint Surg Am*. 1957;39A:631-644.
78. Gallie WF. Fractures and dislocations of the cervical spine. *Am J Surg*. 1939;46:495-499.
79. Brooks AL, Jenkins EB. Atlantoaxial arthrodesis by the wedge compression method. *J. Bone Joint Surg Am*. 1978;60A:279-284.
80. Callahan RA, et al. Modified Brooks fusion for an os odontoideum associated with an incomplete posterior arch of the atlas: a case report. *Spine*. 1983;8:107-108.
81. DeAndrade JR, McNab I. Anterior occipito-cervical fusion using an extra-pharyngeal exposure. *J Bone Joint Surg Am*. 1969;51A:1621-1626.
82. Böhler J. Fractures of the odontoid process. *J Trauma*. 1965;5:386-391.
83. Kelly DL Jr, Alexander E Jr, Davis CH Jr, Smith JM. Acrylic fixation of atlanto-axial dislocations. *J Neurosurg*. 1972;36:366-371.
84. Holness RO, Huestis WS, Howes WJ, Langille RA. Posterior stabilization with an interlaminar clamp in cervical injuries: technical note and review of the long term experience with the method. *Neurosurgery*. 1984;14:318-322.
85. Roy-Camille R, Lapresle P, Mazel C. Les fractures de l'odontöide. In: Roy-Camille R, ed. *Rachis Cervical Superieur*. Paris, France: Masson; 1986:99-118.
86. Borne GM, Bedou GL, Pinaudeau M, Cristino G, Hussein A. Odontoid process fracture osteosynthesis with a direct screw fixation technique in nine consecutive cases. *J Neurosurg*. 1988;68:223-226.
87. Estridge MN, Smith RA. Transoral fusion of odontoid fracture: case report. *J Neurosurg*. 1967;27:462-465.
88. Thompson H. Transpharyngeal fusion of the upper cervical spine. *Proc R Soc Med*. 1970;63:893-896.
89. Bonney G. Stabilization of the upper cervical spine by the transpharyngeal route. *Proc R Soc Med*. 1970;63:896-897.
90. Fang HSY, Ong GB, Hodgson AR. Anterior spinal fusion: the operative approaches. *Clin Orthop*. 1964;35:16-33.
91. Greenberg AD, Scoville WB, Davey LM. Transoral decompression of atlanto-axial dislocation due to odontoid hypoplasia: report of two cases. *J Neurosurg*. 1968;28:266-269.
92. Scoville WB, Sherman IJ. Platybasia: report of ten cases with comments of familial tendency, a special diagnostic sign, and the end results of operation. *Ann Surg*. 1951;133:496-502.
93. Baker LD, Ferlic DC, Heywood HD. Odontoid process fractures. *Gen Prac*. November 1966;34:152-158.
94. Griswold DM, Albright JA, Schiffman E, Johnson R, Southwick WO. Atlanto-axial fusion for instability. *J Bone Joint Surg Am*. 1978;60A:285-292.
95. Hentzer L, Schalimtzek M. Fractures and subluxations of the atlas and axis: a follow-up study of 20 patients. *Acta Orthop Scand*. 1971;42:251-258.
96. Horlyck E, Rahbek M. Cervical spine injuries: a clinical and radiological follow-up study, in particular with a view to local complaints and radiological sequelae. *Acta Orthop Scand*. 1974;45:845-853.
97. Landells CD, Van Peteghem P. Fractures of the atlas: classification, treatment and morbidity. *Spine*. 1988;13:450-452.
98. deMourgues G, Fischer L, Comtet J, Schnepp J, Caltran M. Fractures de l'apophyse odontöide de l'axis: à propos d'une série de 80 fractures. *Acta Orthop Belg*. 1972;38:137-146.
99. Nachemson A. Fracture of the odontoid process of the axis: a clinical study based on 26 cases. *Acta Orthop Scand*. 1960;29:185-217.
100. Pringle RG. Fracture of the dens (odontoid process) of the axis. *J Bone Joint Surg Br*. 1974;56B:200-201. Proceedings and Reports of Universities, Colleges, Councils and Associations.
101. Ramadier JO, Aléon JF, Servant J. Fractures de l'apophyse odontöide 94 cas dont 61 traites par arthrodese. *Int Orthop*. 1977;1:113-119.

102. Roberts A, Wickstrom J. Prognosis of odontoid fractures. *Acta Orthop Scand*. 1973;44:21-30.
103. Seljeskog EL. Non-operative management of acute upper cervical injuries. *Acta Neurochir*. 1978;41:87-100.
104. Schweigel JF. Management of the fractured odontoid with halo-thoracic bracing. *Spine*. 1987;12:838-839.

CHAPTER 7

Management of Nonodontoid Upper Cervical Spine Injuries

Volker K. H. Sonntag, MD, and Mark N. Hadley, MD

One-quarter of all cervical spinal cord and vertebral column trauma occurs between the occiput and the third cervical vertebra (C3) (Table 1).[1-5] About 5% of cervical injuries in adults result in fracture of the atlas,[4,6,7] 18% involve the axis,[4,8,9] and 2% affect C3.[4,5] Among patients up to the age of 16 years, upper cervical spinal trauma accounts for 60% of all spine injuries.[10-12] Fractures and subluxations of the occiput through C2 are particularly prevalent among the youngest pediatric patients (zero to nine years of age) where 50% of spinal injuries involve the three upper cervical vertebrae.[10-12]

Anatomy

Injury to the upper cervical spine is more prevalent among infants and young children due to specific anatomic and physiological features unique to the immature spine and its associated supporting structures.[10-13] Infants have immature neck musculature; underdeveloped, lax ligaments; incompletely ossified wedge-shaped vertebrae; shallow horizontally oriented facet joints; and an absence of uncinate processes that contribute to increased physiologic mobility of the spine. These features, in conjunction with the infant's relatively large head compared to the torso, place the relative fulcrum of the cervical spine at the atlas-axis level and account for the vulnerability of these levels to injury.[10] With age and development the vertebral segments mature, and the relative fulcrum drops to the lower cervical spinal level of C5-C6—the most common level of cervical spine injury in adults.[10]

Development of the immature spinal column and support structures occurs in two stages. Ossification of the vertebral segments, development of the uncinate processes, and changes in facet orientation occur by age eight or nine. Maximal strength and stability of the facet joints, ligaments, and musculature is achieved by about age 14. Adolescents 14 years of age and older sustain spine injuries similar to those that occur in adult patients.[10-12]

The unique anatomy, orientation, and articulations of the atlas and axis predispose them to fracture and subluxation even among adults.[4,5,6,7,9,14-17] The atlas is a thin ring with broad articulation plates for the occiput above and the axis below. The odontoid process of the axis extends superiorly through the ring of the atlas and is secured to the skull base and atlas by several stout ligaments (apical, alar, transverse). In addition, a synovial joint between the dens and the arch of C1 allows for significant rotation, flexion, and extension.[18] Direct loading-compression forces can result in compression of the ring of C1 and, if sufficient force is present, can

---

The views of the authors are their own and are not to be construed as official or reflecting the position of the Department of the Air Force or the Department of Defense.

cause bursting of the ring of the atlas.[7,16,17] Force vectors that are not direct loading injuries can cause a variety of fracture and fracture-dislocation injuries of the atlas or the vulnerable odontoid process.[4,7,8,9,14,15] Frequently, C1-odontoid fractures will occur together.[6,7]

The most common fracture of the second cervical vertebra involves the odontoid process.[4,8,9,19-22] The next most common axis injury is the hangman's fracture, which results in a break of the posterior arch of the axis bilaterally at the pars interarticularis.[4,5,8,9,23] In addition, a variety of miscellaneous fractures of the axis have been described and include isolated fractures of the ring, body, lateral masses, and spinous process.[8,9,14,15]

C3 fractures are much less common than those that affect C1 or C2.[1,4,5] In the authors' experience, one-half of these have been associated with C2 injuries. Isolated C3 fractures include compression-wedging of the body, but posterior element and spinous process injuries are more typical.

Certain congenital anomalies of the skull base and/or proximal cervical vertebral segments and several systemic disease processes may increase the vulnerability of selected patients to upper cervical spinal injuries.[10,24-26] These include Down's syndrome, occipitalization of the atlas, os odontoideum, Warfarin syndrome, and Conradi's syndrome. Adults with rheumatoid arthritis often develop marked progressive occipital C1-C2 instability.[24,27] In patients with basilar invagination and previous subluxation, relatively mild trauma can lead to marked upper cervical spinal instability.[24,26,27]

Evaluation of the Upper Cervical Spine

Radiographic examination of the upper cervical spine begins with anteroposterior and lateral roentgenograms. To assess the upper cervical spine adequately, particularly if the patient has skull base or superior cervical spine pain or if the initial lateral radiographs are suspicious for injury, an open-mouth view of the odontoid process and the C1-C2 articulations should be obtained. The pillar view of the odontoid process (oblique radiograph) will reveal the integrity of the dens in patients who will not (or cannot) cooperate for the performance of the open-mouth radiograph. Approximately 15% of patients with a high cervical fracture will have a second vertebral column fracture, an incidence that warrants a complete spinal column radiographic survey.[3,4,22]

Areas of suspected pathology identified on the plain radiographs should be studied with thin-section computerized tomography (CT).[4,28,35,37] This is particularly true for C1 and C2 fractures because the precise fracture subtype is often difficult to discern on plain x-rays.[6-9] In addition, a number of fractures involve *both* the atlas and the axis, and these are difficult to identify without CT images.[6,7,36] The CT evaluation is followed by dynamic flexion and extension radiographs, myelography, angiography, three-dimensional CT, and magnetic resonance (MR) imaging studies as necessary. MR imaging is rarely used as the initial diagnostic study for patients with spinal injuries. When obtained, it is less useful for evaluation of bony pathology than to demonstrate abnormalities of the spinal cord, integrity of the disks, and the presence of spinal hematomas.

A subgroup of pediatric spine-injured patients will present with clinical signs of a spinal cord injury without radiographic abnormalities (SCIWORA).[10-13] These patients must be immobilized and fully evaluated with radiographic studies to identify injuries that may not be seen on standard radiographs. The level of cervical spine to be studied with CT is determined by the level of neurological injury. Dynamic studies should follow CT in these patients in an attempt to document instability and subluxation. If these studies are normal, immobilization should be maintained, and patients should be evaluated and followed according to the

SCIWORA management principles outlined by Hadley, et al[10,11] and by Pollack, et al.[13]

General Principles of Initial Management

In the patient with an unreduced fracture-dislocation, every attempt should be made to reduce the injury early in the patient's hospital course before CT scanning is performed.[1,4,5,37] In the upper cervical spine reduction of dislocations is usually easy and is accomplished with neutral anatomic positioning and immobilization. Occasionally, a fracture-dislocation will persist (typically at C2-C3) and traction with Gardner-Wells tongs (GWT) will be required.

We treat patients with cervical spine injuries who require GWT in the intensive care unit (ICU) on a Stokes bed. The ICU setting also allows for prompt treatment of respiratory insufficiency, spinal shock, and any associated injuries. Immobilization of the head and neck with respect to the torso can be a problem despite GWT when treating fracture-dislocation of the upper cervical spine, where only a small amount of weight is needed for reduction. This is particularly true for the combative or uncooperative patient. A difficult patient with upper cervical spinal instability may be further immobilized in a rigid collar with sand bags placed at both sides of the head and neck (in addition to GWT). We usually attempt to immobilize such patients with rigid external stabilization (halo vest) early in the hospital course to prevent subluxation and potential neurological injury (even if they are candidates for operation).[4,5,29]

Specific Injuries of the Upper Cervical Spine

Fractures of the Atlas

The first cervical vertebra, the atlas, is uniquely positioned between the skull and the remainder of the vertebral column and is vulnerable to a variety of injuries. Fractures of C1 comprise between 3% and 13% of all cervical spine injuries in most series.[1,4,7,16,17,36] In the past 12 years we have seen 57 atlas fractures, representing 4.5% of

TABLE 1
Relative Frequency of Upper Cervical Spine Fracture in a Series of 1,280 Cervical Spine Fractures

	Number		Total (%)
Atlas Fx	57		4.5
Isolated		32	2.5
Combination		25	2.0
Axis Fx	229		18
Odontoid Type I		0	0
Odontoid Type II		87	6.8
Odontoid Type III		49	3.8
Hangman's		46	3.7
Miscellaneous		47	3.7
Cervical Three Fx	23		1.8
Isolated		12	0.9
Combination		11	0.9
Atlanto-Axial			
Subluxation without Fx	7		0.5
Os Odontoideum		5	0.4
Rheumatoid		2	0.1

Fx = fracture

all patients treated for cervical vertebral column injuries (Table 1).

Thirty-four patients were male with a median age of 40 years (range, 14 to 82 years), and 23 patients were female with a median age of 42 years (range, 17 to 86 years). Thirty-two patients had isolated C1 fractures, and 25 sustained combination C1-C2 fractures. Forty-four percent of patients with a C1 fracture also had a fracture of the axis. Five patients (9%) sustained an additional noncontiguous cervical spine fracture, and 12 patients (21%) had associated head injuries. Motor vehicle accidents were the most common cause of injury, followed by falls and motorcycle accidents. Additional patients sustained an atlas fracture from miscellaneous causes including diving, hang gliding, skateboarding, and other sports-related injuries.

None of the 32 patients with an isolated C1 fracture sustained neurological injury, although several complained of dysesthesias at the base of the skull and neck at the time of presentation. The majority of isolated C1 injuries (56%) consisted of acute bilateral or multiple fractures of the ring of the atlas. There were 10 unilateral ring fractures (31%) and four isolated lateral mass fractures (13%). In 12 of the isolated atlas fractures there was no C1-C2 dislocation as determined by anteroposterior (AP) open-mouth view radiographs. Fifteen of the fractures had less than 6.9 mm of lateral displacement of C1 and C2 (determined by measuring and summing the spread of the lateral masses of C1 beyond the margins of C2 on the AP x-ray), and five fractures were displaced by more than 6.9 mm. These radiographic features are important when determining the appropriate treatment of isolated atlas fractures.[4,7,17]

The treatment of atlas fractures is almost exclusively nonsurgical and depends on the type of injury and the presence of associated axis or other cervical vertebral body fractures.[4,7] For isolated C1 fractures, uncomplicated by an axis fracture or other associated cervical spine fractures (for which more rigid external immobilization or even surgery may be required), Spence et al have provided criteria that help determine appropriate therapy.[4,16,17] They have stated that if the sum of the spread of the lateral masses of C1 over C2 as determined on the AP C1-C2 radiograph exceeded 6.9 mm, then the likelihood of transverse ligament disruption was great. In cadaver studies, this degree of dislocation was associated with transverse ligament disruption and C1-C2 instability. The authors concluded that injuries of this magnitude required a more aggressive approach and advocated surgical stabilization of C1 and C2.[17]

Isolated atlas fractures with spread of the lateral masses less than 6.9 mm on the AP x-ray can be effectively treated with less rigid cervical support (typically a Philadelphia collar) for a duration of 8 to 12 weeks. In spite of Spence's suggestions we believe that operation is unnecessary even in patients whose fractures have a total lateral displacement exceeding 6.9 mm. We advocate rigid external immobilization for these fractures,[4,7] which may be most effectively accomplished with the halo vest for a duration of 10 to 14 weeks. Periodic clinical and radiological follow-up is essential to document patient compliance and adequate alignment and healing. Dynamic flexion and extension radiographs are performed following halo vest removal to confirm stability.

Table 2 shows the treatment used for the 32 isolated C1 fractures in our series. The form of external immobilization employed depended on the degree of C1-C2 lateral mass dislocation. No patient required surgical stabilization or fusion. The median length of treatment for the group was 12 weeks with a range of 8 to 16 weeks. Three of 32 patients were lost to follow-up. None of the remaining 29 patients had evidence of nonunion or instability on follow-up radiographs (including dynamic studies). No patient developed delayed neurological deficit although three patients complained of intermittent neck pain.

TABLE 2
Treatment of Isolated Axis Fractures

Isolated Atlas Fx

Nondisplaced	(N = 12)	1 Soft Collar 10 Rigid Collar 1 SOMI Brace
Displaced < 6.9 mm	(N = 15)	8 Rigid Collar 3 SOMI Brace 4 Halo Vest
Displaced ≥ 6.9 mm	(N = 5)	5 Halo Vest
		(Median TX = 12 weeks) (Range 8 to 16 weeks)

From Sonntag VKH, Hadley MN: Management of upper cervical spinal instability. In: Wilkins RH, ed. *Neurosurgery Update.* New York: McGraw-Hill. In press. Reprinted with permission of McGraw-Hill.

Axis Fractures

We treated 229 acute axis fractures between 1976 and 1988.[5,8] These represented 18% of the total acute cervical spine injuries during this period (Table 1). Odontoid fractures were the most common type encountered and represented 60% of the total. There were no odontoid Type I fractures in this series. Eighty-seven patients had odontoid Type II fractures; 49 had odontoid Type III fractures. There were 46 hangman's fractures and 47 miscellaneous axis fractures (nonodontoid-nonhangman's fractures). Males outnumbered females 2:1, and the median age was 37 years for males and 41 years for females. The most common causes of injury were motor vehicle accidents (65%),[34] followed by falls (15%), diving injuries (6%), and miscellaneous accidents (14%).[4,5,7,8]

Thirteen patients with axis fractures sustained neurological injury. Of these, three had odontoid Type II fractures, four had Type III fractures, two had hangman's fractures, and four had miscellaneous axis fractures. Fifteen patients in this series died, most as a result of severe cardiopulmonary compromise or severe head injury.

Several types of axis fractures are best treated by nonoperative means.[4,8,9] These include hangman's fractures, odontoid Type III fractures, and miscellaneous axis fractures. Odontoid fractures are the subject of another chapter and will not be discussed here except as they occur with other upper cervical spine fractures.

Hangman's fractures (Figure 1) involve the pars interarticularis of the axis bilaterally.[4,9,23,30] Of 46 patients with hangman's fractures that we have treated, four died early in the their hospital course due to severe head injury or multiple trauma. The remaining 44 patients were treated with rigid external immobilization in either a halo vest or SOMI brace for periods of 10 to 16 weeks (Figure 2).

Two patients (4.5%) failed nonoperative therapy and required surgical stabilization. Both were initially treated with a halo vest and both had marked C2-C3 instability. One patient underwent a posterior wiring and fusion procedure of C1-C2-C3. The second patient had a C1 ring fracture, C2 hangman's fracture, and a C3 posterior arch fracture in addition to 4 mm C2-C3 subluxation (Figure 3). He was treated with an anterior C2-C3 discectomy and anterior autologous iliac crest bone graft fusion, secured with C2-C3 Caspar plating (Figure 4). No other patient treated nonoperatively for a hangman's fracture had posttreatment instability. The two patients treated with operation had no evidence of

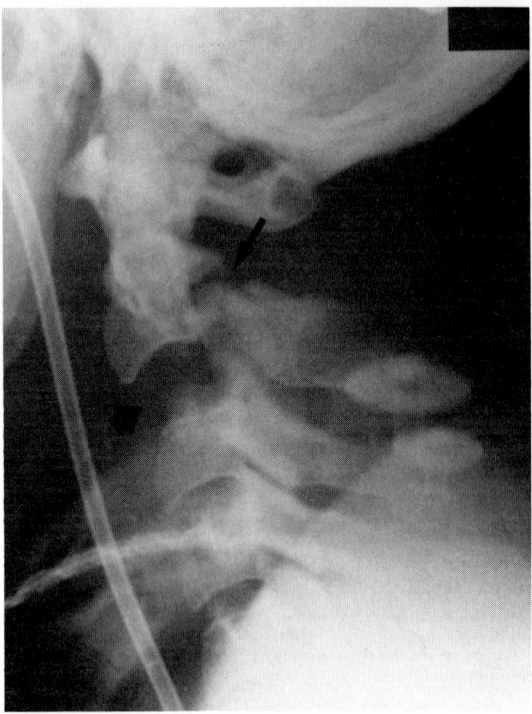

Figure 1. Hangman's fracture with marked C2-C3 dislocation (broad arrow).

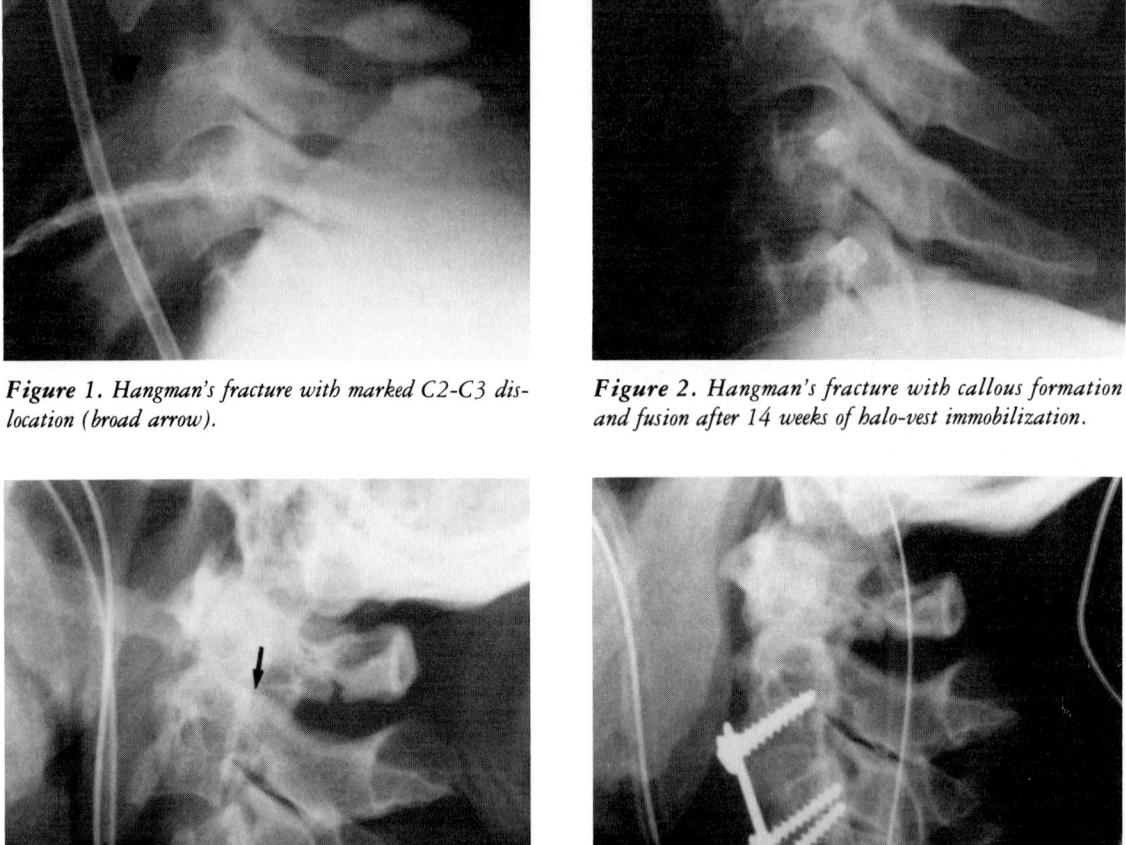

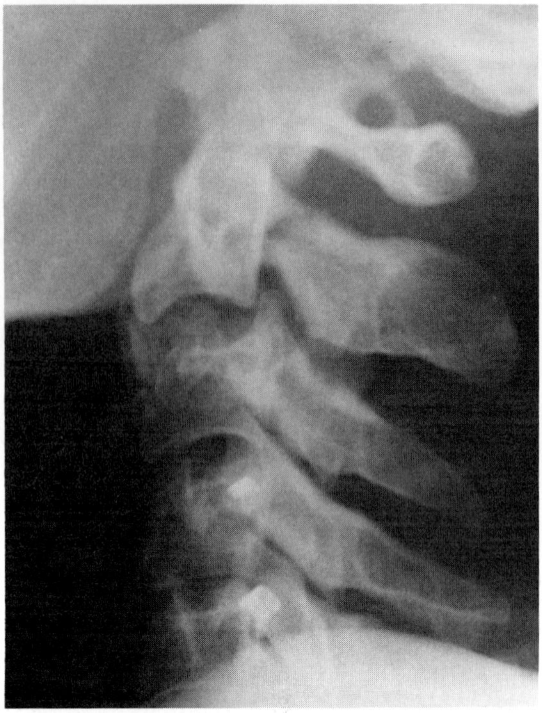

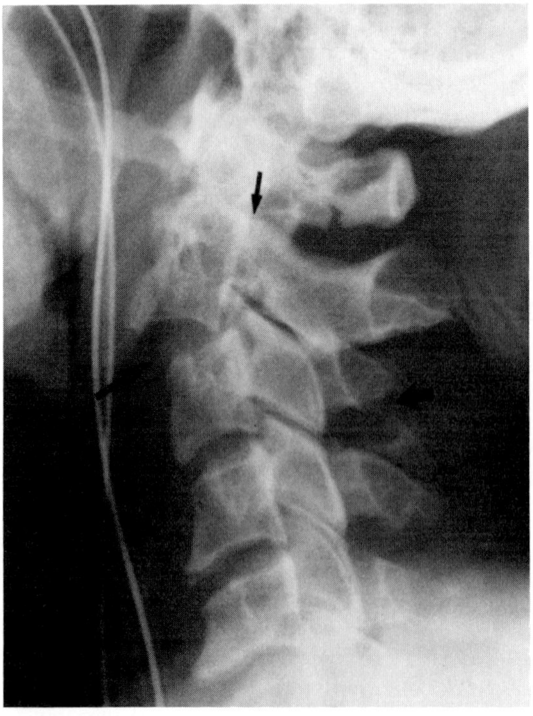

Figure 2. Hangman's fracture with callous formation and fusion after 14 weeks of halo-vest immobilization.

Figure 3. Patient with C1 arch fracture, hangman's fracture, C3 posterior element fracture, and marked C2-C3 instability.

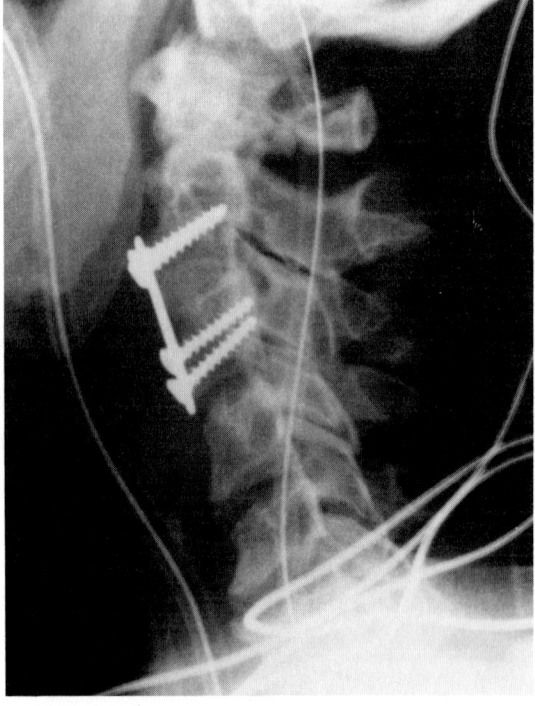

Figure 4. Postoperative radiograph revealing C2-C3 anterior fusion with plating.

nonunion or instability at the time of the latest follow-up.

Miscellaneous fractures of the axis are all axis fracture subtypes other than hangman's and odontoid fractures.[4,9,14] These include C2 body, lateral mass, lamina, and spinous process fractures (Figure 5). The treatment of patients with miscellaneous fractures must be individualized and depends on the severity of the fracture and the presence of associated C2-C3 subluxation.[4,5,14] Clearly, an isolated spinous process or lamina fracture will not require the same type of immobilization or duration of therapy needed to treat a C2 body or lateral mass fracture with a 3 mm C2-C3 subluxation.

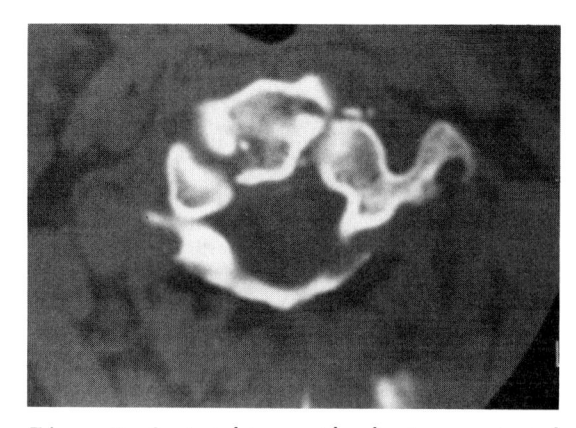

Figure 5. Computed tomography showing comminuted fracture of C2 body.

Of 47 patients with miscellaneous axis fractures in our series, three died. Of the remaining 44 patients, 36 were treated in a halo vest, 4 in a SOMI brace, and 3 in a rigid Philadelphia collar. One patient was treated with operation consisting of posterior wiring and fusion of C1-C3 for a C2 lateral mass fracture and 5 mm subluxation of C2 on C3. Only one patient treated nonoperatively had instability with nonunion. She had a C2 body fracture with a 4 mm C2-C3 subluxation. She was ultimately treated with C2-C3 wiring and fusion procedure. No other patient had evidence of nonunion or instability at last follow-up.

Of 86 patients with hangman's, odontoid Type III, or miscellaneous fractures of the axis who were treated nonoperatively for whom follow-up is available, 3 had persistent instability with nonunion after treatment (3% nonunion rate). All three patients (two hangman's and one miscellaneous fracture) had pronounced subluxation and instability at C2-C3. The presence of marked instability and subluxation at the C2-C3 level may be an indication for early operative treatment in patients with acute axis fractures.

Atlas-Axis Combination Fractures

Twenty-five patients presented with atlas-axis combination fractures.[5,6] These patients represented 2% of the total population of patients with acute cervical spine injuries treated over a period of 12 years (Table 1). Sixteen patients were male with a median age of 40 years, and nine patients were female with a median age of 51 years. Combination C1-C2 injuries accounted for 44% of all acute atlas fractures (n = 57) during this period and 11% of all axis fractures (n = 229). The causes of combined C1-C2 injury are similar to those described for isolated C1 or C2 fractures.

The classification of combination atlas-axis injuries is based on the type of axis fracture present.[6] The most common type of C1-C2 combination fracture in our review was a C1-odontoid Type II injury (40%), followed by C1-miscellaneous C2 fractures (nonodontoid, nonhangman's fractures), C1-odontoid Type III fractures, and C1-hangman's fractures. C1-odontoid Type II fractures were present twice as frequently as C1-odontoid Type III fractures.

Each of the three patients with C1-hangman's fracture combinations had associated multiple fractures of the posterior arch of the atlas. The C1 fractures in the remaining atlas-axis fracture combinations were divided among multiple ring fractures, unilateral C1 ring fractures, or lateral mass fractures.

Three patients (12%) with acute combination C1-C2 fractures had neurological deficits upon admission. Two of these patients had signs consistent with central spinal cord injury due to C1-C2 body fractures (combination C1-miscellaneous C2 fractures). The third patient had a complete neurological injury at the C2 level from a combination C1-odontoid Type II fracture and died from cardiopulmonary complications on the fourth day after injury. He represents the only death in the C1-C2 fracture population.

While much has been written about the treatment of isolated C1 and C2 fractures, little attention has been directed toward the combination C1-C2 fracture injury (Figure 3).[6] Lipson proposed a management strategy employing both nonoperative and operative treatment.[36] He advocated external immobilization in a halo vest for six to eight weeks to allow the atlas fracture to heal, followed by surgical wiring and fusion as definitive treatment of the *axis* fracture dislocation.

More recent experience with the management of patients with *axis* fractures, improved radiographic diagnostic studies, and the knowledge that not all atlas fractures are unstable has led us to conclude that a more refined approach to combination C1-C2 fractures is necessary.[4,6,7,8,9] A unilateral arch fracture of the atlas or an isolated C1 lateral mass fracture does not preclude early surgical wiring of C1 to C2 in the treatment of combination C1-C2 fracture injuries. If the atlas fracture is a bursting type (bilateral or multiple arch fractures), then C1 cannot be incorporated in the wiring and an occiput-to-C2 wiring and fusion procedure should be considered. One can then avoid the additional immobilization of patients for six to eight weeks *prior* to definitive surgical therapy of their combination C1-C2 injury as advocated by Lipson.[36]

The decision to perform early surgery (within 3 to 12 days of injury) on patients with combined C1-C2 fractures is based upon the type of axis fracture present. Several reviews of patients with isolated axis fractures have demonstrated that Type III odontoid fractures, hangman's fractures, miscellaneous C2 fractures, and many Type II odontoid fractures heal with 8-14 weeks of external immobilization alone.[4,8,9,22]

Odontoid Type II fractures with dens dislocations of 6 mm or greater have a high incidence of nonunion with rigid external immobilization, regardless of the patient's age, the direction of dens dislocation, or the degree of neurologic impairment.[4,8,9,22] Therefore, if the axis fracture component of the C1-C2 combination injury is an odontoid Type II fracture with 6 mm or greater dens dislocation, early operative intervention should be considered. All other axis fractures (hangman's, odontoid Type III, and miscellaneous fractures) encountered in combination with a C1 fracture should be initially managed with rigid external immobilization. We favor the halo vest for its superior immobilization characteristics[4,29,31,32]; however, the SOMI brace was effective in the treatment of two patients in this series.

The type of *atlas* fracture present will dictate whether C1 and C2 will be the only levels included in the wiring and fusion, as is the case with unilateral arch or lateral mass fractures, or whether the atlas injury is unsuitable for a direct wiring procedure, as occurs with bilateral or multiple ring fractures, and requires an occiput-to-C2 wiring and fusion.[6,7] The treatment of the 25 combination C1-C2 fracture patients in our series was determined by the type of C2 fracture present. Nonoperative therapy was the initial treatment in 84% of patients (Table 3) and consisted of immobilization in a halo vest or a SOMI brace for 10 to 22 weeks. Early surgical reduction and internal fixation were performed in four patients who had combination C1-Type II odontoid fractures with dens dislocation of 6 mm or greater. In the group treated with early open reduction and internal fixation, the integrity of the ring of the atlas was considered when determining the extent of the wiring and fusion procedure. Three patients had unilateral C1 arch or lateral mass fractures and underwent wiring and fusion of C1 and C2. The one patient with a multiple ring fracture of the atlas underwent an occiput to C2 wiring and fusion.

TABLE 3
Treatment of Combination C1-C2 Fx

C1-Hangman's Fx	(N = 3)	3 Halo vest
C1-Odontoid Fx	(N = 9)	5 Halo vest +
		4 ORIF
C1-Odontoid Type III Fx	(N = 5)	1 SOMI brace
		4 Halo vest
C1-Miscellaneous Fx	(N = 7)	1 SOMI brace
		6 Halo vest
		(Median TX 12 weeks)
		(Range 10–22 weeks)

+ one patient with nonunion required late surgical fusion

From Sonntag VKH, Hadley MN: Management of upper cervical spinal instability. In: Wilkins RH, ed. *Neurosurgery Update*. New York: McGraw-Hill. In press. Reprinted with permission of McGraw-Hill.

Third Cervical Vertebra

Isolated fractures of the third cervical vertebra are extremely uncommon.[1,4,5] We identified 12 isolated C3 fractures out of 1,280 acute cervical fractures (0.9%) (Table 1). These were primarily chip fractures of the body or isolated laminar or spinous process fractures. We treated another 11 patients who sustained fractures of C3 in addition to the axis. The third cervical vertebra appears to be partially protected from injury: it occupies a unique position between the more vulnerable axis and the relative fulcrum of the head with respect to the C5-C6 level of the cervical spinal column where the greatest flexion and extension occur.

The treatment of C3 fractures must be individualized according to the type of fracture and the presence of associated fractures or fracture-dislocations. We have treated these fractures nonoperatively with external immobilization. The majority of the isolated C3 fractures affected only the spinous process or lamina. Of two C3 body fractures one was a stable chip fracture of the inferior aspect of the body, the second a body compression fracture with 3 mm of C3-C4 subluxation, which was effectively treated with a halo vest.

Eleven patients in our review of 1,280 cervical fractures had combined C2-C3 fractures. The treatment of these patients requires consideration of all of the fractures. Nine of 11 patients were satisfactorily treated with halo vest immobilization. One patient with a Type II odontoid fracture with 6 mm dislocation and a C3 lateral mass fracture was treated with early operative posterior wiring and fusion of C1-C2-C3. The other patient had a C1-C2 (hangman's) and C3 posterior arch fracture with 4 mm C2-C3 subluxation and was treated with a C2-C3 discectomy and anterior fusion and plating (Figures 3 and 4).

Traumatic Atlanto-Axial Instability

Operative treatment is indicated for traumatic instability at C1-C2 complicated by os odontoideum or rheumatoid arthritis. Rheumatoid patients must be evaluated to rule out basilar invagination and/or a ventral compressive lesion at the skull base-odontoid process.[24,26,27,33] We have found MR imaging in neutral, flexion, and extension to be particularly useful in these patients. Two patients with rheumatoid arthritis without basilar invagination who had traumatic C1-C2 subluxation and five patients with acute instability with os odontoideum were treated with C1-C2 wiring and fusion procedures.

These patients were immobilized in the halo vest for 12 to 18 weeks followed by a SOMI brace and/or rigid cervical collar for four to eight weeks. Patients without fractures as a cause of C1-C2 instability are difficult to fuse and require longer periods of postoperative external immobilization.

Surgical Techniques

When operation is indicated for axis fractures, combination C1-C2 fractures, or posttraumatic atlanto-axial instability, we prefer a posterior atlas-axis wiring and autologous iliac crest bone graft to achieve stability. If an unstable atlas fracture (multiple ring) complicates the axis fracture-dislocation, then the occiput is included in the C1-C2 wiring and fusion. If the axis fracture is associated with significant C2-C3 subluxation, C3 is incorporated in the stabilization construct.

Preoperatively, we place the patient in a halo vest. This provides immobilization of unstable fractures, particularly in combative or uncooperative patients; it achieves the best possible alignment of the fracture before operation, thereby reducing the amount of intraoperative manipulation; and it immobilizes the head and neck with respect to the torso, effectively eliminating the potential for neurological injury during operative positioning. Once the patient is positioned and draped, the strut bars of the halo vest support the surgeon's hands and wrists when working with high speed tools or microsurgical instruments, but do not obstruct vision or working space.

For the posterior wiring and fusion procedure, the patient is placed in the prone position, and a posterior-midline incision is made down to the spinous process of the axis. For a C1-C2 wiring and fusion procedure, the paraspinous musculature is dissected from the posterior arches of the atlas and axis and retracted laterally. A double-strand twisted 24-gauge stainless steel wire loop is placed under the lamina of the atlas and is secured around the spinous process of the axis (Figure 6). We

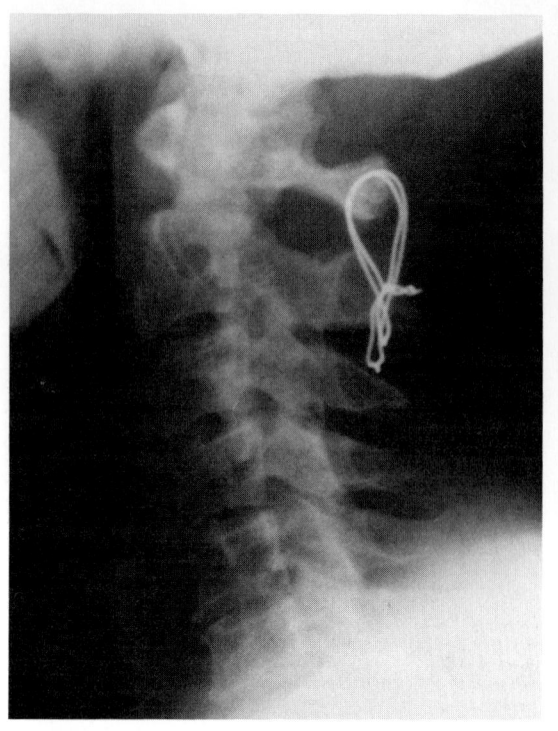

Figure 6. Postoperative radiograph showing sublaminar wiring of C1 with attachment around the spinous process of C2. A bone graft was not interposed between C1 and C2 in this case.

often employ an iliac crest bone plug as a fulcrum between the posterior arches of the atlas and axis to facilitate proper C1-C2 alignment. This is particularly helpful when treating posteriorly displaced Type II odontoid fractures or patients with os odontoideum. The two free ends of the stainless steel wire also are secured around the spinous process of the axis over the bone plug, securing it into position (Figure 7). This technique reduces the amount of posterior distraction and downward angulation of the arch of C1 required to bring the dens into anatomic position for proper bony fusion. The procedure is completed by placing multiple chips of cancellous bone obtained from the iliac crest over the roughened surfaces of C1, the bone plug, and C2.

In selected patients, the occiput must be incorporated into the stabilization procedure. This is performed by exposing the posterior skull base and foramen magnum. Two small

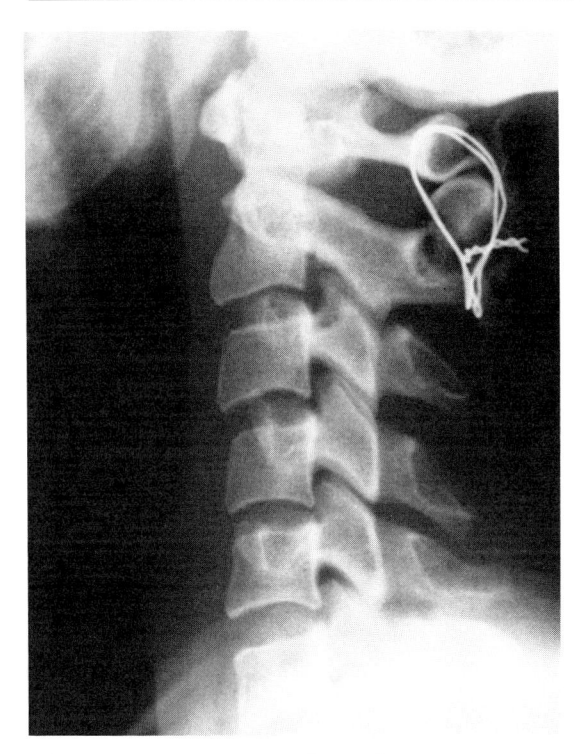

Figure 7. Postoperative radiograph revealing C1-C2 wiring with interposed iliac bone graft between C1 and C2 posteriorly.

holes are made in the skull base, above and on each side of the foramen magnum, with a high-speed drill. These two holes are connected, removing bone between them to create a new bony ring above the foramen magnum. This is done to create a superior bony arch from which to wire, necessitated by a fractured-unstable posterior arch of C1. The posterior arch of C1 is removed in the midline, leaving the lateral aspects of the ring of the atlas intact. The 24-gauge twisted wire loop is passed under the arch made in the skull base in the extradural space and is looped over the spinous process of C2. The wire ends are secured around the spinous process of C2, similar to the procedure described above, incorporating a larger iliac crest bone plug, which is positioned between the bony arch created at the skull base and the arch of C2.

The procedure is completed by roughening the exposed surfaces of the occiput and the lateral arches of the atlas and the axis and by placing chips of cancellous bone obtained from the iliac crest in the operative site to encourage fusion at these levels. Halo-vest immobilization is generally maintained for 10 to 12 weeks postoperatively. Patients with atlanto-axial instability without fracture are immobilized for longer periods as previously outlined. The halo device is removed when dynamic flexion and extension radiographs confirm stability.

Summary

Upper cervical spinal cord and vertebral column injuries are common following trauma. Twenty-five percent of all cervical spinal injuries occur between the occiput and C3. While pediatric patients have a lower incidence of spine injury in general, they are remarkably susceptible to injury at the upper three cervical levels. Several anatomic and physiological factors that account for the high frequency of injury at these superior cervical levels in both children and adults are reviewed.

The management of upper cervical spine injuries begins with immobilization and a comprehensive radiological assessment. Standard radiographs and CT studies are essential for determining the precise nature of each injury and for guiding subsequent therapy. The optimal treatment of each injury must be individualized. Specific guidelines are proposed to help determine the choice of operative or nonoperative management. Irrespective of the form of treatment, careful follow-up is necessary to monitor therapy and to optimize outcome.

References

1. Bohlman HH. Acute fractures and dislocations of the cervical spine: An analysis of three hundred hospitalized patients and review of the literature. *J Bone Joint Surg Am.* 1979;61A:1119-1142.
2. Heiden JS, Weiss MH, Rosenberg AW, Apuzzo MLJ, Kurze T. Management of cervical spinal cord trauma in Southern California. *J Neurosurg.* 1975;43:732-736.

3. Reiss SJ, Raque GH Jr, Shields CB, Garretson HD. Cervical spine fractures with major associated trauma. *Neurosurgery.* 1986;18:327-330.
4. Sonntag VKH, Hadley MN. Nonoperative management of cervical spine injuries. *Clin Neurosurg.* 1988;34:630-649.
5. Sonntag VKH, Hadley MN. Management of upper cervical spinal instability. In: Wilkins R, ed. *Neurosurgery Update.* New York NY: McGraw-Hill. In press.
6. Dickman CA, Hadley MN, Browner C, Sonntag VKH. Neurosurgical management of acute atlas-axis combination fractures: a review of 25 cases. *J Neurosurg.* 1989;70:45-49.
7. Hadley MN, Dickman CA, Browner CM, Sonntag VKH. Acute traumatic atlas fractures: management and long-term outcome. *Neurosurgery.* 1988;23:31-35.
8. Hadley MN, Dickman CA, Browner CM, Sonntag VKH. Acute axis fractures: a review of 229 cases. *J Neurosurg.* 1989;71:642-647.
9. Hadley MN, Sonntag VKH. Acute axis fractures. *Contemp Neurosurg.* 1987;9:1-6.
10. Hadley MN. Pediatric spine injuries. In Camins, O'Leary, eds. *Disorders of the Cervical Spine.* Baltimore, Md: Williams & Wilkins. In press.
11. Hadley MN, Zabramski JM, Browner CM, Rekate H, Sonntag VKH. Pediatric spinal trauma: a review of 122 cases of spinal cord and vertebral column injuries. *J Neurosurg.* 1988;68:18-24.
12. Ruge JR, Sinson GP, McLone DG, Cerullo LJ. Pediatric spinal injury: the very young. *J Neurosurg.* 1988;68:25-30.
13. Pollack IF, Pang D, Sclabassi R. Recurrent spinal cord injury without radiographic abnormalities in children. *J Neurosurg.* 1988;69:177-182.
14. Hadley MN, Browner C, Sonntag VKH. Miscellaneous fractures of the second cervical vertebra. *BNI Quarterly.* 1985;1:34-39.
15. Hadley MN, Browner CM, Liu SS, Sonntag VKH. New subtype of acute odontoid fractures (Type IIA). *Neurosurgery.* 1988;22:67-71.
16. Sherk HH, Nicholson JT. Fractures of the atlas. *J Bone Joint Surg Am.* 1970;52A:1017-1024.
17. Spence KF Jr, Decker S, Sell KW. Bursting atlantal fracture associated with rupture of the transverse ligament. *J Bone Joint Surg Am.* 1970;52A:543-549.
18. Panjabi MM, Thibodeau LL, Crisco JJ III, White AA III. What constitutes spinal instability? *Clin Neurosurg.* 1988;34:313-339.
19. Apuzzo MLJ, Heiden JS, Weiss MH, Ackerson TT, Harvey JP, Kurze T. Acute fractures of the odontoid process: an analysis of 45 cases. *J Neurosurg.* 1978;48:85-91.
20. Dunn ME, Seljeskog EL. Experience in the management of odontoid process injuries: an analysis of 128 cases. *Neurosurgery.* 1986;18:306-310.
21. Ekong CEU, Schwartz ML, Tator CH, Rowed DW, Edmonds VE. Odontoid fracture: management with early mobilization using the halo device. *Neurosurgery.* 1981;9:631-637.
22. Hadley MN, Browner C, Sonntag VKH. Axis fractures: a comprehensive review of management and treatment in 107 cases. *Neurosurgery.* 1985;17:281-290.
23. Seljeskog EL, Chou SN. Spectrum of the hangman's fracture. *J Neurosurg.* 1976;45:3-8.
24. Hadley MN, Sonntag VKH, Spetzler RF. The transoral approach to the superior cervical spine: a review of 53 cases of extradural cervicomedullary compression. *J Neurosurg.* 1989;71:16-23.
25. Menezes AH, Osenbach R. Spinal cord injuries in the young child (below age 3 years). Presented at Congress of Neurological Surgeons; September 1988; Seattle, Wash.
26. Menezes AH, VanGilder JC, Graf CJ, McDonnel DE. Craniocervical abnormalities: a comprehensive surgical approach. *J Neurosurg.* 1980;53:444-455.
27. Stevens JM, Kendall BE, Crockard HA. The spinal cord in rheumatoid arthritis with clinical myelopathy: a computed myelographic study. *J Neurol Neurosurg Psychiatry.* 1986;49:140-151.
28. Brant-Zawadzki M, Miller EM, Federle MP. CT in the evaluation of spine trauma. *AJR.* 1981;136:369-375.
29. Browner CM, Hadley MN, Sonntag VKH, Mattingly LG. Halo immobilization brace care: an innovative approach. *J Neurosci Nurs.* 1987;19:24-29.
30. Bohlman HH, Boada E. Fractures and dislocations of the lower cervical spine. In: Cervical Spine Research Society, ed. *The Cervical Spine.* Philadelphia, Pa: JB Lippincott Co;1983:232-267.
31. Johnson RM, Owen JR, Hart DL, Callahan RA. Cervical Orthoses: a guide to their selection and use. *Clin Orthop.* 1981;154:34-45.
32. Wolf JW Jr, Johnson RM. Cervical orthoses. In: The Cervical Spine Research Society, ed. *The Cervical Spine.* Philadelphia Pa: JB Lippincott Co; 1983:54-61.
33. Hadley MN, Sonntag VKH, Amos MR, Hodak JA, Lopez LJ. Three-dimensional computed tomography in the diagnosis of vertebral column pathological conditions. *Neurosurgery.* 1987;21:186-192.
34. Hadley MN, Sonntag VKH, Grahm TW, Masferrer R, Browner C. Axis fractures resulting from motor vehicle accidents: the need for occupant restraints. *Spine.* 1986;11:861-864.
35. Keene GCR, Hone MR, Sage MR. Atlas fracture: demonstration using computerized tomography. *J Bone Joint Surg Am.* 1978;60A:1106-1107.
36. Lipson SJ. Fractures of the atlas associated with fractures of the odontoid process and transverse ligament ruptures. *J Bone Joint Surg Am.* 1977;59A:940-943.
37. Sonntag VKH. The early management of cervical spine injuries. *Ariz Med.* 1982;39:644-647.

CHAPTER 8

Stabilization of Fractures and Subluxations of the Lower Cervical Spine

Paul R. Cooper, MD

Although thousands of fractures and dislocations of the middle and lower cervical spine are treated by neurosurgeons and orthopedic surgeons each year, there is surprisingly little agreement on the optimal management of these injuries. On the most basic level there are those[1] who claim that operation is rarely necessary to achieve stability and that the outcome of patients managed with prolonged skeletal traction is equal or superior to patients treated with operation. Other authorities (among them a number of surgeons) claim that operative reduction or decompression has no effect on the length of hospitalization or neurologic outcome. While there are data to refute some of these contentions, there is no evidence to support the superiority of operative therapy.

Even among those who agree that operative therapy is to be preferred over prolonged bed rest or external immobilization in the halo vest or similar orthoses, there is disagreement on such basic issues as the effect of timing of operation on outcome, and whether therapy is best accomplished with an anterior or posterior approach.

In this chapter the efficacy of nonoperative management as well as the claims of its partisans are reviewed and discussed. Specific types of cervical spine fractures and dislocations are classified according to the mechanism of injury, and principles of treatment are addressed. It is assumed that the reader will have read the sections on initial care and management and diagnostic imaging; only the briefest reference is made to these subjects. In the last section, specific operative techniques used by this author, as well as a selection of the most important techniques described in the literature, are discussed in detail.

Management of Lower Cervical Spine Injuries with Bed Rest and Traction

One can understand why physiatrists and other nonsurgeons are biased against operative therapy if one examines the surgical management of patients with spinal cord injuries earlier in this century or even as recently as 25 years ago. The operative mortality in patients with severe neurological deficits was high.[2] The most commonly performed operation was laminectomy, which not only had no beneficial effect on outcome but was associated with exacerbation of neurological deficit in the short term and increased instability and deformity in the long term.

In the past 10-15 years there have been significant advances in our understanding of the biomechanics of these injuries[3]; the application of this knowledge as well as the use of instrumentation[4-6] have made operative treatment safer and more effective than in the past. Those who oppose operation may not be won over by these advances and their point of view may not be entirely invalid. However, examination of their arguments in the next four subsections may be enlightening.

Type of Management and Stability

Bedbrook[1] and others[7-11] believed that operation was infrequently needed to produce stability. Only eight patients with cervical spine injuries reported by Bedbrook[1] underwent operative treatment for severe dislocation or locked facets, and even in retrospect he was not convinced that operation was truly necessary. He presented data collected from the literature to show that more than 90% of patients with facet dislocations are stabilized as a result of 8-10 weeks of bed rest in traction. However, 10 weeks of bed rest is hardly benign therapy and almost certainly carries with it a higher morbidity than operative stabilization.

Dorr et al[12] could not discern a superior outcome in patients who had operation for any category of injury except patients with facet dislocations. In their series patients who had operation had less than 9° of angulation at three months after injury, whereas those who were treated with traction had over 17°. Donovan et al[13] also found a statistically significant increase in angulation in patients who were treated without operation compared to those treated with cervical fusion. More than 40% of patients never developed angulation, and of those who did the mean deformity was only 14%; only 2 of 43 patients had a deformity greater than 25° after one year. Norrell,[14] a strong advocate of operative therapy, managed patients with unilateral facet dislocations with closed reduction followed by nonoperative therapy. He gave no data on the long-term outcome of these patients.

From these data there seems little doubt that spinal deformity does not necessarily occur in all patients treated with skeletal traction as the definitive method of management. However, deformity is more common with nonoperative therapy and in some patients may be quite severe. Definitive treatment with skeletal traction necessitates prolonged bed rest, which is almost certainly associated with a higher rate of complications than operative therapy.

Type of Management and Neurological Outcome

It seems logical that stabilization of the spine and decompression of the injured spinal cord should result in improved neurological outcome. There are data in the *experimental* literature suggesting that acute immobilization of the spine after injury improves outcome.[15] Unfortunately there is a paucity of data in the *clinical* literature to support this hypothesis and no prospective randomized controlled study has ever been conducted to determine if stabilization and decompression would beneficially affect outcome.

Rogers[16] contended that myelopathy was more likely to get worse in patients with spinal cord compression from persistent subluxation, although patient data were not provided. Roy-Camille et al[17] performed decompressive operation on an emergency basis on quadriplegics with spinal cord compression but provided no data to support the efficacy of this strategy. Neurological improvement occurs after spinal cord injury in most patients regardless of therapy; in a number of series the percentage of patients sustaining improvement in surgical and nonsurgical groups has been similar.[7,9,12,13,18,19]

In brief, there is no firm evidence that operation to stabilize the spine or decompress the spinal cord and nerve roots in the acute period after injury changes neurological outcome. Decompression of chronic deformities in patients with partial preservation of neurologic function is another issue; in one series,[20] when late fixed deformity was corrected through anterior decompression and posterior stabilization, neurological improvement occurred in all eight patients.

Type of Management and Length of Hospitalization

Proponents of operative management of patients with cervical spine injuries assert that (1) operation will allow patients to be mobilized sooner, and (2) hospital stays in patients so treated will be shorter than is the case for those treated with bed rest and traction. Born et al,[21] Norrell and Wilson,[22] and others[23-25] all contended that operative management shortened hospital stay, but provided no data to support this contention. Aebi et al[26] stated that 65% of patients on their unit who had incomplete neurological deficit were hospitalized for less than 28 days including the time for rehabilitation.

On our spinal cord injury unit we have managed almost all patients with operative stabilization. Analysis of hospital stay in our patients treated with posterior stabilization with Roy-Camille plates over the past three years shows a hospitalization time of 20 days in patients with complete spinal cord injuries and 13 days in patients with incomplete injuries. This is a fraction of the time needed to achieve spinal stability in patients managed solely with bed rest and traction. Moreover, patients stabilized with posterior cervical plates are mobilized immediately after operation and, in most cases, are able to sit in a chair the day after operation.

Rogers[16] examined the length of time from injury to return to work in patients treated with and without operation. Operated patients began working in 5.4 months, more than three months sooner than patients treated with bed rest and traction. In spite of this, Bedbrook[1] has stated that "early mobilisation has little to commend it, since, in well-disciplined units, mobilisation and physical restoration can be practised equally well whilst the patient is in bed." This statement is simply not supported by our own experience or that of others who have access to modern rehabilitation units where the goal is early mobilization and return to independent functioning.

In summary, there is now little doubt that operative stabilization results in shorter stay than management in bed with traction. Hospital stay in operated patients is most closely correlated with pulmonary and septic complications common to patients with cervical spinal cord injury.

Type of Management, Mortality, and Complications

In our experience and that of others,[26] neurological deterioration as a result of operation is rare; nonneurological operative complications are few and have little influence on the patient's ultimate outcome. Although Bohlmann[2] reported exacerbation of neurological deficit in several patients in his series, all had laminectomy as their operative procedure. For the most part mortality is related to gastrointestinal hemorrhage, associated injuries in patients with multiple-system trauma, and respiratory complications common to quadriplegics.

The 42% overall mortality reported by Bohlmann[2] in 1979 in operative and nonoperative patients was related to these factors and was even higher when nonoperative patients were considered separately. A recent series reports a more respectable mortality of 9%.[26] The mortality rate on our unit over the past two years has been less than 3%.

In short, operative morbidity and mortality of cervical spinal cord injury are related to the complications inherent to the injury and not to operative treatment.

Halo Vest Immobilization as the Definitive Treatment of Fractures and Subluxations

The use of the halo vest represented a real advance in the management of cervical spine fractures and subluxations when it was first described 20 years ago.[27] In a sense, it formed the middle ground between operative therapy on the one hand and prolonged bed rest and cervical traction on the other. It enabled patients to to get out of bed or ambulate while the cervical spine was being immobilized, and enabled the unstable spine to heal without the necessity for operation.

The halo vest provides excellent immobilization in the upper cervical spine for fractures of C1 and C2. Movement occurs at all cervical motion segments in the halo vest, but motion is limited to 20-35% of normal when measured in the sagittal plane.[28] This movement tends to occur when the patient moves between an upright and a recumbent position. Although limitation of movement in the lowest segments of the cervical spine is no less than that which occurs at higher levels,[28] our patients have experienced a higher redislocation rate at these lowest motion segments. This may be secondary to a "snaking" motion[29] of the cervical spine in the halo. Although there is little movement of the entire cervical spine in the halo vest, movement at individual motion segments may occur as one segment flexes and an adjacent one extends.

In spite of a low complication rate and a low redislocation rate reported by a number of authors,[30-32] it has become apparent that the halo vest is not a panacea in the management of cervical spinal instability. Even with careful patient selection at least 10-15% of patients fail halo vest therapy and require operative stabilization.[32,33] If patients who have injuries between C3-T1 are analyzed, almost one-quarter will fail halo vest treatment.[33] Over the past five years we have used the halo vest less frequently than formerly. Although the halo vest will frequently provide adequate immobilization and healing, there are certain bony injuries which are markedly unstable; other lesions involving the posterior ligamentous complex at the facet joint can almost be predicted to fail halo vest treatment (Figures 1a-c). In other injuries which were apparently minimally unstable, the use of the halo vest was associated with loss of reduction during immobilization or progressive angulation and subluxation in the postimmobilization period.

The availability of both anterior and posterior instrumentation for the cervical spine has made operative stabilization safe and extremely effective. As a result, the halo vest is a less attractive option. The entire issue of stability is resolved with one operation, and the specter of resubluxation during halo vest immobilization or failure of the halo vest to stabilize a fracture or subluxation after three or more months of treatment no longer exists. In addition, patients are spared disfiguring forehead scars as well as the social embarrassment and annoyance of wearing the apparatus for an extended period of time.

Inherent Problems of the Halo Vest

Contraindications to the use of the halo vest center around the type of bony and ligamentous injury sustained by the patient. In a sense the contraindications to the use of the halo vest are the indications for operative stabilization. These indications are discussed in a separate section. This discussion centers on factors other than the bony and ligamentous injury that represent contraindications to the use of the halo vest.

In spite of the fact that most varieties of halo vests are "fitted" around the trunk, conformity to the body is imperfect and movement may occur as a result of a loose fit. A thermoplastic Minerva body jacket has been designed which, when heated, may be molded to the exact contours of the thorax.[28] Mean sagittal movement at all cervical motion segments is one-half or less than that seen with the halo connected to a plastic body jacket.

Body habitus in patients with preexisting kyphosis, kyphoscoliosis, or a barrel chest deformity associated with chronic respiratory disease will frequently make fitting of the plastic molded vest difficult or impossible. Elderly or very petite patients will occasion-

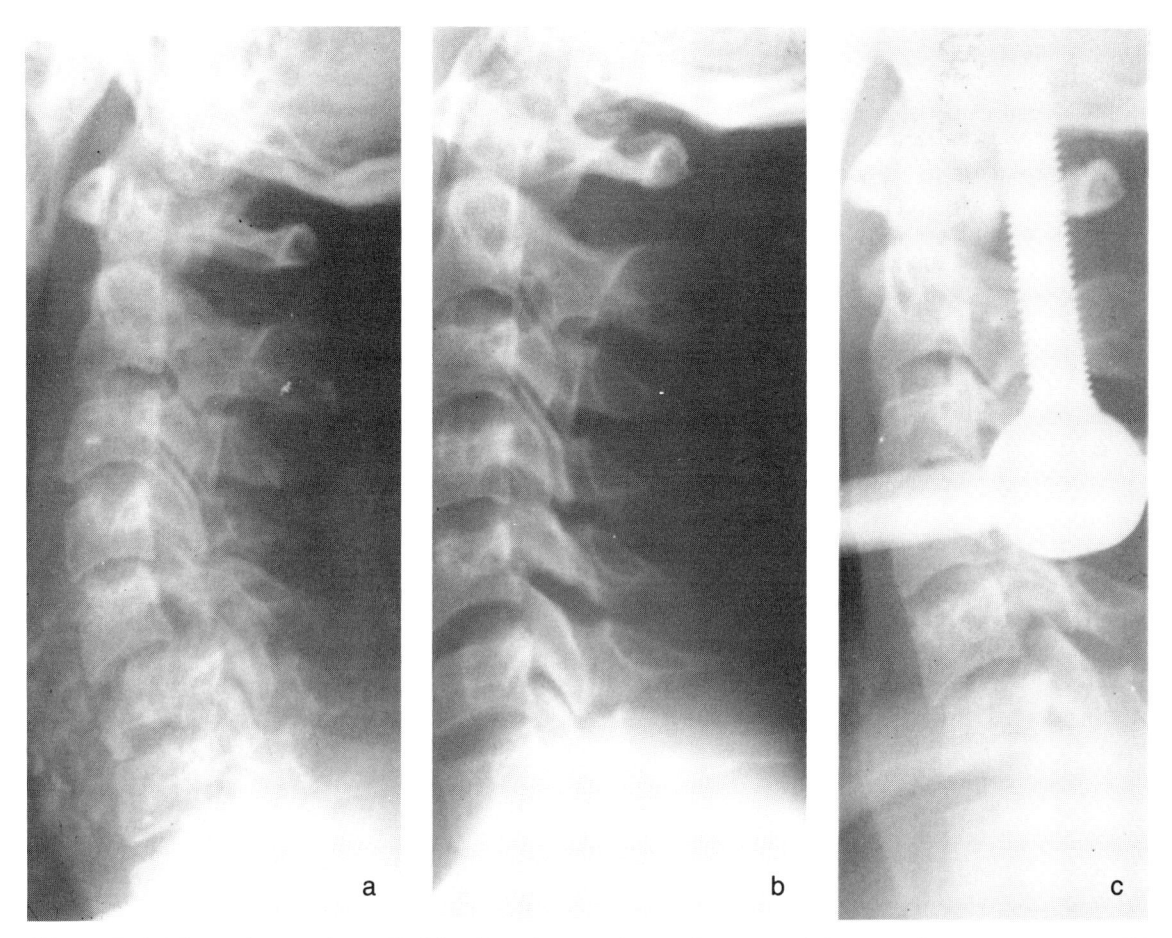

Figure 1. (a) *Lateral x-ray shows C5-C6 subluxation secondary to ligamentous injury. No fractures were seen on CT scans.* (b) *Reduction of subluxation following cervical traction.* (c) *Recurrent subluxation in halo vest.*

ally not be able to support the extra weight of the halo vest. Unreliable patients may sometimes unbuckle the vest or even manipulate the halo pins or connections between the vest and halo.

Occasionally a patient will refuse to wear the halo vest in spite of the alternative of operative therapy. The use of the halo vest should be discontinued in quadriplegics with loss of protective sensation who experience skin breakdown in spite of careful fitting of the vest. The halo vest should also be discontinued in all patients who lose reduction on more than one occasion, or who experience deterioration of neurological function at any time.

Contraindications to the Use of the Halo Vest

Purely ligamentous injuries heal poorly in the halo vest. This is particularly true for injuries involving the posterior ligamentous complex securing the facet joints.[30,34] Redislocation is common, and it is unlikely that the healing of ligaments achieved in the halo vest is ever sufficient to withstand physiologic loads.[25] Moreover, late and progressive angulation may occur after the device has been removed as a result of incomplete ligamentous healing. The presence of injury to these ligaments is a clear indication for operative stabilization.[2]

Specific Injuries: Their Mechanisms and Principles of Management

Several schema classifying injuries of the cervical spine have been proposed.[3,8,16,35,36] The most useful are based on the mechanism of the injury and do not merely describe the injury itself. The most elaborate of these (and perhaps the best) is the one formulated by Allen[3] in 1982, defining six major groups of injuries: (1) vertical-compressive, (2) distractive-flexion, (3) compressive-flexion, (4) compressive-extension, (5) distractive-extension, and (6) lateral-flexion. Donovan et al[13] and Dorr et al[12] presented classification schemes similar to that of Allen's. The classification formulated by Ducker et al[37] is especially useful because it is simple and combines the mechanistic approach of Allen along with a description of the injury. Although five categories of injury are proposed, one for gunshot and penetrating wounds is not discussed here. The other four categories form the basis for the discussion that follows in this section and include the following: (1) flexion-dislocation, (2) flexion-compression, (3) compression-burst, and (4) extension. While these divisions are conceptually useful, patterns of fractures and subluxations of the cervical spine are complex, and injuries frequently encompass two or more categories.

Flexion-Dislocation Injuries

Mechanism and Pathologic Anatomy of Facet Subluxations

These lesions correspond to the distractive-flexion injury described by Allen et al.[3] They make up over one-half of all cervical injuries[1] and are potentially the most unstable injuries to affect the cervical spine. When flexion is combined with rotation, unilateral facet dislocation occurs on the side opposite the direction of rotation,[38] although in a cadaver study[39] Maiman et al were unable to produce the lesion by the application of flexion and rotation forces. The capsule of the involved facet joint is disrupted along with the interspinous ligament,[40] but the annulus and posterior longitudinal ligament are generally not injured.[41] Dislocation in the sagittal plane is generally less than one-half the anteroposterior dimension of the vertebral body (Figures 2a,b).[1,41]

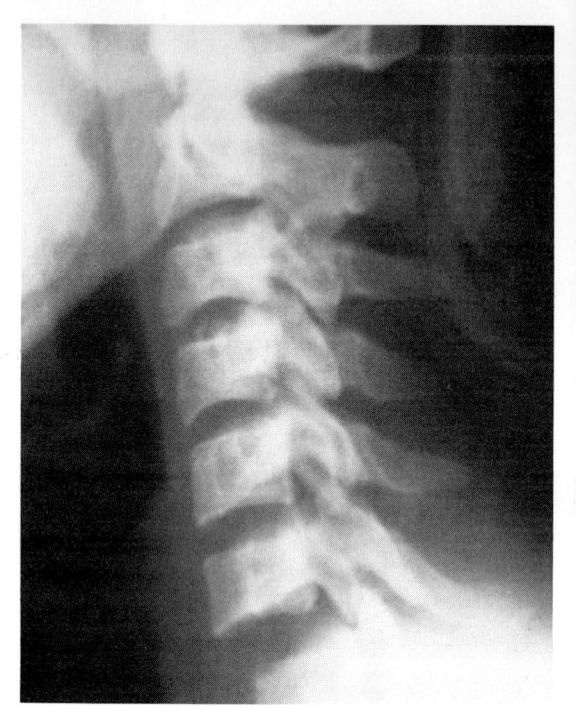

Figure 2a. Lateral cervical spine x-ray of a patient with a unilateral jumped facet at C6-C7 (arrow).

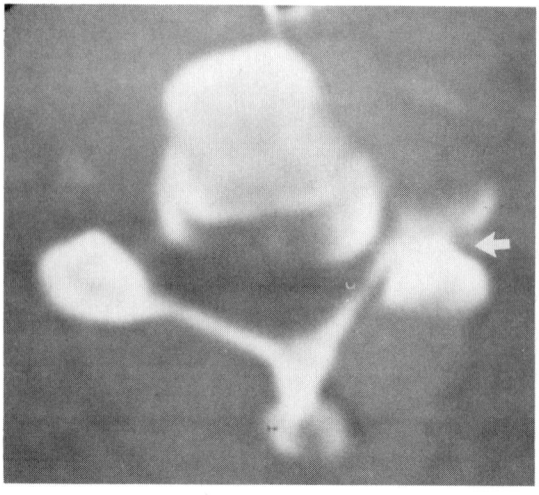

Figure 2b. CT scan of another patient with a similar injury shows a jumped facet on the left (arrow).

Bilateral facet dislocation occurs as a result of severe ligamentous injury to both joint capsules, the posterior ligamentous complex, the intervertebral disc, and the posterior longitudinal ligament,[14,42] although the anterior longitudinal ligament may be spared.[37,43] The facets will lock in a subluxed position as the superior facet of the inferior vertebra dislocates to a position posterior to the inferior facet of the superior vertebra (Figures 3a-c). The mechanism is probably hyperflexion and distraction[3,42] as the upper vertebra is translated forward on the lower.[17] Subluxation is severe and is usually greater than one-half the anteroposterior diameter of the vertebral body.[1,41]

These facet dislocations are sometimes associated with fractures of either the superior or inferior articulating facet[17] as a result of "sudden forced hyperextension or contralateral flexion . . . exerted on the unstable articular process."[38] Fractures through the pedicle and base of the lamina occur frequently with this lesion[17] as a result of the forced rotation.[38] Fractures in these two loca-

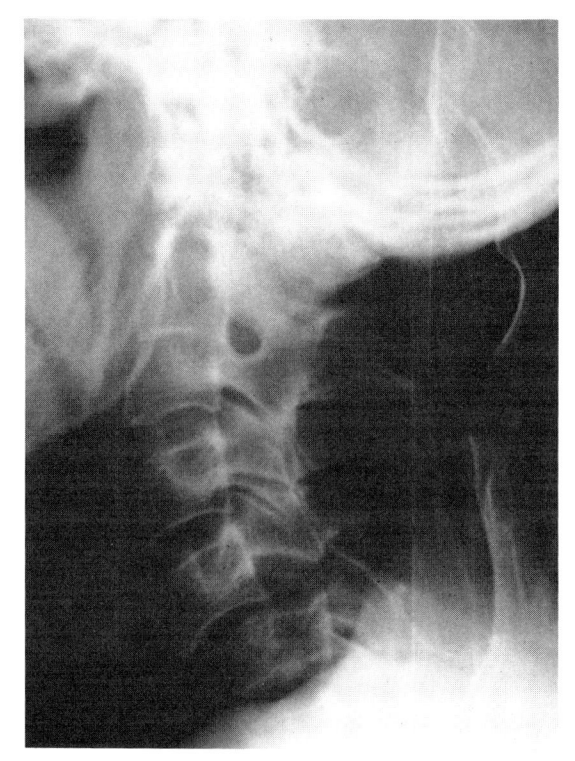

Figure 3a. Lateral cervical spine x-rays of a patient with bilateral jumped facets.

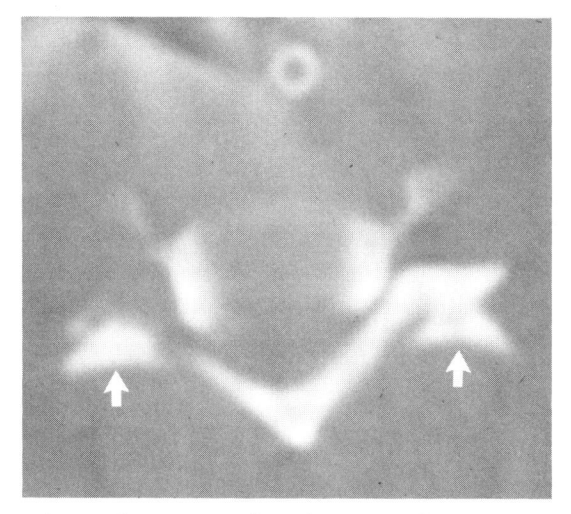

Figure 3b. CT scan of another patient shows bilateral jumped facets. Arrows point to the exposed articular surface.

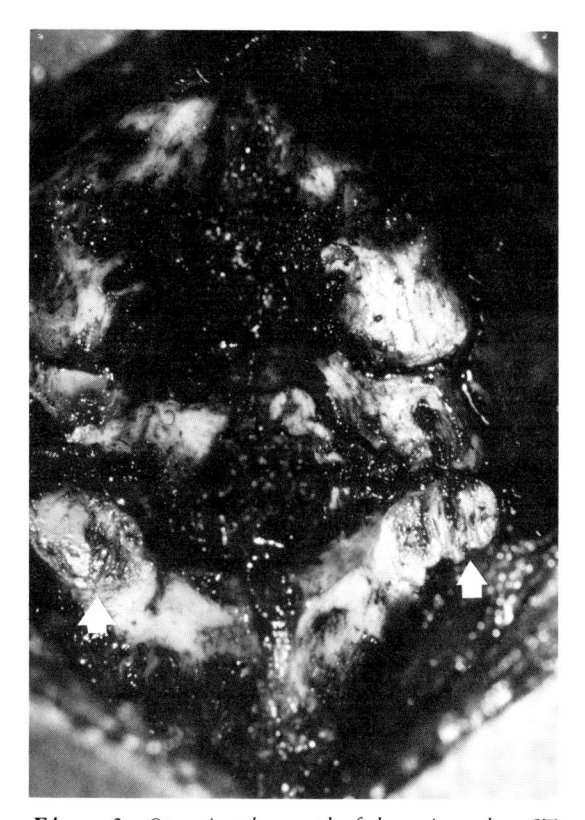

Figure 3c. Operative photograph of the patient whose CT scan is shown in Figure 3b. Arrows point to the superior facets of C5 which are totally exposed.

tions will, in effect, separate the lateral mass from both the anterior and posterior elements.

Stability of Facet Dislocations

Surprisingly there has been considerable disagreement in the literature on the stability of these lesions. In a review of more than 400 cases of facet dislocations from his own and several large series, Bedbrook[1] concluded that 90% of injuries were stable. It is not clear whether he believed they were stable acutely or over the long term. In any event, this figure is inconsistent with this author's experience and what most others have written about these lesions.[14,40,44] Indeed Nieminen[45] noted instability in almost 50% of patients with bilateral subluxations treated without operation, and O'Brien et al noted a 37.5% instability rate in neurologically incomplete patients treated with the halothoracic brace.[40]

In short, the ligamentous disruption necessary to produce bilateral facet dislocations is so profound that stability is extremely unlikely in the acute period after injury. Healing of ligaments is generally imperfect even in those patients who may gain some stability after removal of immobilizing orthoses. Progressive deformity in the postimmobilization period frequently occurs.

The problem of the unilateral facet dislocation is more complex than bilateral facet dislocations. The ligamentous instability of unilateral facet dislocation is less profound and involves the ligaments of only one facet and the posterior interspinous ligament. Indeed the stability of some of these lesions is attested to by the difficulty in reduction. Although these lesions are frequently stable in their unreduced position in the early postinjury period, if left unreduced, they may progressively deform. When the dislocations are reduced, resubluxation is common when patients are moved or the weight is reduced in traction. These injuries are particularly prone to resublux in the halo vest, which provides less stability than skeletal traction.

Reduction of Facet Subluxations and Neurological Outcome

Although there is general agreement that reduction of facet dislocations using cervical traction is a desirable goal, it is not at all clear that this has a beneficial effect on neurological functioning in either the short or long term. Of patients with unilateral facet subluxations, more than one-quarter have root injury and another one-quarter have incomplete spinal cord lesions.[40] The neurological deficit in this situation should be ameliorated by the decompression that occurs with reduction. Although almost two-thirds of patients with bilateral facet subluxations have a complete spinal cord lesion,[40] the incomplete spinal cord lesion or root injury in the remaining patients should also be improved with reduction.

Indeed, Ducker et al[37] and Roy-Camille et al[17] believed that persistent spinal cord compression caused by unreducible subluxation was an indication for acute operative decompression. None of these authors presented any statistical basis for this belief. However, Maiman et al[42] noted that "little neurological improvement occurred as a result of reduction." In addition, delay in reduction did not affect neurological outcome. However, they did note improvement in neurological function in patients with complete myelopathy as a result of root recovery, presumably from restoration of the size of the neural foramina. Lind et al,[32] in a similar analysis, compared neurological improvement in patients who were reduced and in those who were left in a subluxed position, and could find no difference between the two groups. Stauffer[46] reached similar conclusions.

The *long-term* outcome of patients with unreduced facet subluxations has not been investigated from the point of view of progressive deformity, the development of facet arthritis with pain and limitation of movement, and late neurological deterioration from spinal cord or root compression. Until these data are available, it seems reasonable to make an attempt to reduce all facet dislocations, whether unilateral or bilateral, regardless of the patient's neurological function.

Reduction/Manipulation of Facet Dislocations

After the insertion of a halo ring or Gardner-Wells tongs, we apply 10 lbs of weight while the patient's head is kept in a neutral position. Ideally we will gradually increase the weight by 10-lb increments every 1-2 hours until reduction has been achieved or 50-60 lbs has been applied. Neurological examination is performed just before and after weight is increased. In practice the attempt at reduction frequently takes longer and is delayed by the inability to obtain lateral radiographs of the cervical spine at the exact moment they are needed, before the application of the next set of weights.

Caution must be exercised in the application of weights as it is easy to overdistract vertebrae at the site of the injury because of failure of supporting ligamentous structures, with resultant exacerbation of neurological deficit.[40,42] In persistent facet dislocations the application of distraction by itself is frequently not sufficient to achieve reduction. This accounts for the fact that almost one-half of patients with either unilateral or bilateral facet subluxations cannot be reduced with conventional traction methods, even with weights of more than 50 lbs.[40] Approximately the same percentage of patients with unilateral and bilateral dislocations failed reduction.

In patients who cannot be reduced with the application of a considerable amount of traction, lateral roentgenograms reveal that flexion of the neck might allow the overriding but distracted facets to assume their normal anatomical position. Cotler et al[47] describe a technique for the reduction of locked facets using manipulation. They first remove several springs of the Stryker Frame beneath the patient's shoulders to increase the flexion of the neck. This can also be accomplished using a pillow or folded sheet beneath the patient's head. For unilateral facet dislocations, when the facets are distracted, the tongs are grasped and traction is maintained manually while the head is rotated toward the dislocated side to 30-40° beyond the midline. If successful, they reduce the traction to 10-20 lbs.

A similar maneuver rotating the head to both sides is described by these same authors for the reduction of bilaterally locked facets. They also use muscle relaxants or even general anesthesia to aid in reducing these subluxations. Their statement that "this rotational manipulation is an extremely dangerous maneuver" appears to this author to be a gross understatement. Nevertheless their data reveal that no patient deteriorated as a result of manipulation. Bedbrook[1] performed similar manipulation in 500 *complete* cases and noted deterioration on only one occasion.

If one accepts the fact that facet dislocations are inherently unstable injuries which will eventually require operative treatment, one might reasonably ask how important it is to achieve nonoperative reduction. Couldn't reduction be achieved just as easily at the time of stabilization? In this author's opinion, operative reduction is easily achieved when performed in the first week after injury and vigorous attempts to reduce facet dislocations with large amounts of traction are not indicated. Although manipulation in traction using flexion or rotational maneuvers may increase the number of patients who can be reduced, there is no demonstrated benefit in terms of improved neurological functioning; the risks of exacerbating neurological deficit are real and for this reason manipulation should be avoided.

Principles of Operative Stabilization

Operative stabilization of facet subluxations may be performed from an anterior or posterior approach.[42] However, the posterior approach is superior and is preferred by a number of authorities.[6,17,37] A high percentage of these injuries remain subluxed at the time of operation and open reduction must be carried out by direct manipulation of the jumped facets. Although anterior reduction has been described by some authors,[48,49] the ability to visualize and directly manipulate the facet joint from a posterior approach would seem to make this the preferred method.

Even in patients whose facet joints have been reduced preoperatively, posterior stabilization is a more rational approach. Bilateral facet dislocations tend to deform in flexion. Posterior stabilization prevents angulation and flexion deformity more effectively than anterior operations. Anterior cervical fusion necessitates resection of the anterior longitudinal ligament, which is often the only ligamentous structure remaining intact and will thus increase instability in the short term. Because bone grafting has no immediate effect on stability, recurrent angulation, dislocation, and bone graft displacement are common.[50,51] The use of anterior plating procedures[4,48] may minimize these complications, but the results of application of this technique in a large series of patients with facet disruptions has not yet been published.

The disadvantages of the posterior approach are said to be a slower recovery of mobility and frequent extension of the fusion to adjacent levels.[38,50] This author has not observed a slower recovery of mobility with posterior fusion techniques. Extension of the fusion mass can be avoided by appropriate operative technique and will be discussed in a subsequent section.

Cervical disc herniation is surprisingly infrequent considering the degree of ligamentous disruption that occurs in facet disruption. However, the presence of a cervical disc herniation is perhaps the only clear indication for an anterior approach to treat acute facet disruptions.

Chronic Fixed Facet Deformities

Chronic fixed deformities occur as a result of unrecognized subluxations which are not reduced shortly after injury, failure of nonoperative treatment, or unsuccessful operative fixation. It also may occur in patients whose alignment is good after injury in spite of ligamentous injury leading to progressive deformity, which eventually becomes fixed. Restoration of alignment and normal lordosis is frequently impossible, regardless of the operative technique used, as the subluxed facet joints are often fused. Roy-Camille et al[6] prefer an anterior approach to treat these deformities believing that "corpectomy rather than corrective osteotomy" is the correct procedure. In this fashion the posterosuperior portion of the inferior vertebra at the level of the subluxation may be resected and the spinal cord decompressed, after which a bone graft is placed (Figures 4a-c).

Savini et al[52] perform in situ anterior decompression and stabilization when the dislocation measures less than one-third of the sagittal diameter of the vertebral body. When the dislocation is more than one-third

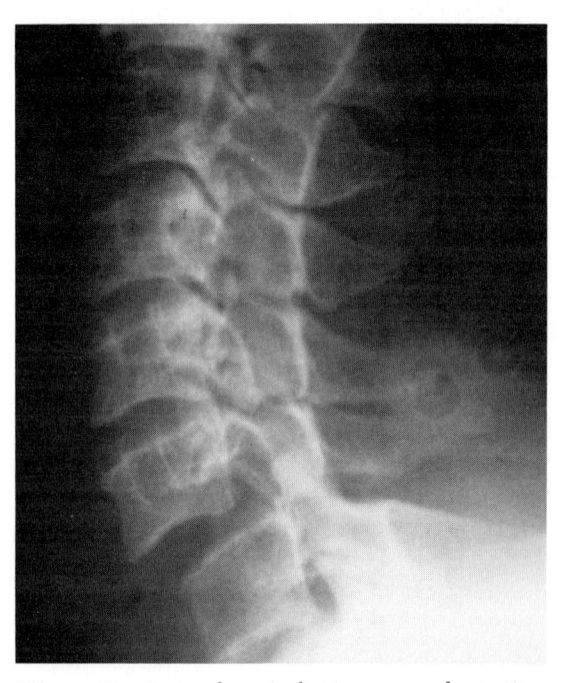

Figure 4a. Lateral cervical spine x-ray of a patient with a fixed flexion deformity secondary to posterior ligamentous injury and locked facets. These films were taken after the patient had been treated in a halo vest for three months. The deformity was irreducible at this time.

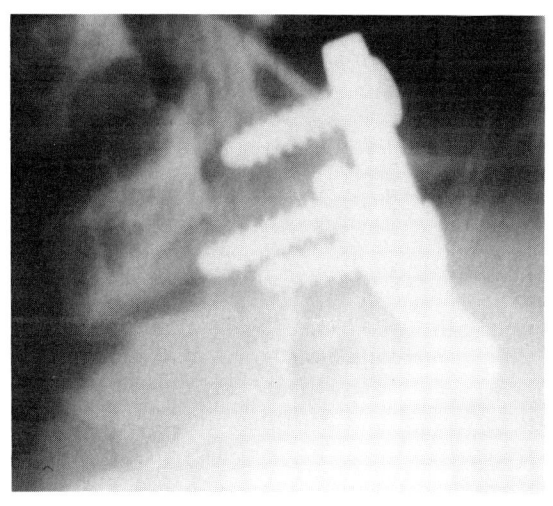

Figure 4b. Roy-Camille plates were placed after the jumped facets were drilled away resulting in slight improvement in angulation.

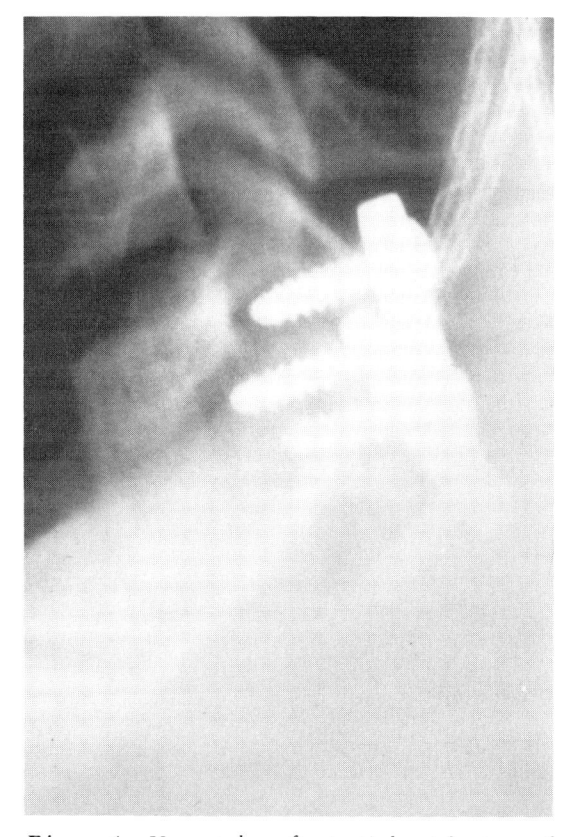

Figure 4c. X-ray taken after partial vertebrectomy of C6 and C7 and placement of an anterior bone graft. The angulation is improved and the patient's neurological deficit cleared.

the diameter of the vertebral body, these authors first perform "release-anterior fusion" followed by posterior reduction and stabilization with plates.

Flexion-Compression Injuries

Flexion-compression injuries are characterized by loss of less than 50-60% of the height of the vertebral body. The integrity of the anterior longitudinal ligament is generally uncompromised except in the most severe injuries.[3] Similarly, the interspinous ligament and ligaments of the facet joint are disrupted in the most severe injuries.[37] An important clue to posterior ligamentous disruption is the finding of an increased interspinous distance on the lateral roentgenogram or widening of the facet joint on the axial computerized tomography (CT) scan.

All patients with flexion-compression fractures greater than one-third of the height of the vertebral body, and those who manifest any evidence of ligamentous instability, should be placed in spinal traction. Extension helps to reduce the deformity and may be achieved by placing the traction apparatus relatively posteriorly, or by putting a folded sheet beneath the patient's shoulders.

Subsequent management depends on the following: (1) the nature of the patient's neurological deficit, (2) the presence of bone, disc, or soft tissue impingement of the spinal canal, (3) the presence of injury involving the interspinous ligament or the ligaments stabilizing the facet joints, and (4) the amount of vertebral body compression.

Patients with compression resulting in loss of one-third of the vertebral body height or less may be managed with rest and physical therapy, provided there is no ligamentous instability.[17] Patients with greater than one-third loss of vertebral body height, who have no impingement on the spinal canal and who demonstrate no ligamentous injury, may be considered stable.[1] They can be managed in a halo vest for a period of 8-12 weeks until there is healing and spontaneous anterior fusion of the vertebral body. Lateral cervical spine films must be taken in flexion and extension when the halo vest is removed to make certain that there is no instability. Occult ligamentous injury is always a possibility and mandates that frequent lateral films be taken in the postimmobilization period for at least one year following the injury to identify the occurrence of angulation.

Anterior spinal compression from disc or bone is unusual in this injury. However, in patients with preservation of neurological function and anterior compression, decompression is essential. If the posterior ligaments at the facet joint and the interspinous ligaments are not injured, anterior decompression and fusion utilizing iliac crest bone graft are indicated. If there is evidence of ligamentous injury, anterior plating must be performed as an adjunct to fusion to minimize the risk of postoperative graft dislodgement and recurrent subluxation.

Decompression is not indicated in patients with complete neurological deficit and compromise of the spinal canal from bone fragments, as neurological improvement is unlikely to result from operation.

In patients with associated ligamentous injury who do not require decompression, stabilization is best achieved from a posterior approach using wiring or, as we now prefer, the posterior plates and screws designed by Roy-Camille.[5] The disc space must be carefully examined on lateral radiographs prior to operation. If there is evidence of injury to the disc above and below the compression fracture, as is frequently the case, the stabilization must include both these motion segments. Thus, for a compression fracture of C6 with injury to both adjacent disc spaces, the fusion must span C5-C7.

Compression-Burst Fractures

Compression-burst fractures occur when there is axial loading of a spine which is maintained in a neutral to very slightly flexed position. This mechanism corresponds to the vertical compressive injury of Allen.[3]

The force is absorbed by the vertebral body, which bursts, breaking into several fragments. The posteroinferior portion of the injured vertebral body along with attached disc may be displaced posteriorly into the spinal canal.[14,17] A fragment breaks off the anterior inferior aspect of the vertebral body producing a "teardrop fracture," a name coined by Schneider (Figure 5).[53] The stabilizing ligamentous structures are generally intact, although in the most severe injuries "there is comminution of the vertebral arch with gross failure of the posterior ligamentous complex."[3] Neurological deficit is common from retropulsion of bone fragments into the spinal canal but some function is frequently preserved.[37]

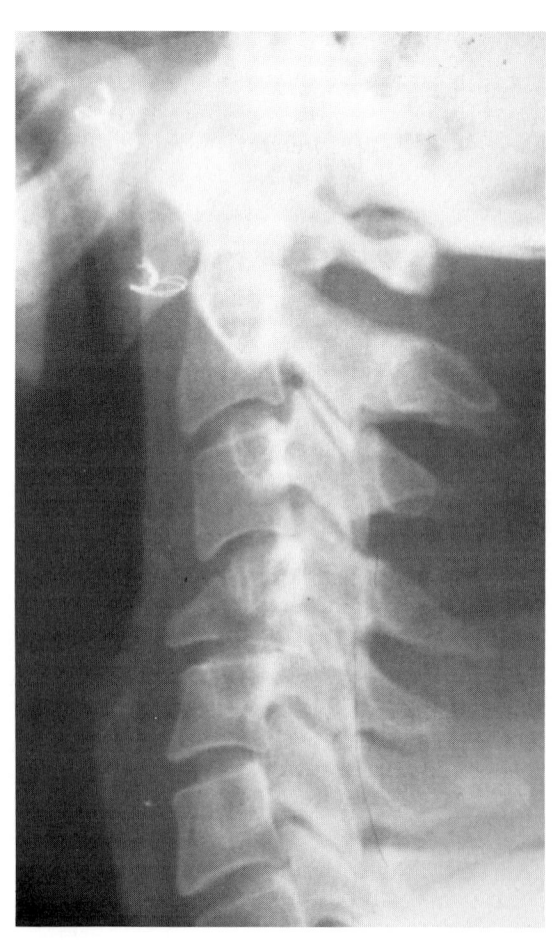

Figure 5. X-ray shows "teardrop fracture" of C4. Note subluxation of C4-C5.

Principles of Operative Stabilization

Although the ligaments generally remain intact in compression-burst fractures, the lesion is unstable anteriorly as a result of injury to the vertebral body. Patients are immobilized in traction to achieve maximum reduction. The subsequent management is controversial. Lind et al[32] documented the successful treatment of seven patients with this lesion using the halo vest for immobilization. Ducker et al[37] also advocated nonoperative management using the halo vest. Others[14,17,51] used an operative approach. Although nonoperative management may be successful, flexion deformity may occur as a result of the vertebral body fracture. This is particularly likely in the minority of cases where there has been posterior ligamentous injury.

We have managed these lesions exclusively with operative stabilization. Fractures may be stabilized from anterior or posterior approaches.[17] We prefer a posterior approach using Roy-Camille plates. Before the plates became available we achieved successful stabilization using interspinous wiring and bone grafts, a method that is still preferred by most North American neurosurgeons. Regardless of whether wiring or plating is used, the surgeon must be aware that there is often disruption to both discs adjacent to the fractured vertebral body and stabilization must immobilize both these motion segments. If this is not done, angulation is virtually predictable.

Anterior vertebrectomy and stabilization is preferred by some[14,51] and is generally satisfactory. We reserve its use for those patients with anterior spinal cord compression with preservation of some neurological function. We now use anterior plating as an adjunct to vertebrectomy, and anterior interbody fusion when anterior decompression is indicated.

Extension Injuries

Extension injuries may occur while the neck is distracted or compressed.[3] In the least severe compression extension injuries, there is a unilateral fracture of the posterior elements and there may also be an anterorotatory vertebral body displacement. With more severe injuries there will be bilateral laminar fractures at one or more contiguous levels and vertebral body displacement with ligamentous failure occurring "posteriorly between the suprajacent and fractured vertebra and anteriorly between the fractured vertebra and the subjacent one."[3] Most injuries are of the least severe variety, with only unilateral fracture of the posterior elements. The majority of patients are neurologically intact or have partial preservation of neurological function.

In less severe distractive extension injuries, failure of the anterior longitudinal ligament occurs with a chip fracture of the anterior and inferior surface of the injured vertebral body as a result of avulsion of the body by the anterior longitudinal ligament. However, no stress is placed on the posterior longitudinal ligament, the facet ligaments, or the interspinous ligament. With more severe distraction-extension injuries there may also be failure of the posterior ligamentous complex, with retrolisthesis of the upper vertebral body into the spinal canal.[3]

Mild distraction-extension injuries are usually stable but the neurological deficit may be profound. In older patients, in particular, the presence of spondylosis will narrow the spinal canal; hyperextension will produce a central spinal cord injury, with relatively greater motor deficit in the upper extremities than in the lower and a variable pattern of sensory loss. Herniation of a cervical disc will occur rarely.[37]

In those extension injuries which do not manifest instability, operation is unnecessary. The treatment of neurological deficit (usually manifest as a central spinal cord injury) in patients with cervical spondylosis and no instability is controversial. With time these patients will usually have neurological improvement. In patients with residual deficit there is no evidence that anterior decompression of osteophytes will alter the course of improvement or the patient's ultimate neurological outcome.

Indications for Operation

Although the halo vest has been used successfully for the management of a variety of cervical spine fractures,[33] the reported incidence of halo vest failure in instability of the lower cervical spine is unacceptably high. The complications of operation are few, the spine is immediately stabilized, and the total treatment time is shortened. In particular the possibility that the patient may still be unstable after three months of immobilization in the halo vest is completely eliminated.

Operation is clearly indicated when facet subluxations cannot be reduced by traction,[2,25,26,54] or when retropulsed vertebral body fragments produce persistent compromise of the spinal canal[25] in patients with residual neurological function below the level of their injury. Operation to remove retropulsed bone fragments compressing the dura mater in patients with no preservation of motor or sensory function is a controversial subject, but this author does not believe that improvement of neurological function occurs as a result of operation in this circumstance.

Other indications for operative stabilization include progressive neurological deficit from spinal instability or persistent compression by bone or soft tissue,[2] the necessity to decompress a root,[54] and chronic progressive deformity or chronic fixed deformity in patients with evidence of incomplete spinal cord or root deficit.

Roy-Camille et al[17] have defined a group of patients with particularly unstable lesions who have injury to the "middle vertebral segment," defined as the posterior vertebral body wall with its attached disc and posterior longitudinal ligament, the pedicles, facets, and the origin of the laminae. These lesions are particularly likely to resublux and undergo progressive deformity if they are not stabilized by operation. Petrie[25] believes that operation is indicated when any two of the following are injured: vertebral body, pedicle, facets, lamina. Other authors have similar indications for operation.[26,54]

Anterior versus Posterior Operation

The relative indications for anterior or posterior operation to stabilize cervical spine injuries are controversial. Prior to the use of instrumentation, anterior decompression and fusion of the unstable cervical spine was fraught with the hazard of recurrent subluxation and bone plug extrusion. However, the advent of instrumentation has made it possible to stabilize the cervical spine from either an anterior or posterior approach for many injuries.

The factors which the surgeon should consider in selecting an anterior or posterior approach include the following: (1) the degree of neurological injury, (2) the presence of persistent spinal cord compression by bone or soft tissue, (3) the type of bony injury, and (4) the skill of the surgeon in utilizing specific operative techniques.

Patients who have partial preservation of neurological function and persistent anterior spinal cord compression should be decompressed from an anterior approach. Even though these patients will undergo anterior bone grafting they should also be stabilized intraoperatively using anterior plates or immediately after operation using a halo vest.

In general, we use posterior stabilization techniques in patients who have complete neurological deficit even if there is persistent anterior decompression. While the patients may also be effectively stabilized from an anterior approach, posterior stabilization is technically simpler and is associated with fewer postoperative complications.[50]

Posterior stabilization is particularly appropriate in patients with posterior ligamentous instability and minimal injury to the vertebral body. While an anterior approach using plating techniques can stabilize the spine in this situation, it makes more sense to stabilize the spine posteriorly, close to the site of injury. In theory, injuries that predominantly involve the vertebral body should be treated anteriorly. In practice, however, vertebral body injuries are quite adequately stabilized through a posterior as well as anterior approach.

Operative Techniques

Posterior Approaches

Interspinous Wiring

Interspinous wiring is the technique most often used in North America to stabilize the cervical spine. It is technically simple, generally effective, and safe.[55] It has the disadvantage of requiring intact posterior elements of the vertebrae to be fused, a situation which is not present in about one-half of all patients with cervical spinal instability.[5] When this occurs an additional level must be incorporated into the fusion construct.[55] While it has been claimed that interspinous wiring provides little rotational stability,[56] we believe that rotational stability is satisfactory if the posterior elements are wired together tightly.

The technique of interspinous wiring has been described by a number of authors.[55-59] Our technique is briefly described. After the patient is turned in traction, the paraspinous muscles are stripped off the posterior elements to be fused and an x-ray is taken both to confirm the appropriate level and the degree of reduction. All soft tissue is removed from the posterior elements, which are then roughened with a curette or high-speed air drill. A towel clip or a right-angle drill is used to make a hole at the most rostral portion of the base of the spinous process to minimize the chance of the wire pulling through the bone of the spinous process.

Heavy stainless steel wire (1 or 1.2 mm in diameter) is passed through the drill hole and the ends are passed around the spinous process of the inferior vertebra to be included in the fusion. The ends of the wire are twisted tightly until there is no movement between the fused vertebrae. Corticocancellous bone grafts taken from the iliac crest are held in place by the ends of the twisted wires, which are used as a spring to wedge the graft between the wire and the posterior elements (Figures 6a-d). Alternatively a second wire may be passed below the interspinous wire and tightened around bone grafts placed on either side of the midline (Figure 7).[55] Patients are placed in a hard cervical collar for three months until bony fusion occurs.

Sublaminar Wiring

Although sublaminar wiring is a safe and effective means of stabilizing the upper cervical spine at C1-C2, it should not be used in the lower cervical spine as the spinal canal is smaller here and the risk of injury to the spinal cord during wire passage is too high.

Facet Fusion

Callahan et al[60] have described a technique of facet wiring and fusion for control of postlaminectomy instability. A twisted strand of two 24-gauge wires is passed bilaterally through the inferior facets of the vertebrae to be fused, and is tied tightly around a bone strut fashioned from an iliac crest graft. Because laminectomy is now infrequently performed for patients with spine injuries there is little need for this technique. Moreover, it is difficult to see how this technique could produce immediate stability, and prolonged external immobilization until bony fusion could take place would seem essential.

Cahill et al[56] proposed a bilateral facet to spinous process fusion to stabilize the cervical spine after trauma. Double braided 22- or 24-gauge wire is passed bilaterally through the inferior facet of the superior vertebra to be included in the fusion and is wired to the spinous process of the subjacent vertebra. Corticocancellous bone is then placed over the roughened posterior elements to assure long-term fusion and stability.

The authors believe that this technique has the advantage of controlling rotational instability. This procedure cannot be used if

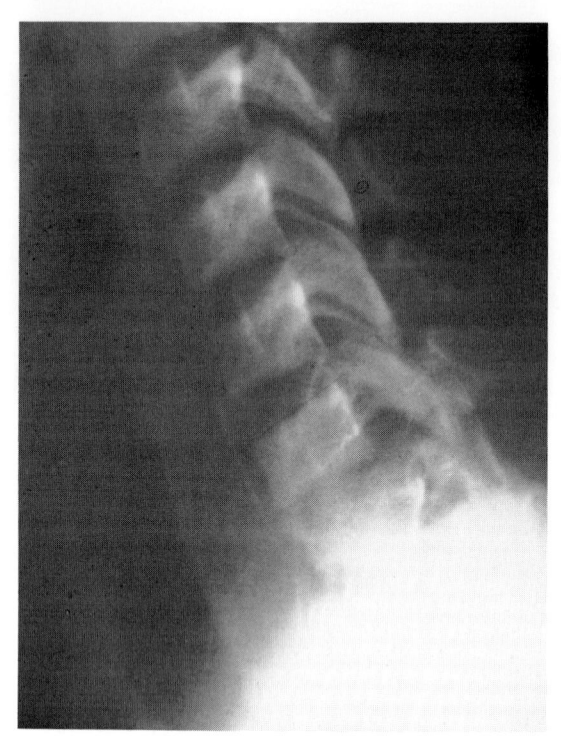

Figure 6a. X-ray of a patient with a C5-C6 subluxation.

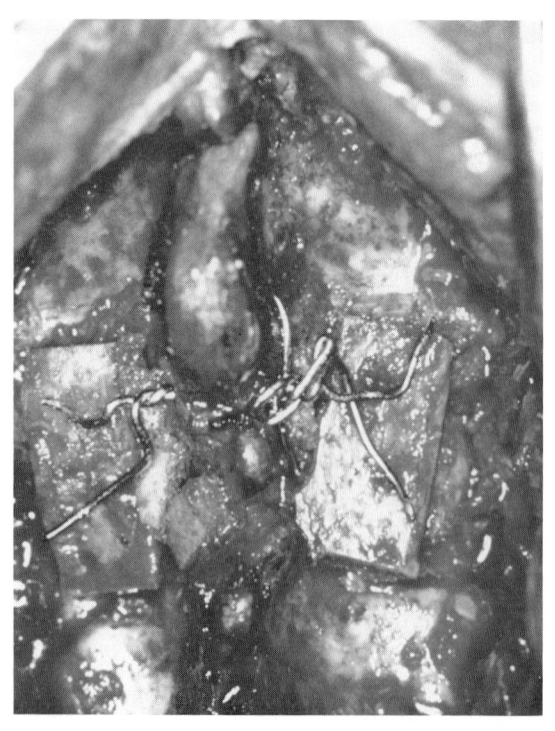

Figure 6b. Operative photograph showing wiring and bone grafts held down by the ends of the interspinous wires.

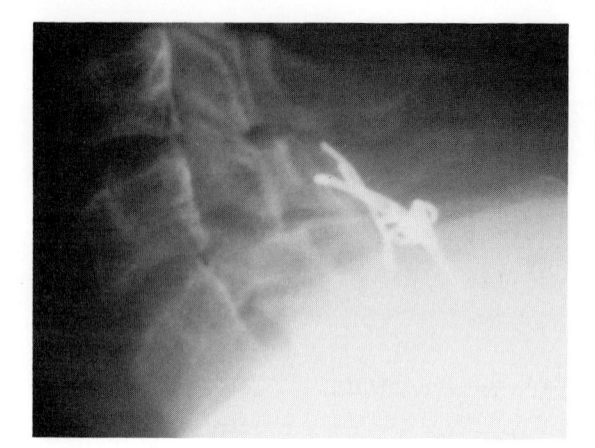

Figure 6c. Postoperative lateral x-ray shows excellent reduction.

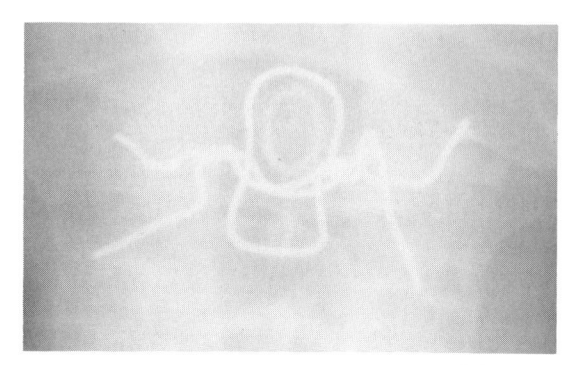

Figure 6d. AP x-ray shows the long ends of the wires holding the graft in place.

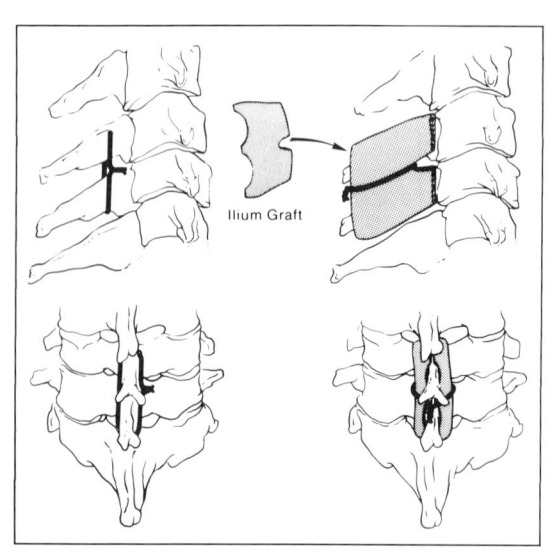

Figure 7. Illustration shows the technique of Benzel et al[56] for interspinous wiring of one or two motion segments. Iliac bone grafts are secured in place with a second wire.

the facet or the inferior spinous process is not intact. The weak point of the technique is dependence of the fusion on a wire which passes through the facet. The bone is thin at the point where the hole is made in the facet and it is quite easy for the wires to pull through, either as they are being passed through the hole or in the postoperative period.

Interlaminar (Halifax) Clamps

Holness et al[61] proposed the use of interlaminar clamps for the posterior stabilization of the upper and lower cervical spine. These clamps consist of two hooks which are connected by a screw. The hooks fit around the two laminae to be stabilized and pull the laminae closer to each other as the screw is tightened. The clamps are used bilaterally and thus provide rotational stability. These clamps, which are commercially available, have not been widely used. They have the disadvantage of requiring intact laminae, the instruments designed to tighten the clamps are poorly designed, and the clamps are awkward to insert.

Posterior Plates and Screws

We have recently described our experience with the plates and screws designed by Roy-Camille.[5] They are simple to insert, require little technical expertise, and provide immediate stability without the necessity for bone grafting. This technique is currently our choice for the posterior stabilization of the cervical spine.

Patients are positioned in the prone position in traction and alignment is confirmed with an intraoperative x-ray. After exposure of the posterior elements to the lateral margins of the lateral masses, the two or three vertebrae to be stabilized are identified and holes are drilled bilaterally in the exact center of the lateral masses to a depth of 10 mm. The holes are angled 10-20° laterally to avoid the vertebral arteries. The plates we use have either two or three holes 13 mm apart for

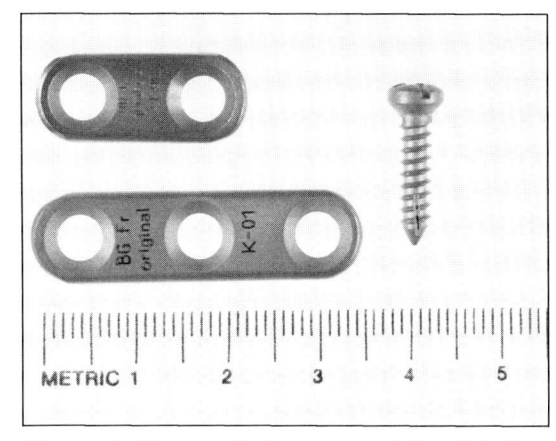

Figure 8. Photograph shows two and three hole Roy-Camille plates and the 3.5 mm diameter screws used to secure them in place.

stabilizing one or two motion segments respectively (Figure 8). Screws 3.5 mm in diameter and 16 mm in length are screwed into the holes made in the lateral masses to secure the plates in place. This technique produces immediate stability without the need for bone grafting (Figures 9a-c). Postoperatively patients are kept in a Philadelphia or similar collar for three months.[5]

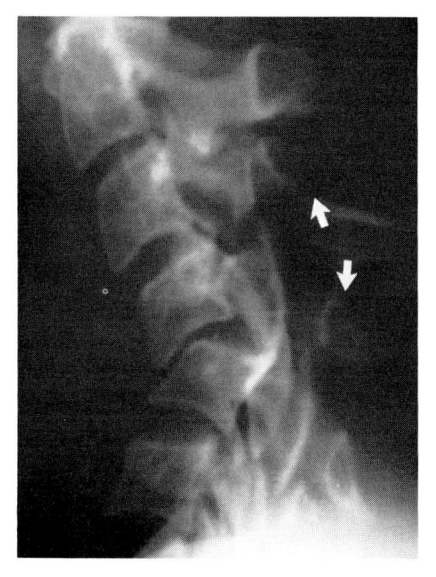

Figure 9a. Lateral x-ray shows severe C4-C5 subluxation in a patient with a complete neurological deficit. Arrows show widened interspinous distance between C3-C4 suggesting instability at this level also.

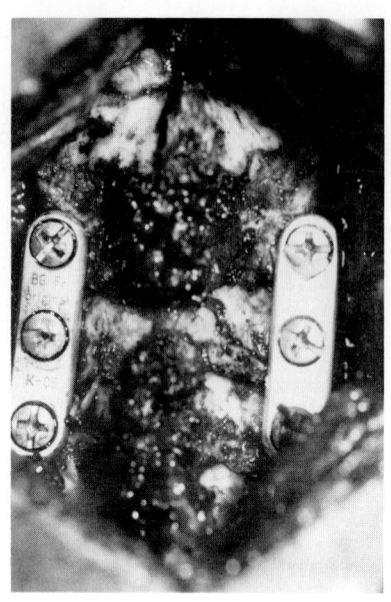

Figure 9b. Operative photograph of three hole plates in situ stabilizing C3-C5.

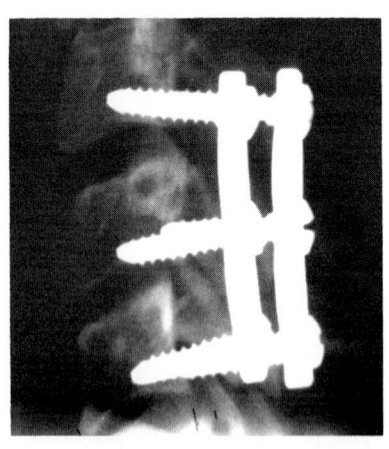

Figure 9c. Postoperative lateral cervical spine x-ray showing excellent alignment after posterior plating.

The use of plates and screws to achieve spinal stability is particularly efficacious in patients with fractures of the spinous processes or laminae, as this technique stabilizes the lateral masses and the presence of intact laminae or spinous processes is unnecessary for its successful application. We have used posterior plating in more than 50 patients. We have failed to achieve long-term stability in only two patients. One patient had ankylosing spondylitis and extremely soft bone and in retrospect should not have been plated. A second patient, an alcoholic, refused to wear his collar in the postoperative period, resulting in screw extrusion.

Posterior Constructs Using Methylmethacrylate

Methylmethacrylate (MMA) has been used with wire or as a supplement to wiring and bone grafting in stabilizing the cervical spine.[35,62] MMA is "not a glue but an inert filler."[59] It adds little strength to fusion constructs in the short term and loses strength over time. Unlike bone, it never becomes incorporated into living tissue and forever remains a foreign body. When used with bone, it has the potential for preventing bony fusion if it gets between the grafts and the posterior elements. The use of MMA in patients with cervical spinal instability as a result of trauma has little to commend it and its use should be avoided.

Anterior Approaches

Bone Grafting without Plating

Anterior cervical fusion may be accomplished using either the Cloward[63] or the Smith-Robinson method.[64] The disadvantage of these procedures is that neither provides immediate stabilization. Indeed, removal of the anterior and posterior longitudinal ligaments and disc has the short-term effect of destabilizing the spine. Excellent external immobilization must be provided in the postoperative period. Even with good immobilization, bone graft extrusion and resubluxation is a distressingly frequent complication (Figures 10a,b).

The Cloward procedure is ill-suited to patients with vertebral body trauma. The drill bits of fixed size are poorly adapted to the performance of vertebrectomies and do not allow for tailoring of the bone plug. In addition, the technique does not allow for a keystone graft to lock the bone plug in the graft site. Drilling a fractured retropulsed, unstable vertebral body with the Cloward drill

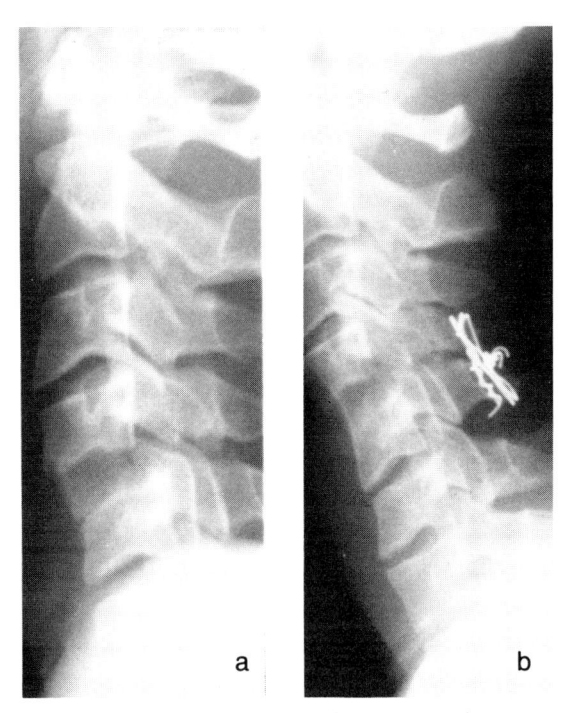

Figure 10. (a) Lateral x-ray of a patient with a recurrent subluxation in spite of an anterior cervical fusion with iliac crest bone graft. (b) Lateral x-ray after posterior wiring to supplement the anterior fusion.

may further push fragments toward the spinal cord and produce additional neurological deficit.

The technique designed by Robinson and Smith[64] and adapted by others over the years is more appropriate for use in patients with cervical trauma, because it allows the amount of bone removal to be tailored to the extent of injury. We advocate total vertebrectomy in patients with fractured or retropulsed vertebral body. Partial vertebrectomy will result in placing a graft in an injured vertebral body and increases the risk of graft extrusion. Total vertebrectomy carried as far laterally as the uncovertebral joints, with removal of the posterior longitudinal ligament, will allow wide visualization of the dural tube and assure that there is no residual spinal cord compression.

The placement of the bone graft is crucial to the success of the operation. The graft must be wedged tightly and countersunk to minimize the chances of extrusion. Locking the bone graft into place as described by Gore[65] and others[66] will provide additional insurance against bone graft extrusion. Regardless of the technique used, external immobilization with a halo vest or other orthosis in the postoperative period is essential to prevent graft displacement and/or resubluxation.

Bone Grafting with Anterior Cervical Plating

The use of anterior cervical plating as an adjunct to bone grafting represents a major advance in stabilizing the cervical spine following trauma. Anterior plates provide immediate internal stabilization of the cervical spine and prevent subluxation and graft extrusion until fusion can take place. Several plates and techniques have been described.[4,67-69] The instrumentation described by Caspar is elegant and ideally suited to safe and accurate placement of anterior cervical plates.[4]

The vertebrectomy is carried out in standard fashion. The remainder of the procedure is carried out using the image intensifier. Intraoperative fluoroscopy is absolutely essential to this procedure, and if the posterior margins of the vertebral bodies to be plated cannot be clearly visualized the procedure cannot be safely performed.

The Caspar set contains distraction pins which are drilled into the vertebral bodies above and below the vertebrectomy, allowing the vertebral bodies to be distracted and the bone graft to be wedged into place, after which distraction is released and the pins removed. A number of plates have been designed for this procedure, but we have preferred to use the A-O plates marketed in this country by Synthes (Figure 11) or the trapezoidal plates designed by Caspar. All the plates contain two sets of parallel holes, a feature which is absolutely essential to prevent rotational movement and screw extrusion with subsequent loosening of the plate.

The plates must be of sufficient length to allow screws to be placed in the center of the

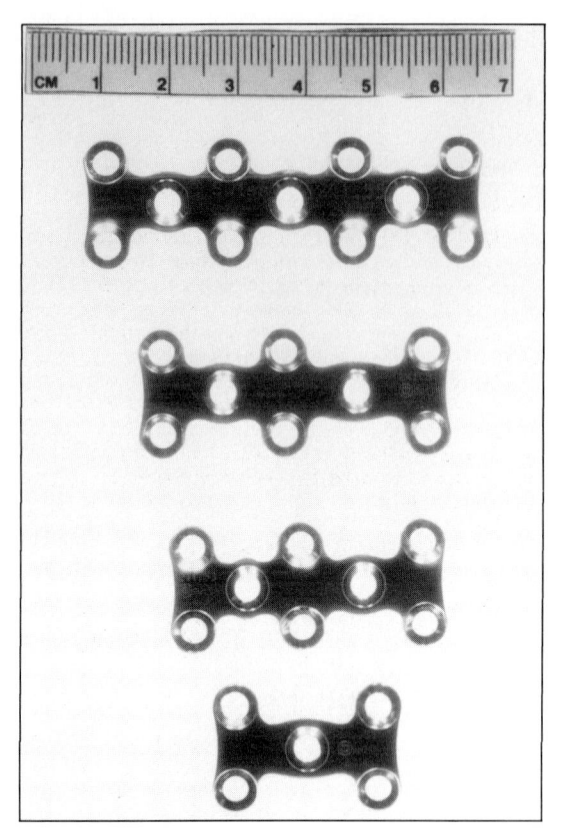

Figure 11. Photograph shows multiple sizes of A-O plates for anterior cervical stabilization.

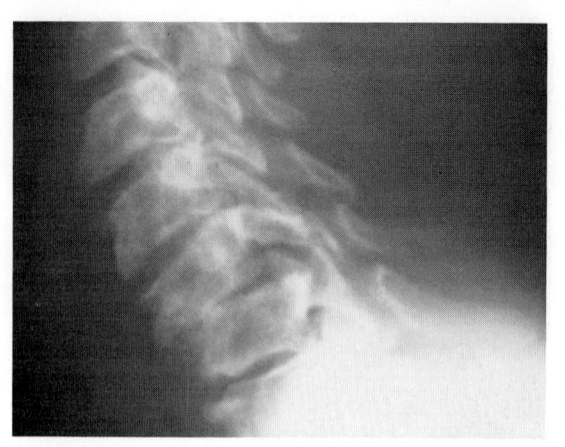

Figure 12a. Lateral x-ray of a patient with a fixed flexion deformity at C6-C7 two months after injury. Subluxation was not present (or was missed) on initial films taken shortly after injury.

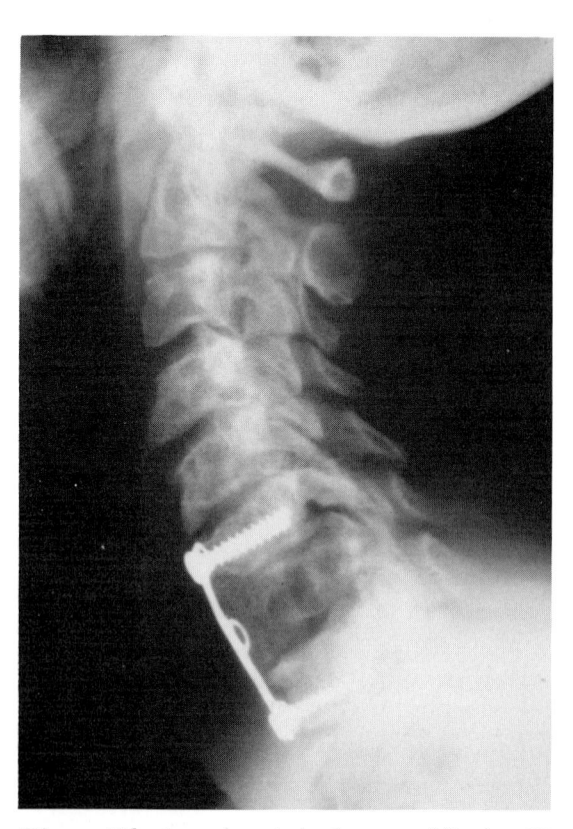

Figure 12b. Lateral cervical spine x-ray following C7 vertebrectomy, bone grafting, and anterior plating from C6 to T1 showing excellent reduction. Two upper and two lower screws are present but are not seen well because they overlap and are superimposed. The screw position is ideal: in the center of the vertebral body and long enough to extend to the posterior cortical margin.

vertebral bodies to be fused, but must not extend above or below the vertebral body to nonfused segments as flexion or extension movement could result in plate movement and screw pull-out. Holes are drilled in the vertebral body directed away from the disc space and angled medially away from the roots and vertebral arteries. They must be of sufficient length to penetrate the posterior cortical bone but not extend into the spinal canal. The screws must be tightened so that the plates are firmly against the anterior margin of the vertebral bodies (Figures 12a,b).

While this is an elegant procedure, it is also technically exacting. Failure to follow these basic principles and the details provided by Caspar[4] may result in neural injury, or screw and plate dislodgement (Figure 13) with injury to the esophagus and adjacent soft tissues in the neck.

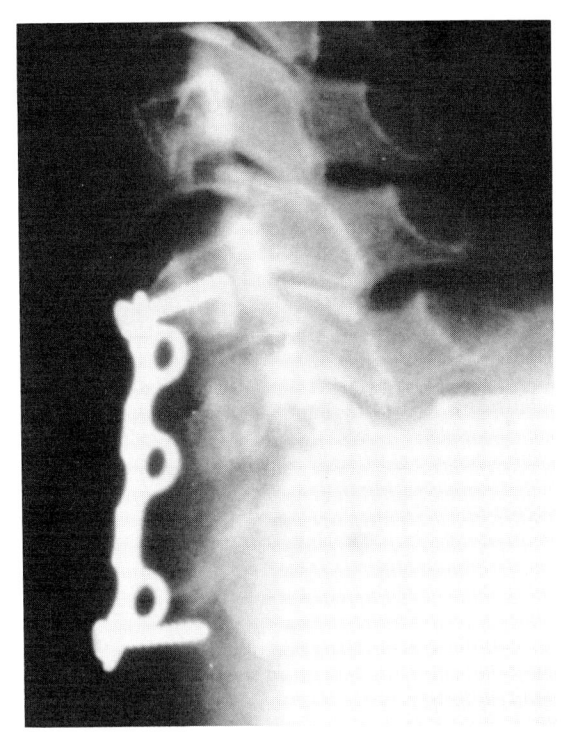

Figure 13. Lateral cervical spine x-ray of a patient who had incorrect placement of cervical plates with screw pullout. Screws are too short to reach the posterior cortical margin of the vertebral body and a single row of screws rather than two parallel rows increase the chances of rotational movement and screw pull-out.

References

1. Bedbrook GM. Spinal injuries with tetraplegia and paraplegia. *J Bone Joint Surg Br.* 1979;61B:267-284.
2. Bohlman HH. Acute fractures and dislocations of the cervical spine: an analysis of three hundred hospitalized patients and review of the literature. *J Bone Joint Surg Am.* 1979;61A:1119-1142.
3. Allen BL Jr, Ferguson RL, Lehmann TR, O'Brien RP. A mechanistic classification of closed, indirect fractures and dislocations of the lower cervical spine. *Spine.* 1982;7:1-27.
4. Caspar W. Anterior cervical fusion and interbody stabilization with the trapezial osteosynthetic plate technique. *Aesculap Scientific Information.* 1985;12:1-36.
5. Cooper PR, Cohen A, Rosiello A, Koslow M. Posterior stabilization of cervical spine fractures and subluxations using plates and screws. *Neurosurgery.* 1988;23:300-306.
6. Roy-Camille R, Saillant G, Mazel C, Gagna G, Caubel P, Ciniglio M. The surgical treatment of post-traumatic vertebral deformities. *Ital J Orthop Traumatol.* 1986;12:419-426.
7. Brav EA, Miller JA, Bouzard WC. Traumatic dislocation of the cervical spine: Army experience and results. *J Trauma.* 1963;3:569-582.
8. Cheshire DJE. The stability of the cervical spine following the conservative treatment of fractures and fracture-dislocations. *Paraplegia.* 1969;7:193-203.
9. Dall DM. Injuries of the cervical spine, II: does anatomical reduction of the bony injuries improve the prognosis for spinal cord recovery? *S Afr Med J.* 1972;46:1083-1090.
10. Frankel HL, Hancock DO, Hyslop G, Melzak J, Michaelis LS, Ungar GH, et al. The value of postural reduction in the initial management of closed injuries of the spine with paraplegia and tetraplegia: part 1. *Paraplegia.* 1969;7:179-192.
11. Guttmann L. The conservative management of closed injuries of the vertebral column resulting in damage to the spinal cord and spinal roots. In: Vinken PJ, Bruyn GW, eds. *Handbook of Clinical Neurology.* New York, NY: American Elsevier; 1976;26:285-306.
12. Dorr LD, Harvey JP Jr, Nickel VL. Clinical review of the early stability of spine injuries. *Spine.* 1982;7:545-550.
13. Donovan WH, Kopaniky D, Stolzmann, Carter RE. The neurological and skeletal outcome in patients with closed cervical spinal cord injury. *J Neurosurg.* 1987;66:690-694.
14. Norrell H. The treatment of unstable spinal fractures and dislocations. *Clin Neurosurg.* 1978;25:193-208.
15. Ducker TB, Salcman M, Daniell HB. Experimental spinal cord trauma, III: therapeutic effects of immobilization and pharmacologic agents. *Surg Neurol.* 1978;10:71-76.
16. Rogers WA. Fractures and dislocations of the cervical spine: an end-result study. *J Bone Joint Surg Am.* 1957;39A:341-376.
17. Roy-Camille R, Saillant G, Judet T, Mammoudy P. Traumatismes récente des cinq dernières vertèbres cervicales chez l'adulte (avec et sans complication neurologique). *Hôp Sem Paris.* 1983;59:1479-1488.
18. Munro D. Treatment of fractures and dislocations of the cervical spine complicated by cervical cord and root injuries: a comparative study of fusion vs. nonfusion therapy. *N Engl J Med.* 1961;264:573-582.
19. Wagner FC Jr, Chehrazi B. Surgical results in the treatment of cervical spinal cord injury. *Spine.* 1984;9:523-524.
20. McAfee PC, Bohlman HH. One-stage anterior cervical decompression and posterior stabilization with circumferential arthrodesis. *J Bone Joint Surg Am.* 1989;71A:78-88.
21. Born JD, Lenelle J, Albert A, Collignon J, Hans P, Bonnal J. Les traumatismes du rachis cervical démarche thérapeutique: facteurs discriminants. *Rev Med Liege.* 1985;40:131-139.
22. Norrell H, Wilson CB. Early anterior fusion for injuries of the cervical portion of the spine. *JAMA.* 1970;214:525-530.
23. Durbin FC. Fracture-dislocations of the cervical spine. *J Bone Joint Surg Br.* 1957;39B:23-38.
24. Forsyth HF, Alexander E Jr, Davis C Jr, Underdal R. The advantages of early spine fusion in the treatment of fracture-dislocation of the cervical spine. *J Bone Joint Surg Am.* 1959;41A:17-36.
25. Petrie GJ. Flexion injuries of the cervical spine. *J Bone Joint Surg Am.* 1964;46A:1800-1806.
26. Aebi M, Mohler J, Zäch GA, Morscher E. Indication, surgical technique, and results of 100 sur-

27. gically-treated fractures and fracture-dislocations of the cervical spine. *Clin Orthop.* 1986;203:244-257.
27. Nickel VL, Perry J, Garrett A, Heppenstall M. The halo: a spinal skeletal traction fixation device. *J Bone Joint Surg Am.* 1968;50A:1400-1409.
28. Millington PJ, Ellingsen JM, Hauswirth BE, Fabian PJ. Thermoplastic Minerva body jacket—a practical alternative to current methods of cervical spine stabilization: a clinical report. *Phys Ther.* 1987;67:223-225.
29. Johnson RM, Owen JR, Hart DL, Callahan RA. Cervical orthoses: a guide to their selection and use. *Clin Orthop.* 1981;154:34-45.
30. Cooper PR, Maravilla KR, Sklar FH, Moody SF, Clark WK. Halo immobilization of cervical spine fractures. *J Neurosurg.* 1979;50:603-610.
31. Garfin SR, Botte MJ, Waters RL, Nickel VL. Complications in the use of the halo fixation device. *J Bone Joint Surg Am.* 1986;68A:320-325.
32. Lind B, Sihlbom H, Nordwall A. Halo-vest treatment of unstable traumatic cervical spine injuries. *Spine.* 1988;13:425-432.
33. Bucholz RD, Cheung KC. Halo vest versus spinal fusion for cervical injury: evidence from an outcome study. *J Neurosurg.* 1989;70:884-892.
34. Whitehill R, Richman JA, Glaser JA. Failure of immobilization of the cervical spine by the halo vest. *J Bone Joint Surg Am.* 1986;68A:326-332.
35. Duff TA. Surgical stabilization of traumatic cervical spine dislocation using methylmethacrylate: long-term results in 26 patients. *J Neurosurg.* 1986;64:39-44.
36. Holdsworth F. Fractures, dislocations, and fracture dislocations of the spine. *J Bone Joint Surg Am.* 1970;52A:1534-1551.
37. Ducker TB, Bellegarrigue R, Salcman M, Walleck C. Timing of operative care in cervical spinal cord injury. *Spine.* 1984;9:525-531.
38. Argenson C, Lovet J, Sanouiller JL, de Peretti F. Traumatic rotatory displacement of the lower cervical spine. *Spine.* 1988;13:767-773.
39. Maiman DJ, Sances A Jr, Myklebust JB, Larson SJ, Houterman CH, Chilbert M, et al. Compression injuries of the cervical spine: a biomechanical analysis. *Neurosurgery.* 1983;13:254-260.
40. O'Brien PJ, Schweigel JF, Thompson WJ. Dislocations of the lower cervical spine. *J Trauma.* 1982;22:70:710-714.
41. Beatson TR. Fractures and dislocations of the cervical spine. *J Bone Joint Surg Br.* 1963;45B:21-35.
42. Maiman DJ, Barolat G, Larson SJ. Mangement of bilateral locked facets of the cervical spine. *Neurosurgery.* 1986;18:542-547.
43. Stauffer ES, Kelly EG. Fracture-dislocations of the cervical spine: instability and recurrent deformity following treatment by anterior interbody fusion. *J Bone Joint Surg Am.* 1977;59A:45-48.
44. White AA III, Southwick WO, Panjabi MM. Clinical instability in the lower cervical spine: a review of past and current concepts. *Spine.* 1976;1:15-27.
45. Nieminen R. Conservative treatment of luxations and subluxations of the lower cervical spine. *Ann Chir Gynaecol Fenn.* 1974;63:57-68.
46. Stauffer ES. Neurologic recovery following injuries to the cervical spinal cord and nerve roots *Spine.* 1984;9:532-534.
47. Cotler HB, Miller LS, DeLucia FA, Cotler JM, Davne SH. Closed reduction of cervical spine dislocations. *Clin Orthop.* 1987;214:185-199.
48. Böhler J, Gaudernak T. Anterior plate stabilization for fracture-dislocations of the lower cervical spine. *J Trauma.* 1980;20:203-205.
49. Reynier Y, Lena G, Diaz-Vazquez P, Vincentelli F, Vigouroux RP. Bilan de 138 fractures du rachis cervical sur une période récente de 5 ans (1979-1983): attitudes thérapeutiques. *Neurochirurgie.* 1985;31:153-160.
50. Capen DA, Garland DE, Waters RL. Surgical stabilization of the cervical spine: a comparative analysis of anterior and posterior spine fusions. *Clin Orthop.* 1985;196:229-237.
51. Stauffer ES. Surgical stabilization of the cervical spine after trauma. *Arch Surg.* 1976;111:652-657.
52. Savini R, Parisini P, Cervellati S. The surgical treatment of late instability of flexion-rotation injuries in the lower cervical spine. *Spine.* 1987;12:178-182.
53. Schneider RC, Kahn EA. Chronic neurological sequelae of acute trauma to the spine and spinal cord, I: the significance of the acute-flexion or "tear-drop" fracture-dislocation of the cervical spine. *J Bone Joint Surg Am.* 1956;38A:985-997.
54. Nieminen R, Koskinen VS. Posterior fusion in cervical spine injuries: an analysis of fifty cases treated surgically. *Ann Chir Gynaecol Fenn.* 1973;62:36-48.
55. Benzel EC, Kesterson L. Posterior cervical interspinous compression wiring and fusion for mid to low cervical spine injuries. *J Neurosurg.* 1989;70:893-899.
56. Cahill DW, Bellegarrigue R, Ducker TB. Bilateral facet to spinous process fusion: a new technique for posterior spinal fusion after trauma. *Neurosurgery.* 1983;13:1-4.
57. Cooper PR. Operative management of cervical spine injuries. *Clin Neurosurg.* 1988;34:650-674.
58. Cooper PR. Stabilization of fractures and subluxations of the middle and lower cervical spine. *Contemp Neurosurg.* 1988;10:1-6.
59. White AA III, Panjabi MM. The role of stabilization in the treatment of cervical spine injuries. *Spine.* 1984;9:512-522.
60. Callahan RA, Johnson RM, Margolis RN, Keggi KJ, Albright JA, Southwick WO. Cervical facet fusion for control of instability following laminectomy. *J Bone Joint Surg Am.* 1977;59A:991-1002.
61. Holness RO, Huestis WS, Howes WJ, Langille RA. Posterior stabilization with an interlaminar clamp in cervical injuries: technical note and review of the long term experience with the method. *Neurosurgery.* 1984;14:318-322.
62. Eismont FJ, Bohlman HH. Posterior methylmethacrylate fixation for cervical trauma. *Spine.* 1981;6:347-353.
63. Cloward RB. The anterior approach for removal of ruptured cervical disks. *J Neurosurg.* 1958;15:602-617.
64. Robinson RA, Smith GW. Anterolateral cervical disc removal and interbody fusion for cervical disc syndrome. *Bull Johns Hopkins Hosp.* 1955;96:223-224. Abstract.
65. Gore DR. Technique of cervical interbody fusion. *Clin Orthop.* 1984;188:191-195.
66. Simmons EH. The surgical correction of flexion deformity of the cervical spine in ankylosing spon-

dylitis. *Clin Orthop*. 1972;86:132-143.
67. Bremer AM, Nguyen TQ. Internal metal plate fixation combined with anterior interbody fusion in cases of cervical spine injury. *Neurosurgery*. 1983;12:649-653.
68. Gassman J, Seligson D. The anterior cervical plate. *Spine*. 1983;8:700-707.
69. Lesoin F, Viaud C, Jomin M. Universal plate for anterior cervical spine osteosynthesis: technical note. *Acta Neurochir*. 1985;77:60-61.

CHAPTER 9

Thoracolumbar Spine Injuries

Thomas J. Errico, MD, and R. David Bauer, MD

Over the last decade, dissatisfaction with the results of nonoperative treatment of the thoracic and lumbar spine fractures led to an increased role for operation. The exquisite definition of the anatomy provided by computerized tomography (CT) imaging resulted in a greater understanding of the pathologic anatomy.[193,197] This, combined with a variety of advances in operative instrumentation led to revolutionary changes in the management of thoracic and lumbar injuries.

This chapter describes the injuries that occur in the thoracic and lumbar spine. The principles of managing these injuries are detailed. Although examples of stabilization procedures are provided, a detailed "how-to-do-it" is beyond our scope here. Copious references enable the reader to learn the details of specific operative techniques.

Clinical Features

Fractures of the thoracic and lumbar spine tend to affect a younger segment of the population. They occur most often due to motor vehicle accidents, winter sports,[1,2] airplane crashes,[3,4,194] industrial accidents, falls, jumps and suicide attempts, and less frequently are due to direct violence.

Upper Thoracic Spine

Considerable violence is necessary to produce a fracture or dislocation of the upper part of the thoracic spine. It is more rigid than other parts of the spine, and is stabilized by the contiguous rib cage which resists lateral bending and extension. In addition, the facets and laminae are oriented so as to restrict motion in the rotatory plane.

The narrower spinal canal in this region, along with the critical vascular supply of the spinal cord, makes it almost inevitable that patients with injuries at this level also sustain a severe concomitant neurologic injury.[5-8] In the thoracic region, approximately 80% of fractures of the upper part of the thoracic spine with spinal cord injury result in complete paraplegia.[5,7,9]

Lumbar Spine

The lumbar spine is the second most mobile region of the spine. It is relatively free to move in flexion, extension, lateral bending, and rotation, all of which increase with caudal progression towards L5.[7,10] The lumbar spine can have its overall configuration changed from lordosis to neutral or slight flexion by the position of the pelvis at the time of impact. Only when the physiologic range of motion is exceeded is it susceptible to injury.

Thoracolumbar Junction

The thoracolumbar junction is the region at greatest risk for injury, and the majority of fractures of the thoracic and lumbar spine occur here. The thoracolumbar junction is the first mobile area distal to the stabilizing influence of the ribs, and acts as the fulcrum of motion for the thorax. It is best seen as a transition zone between the distal end of the relatively long lever arm of the thoracic complex and the highly mobile lumbar spine. It is located in an area where the kyphotic thoracic spine changes to the lordotic lumbar spine[5,11] and the facets begin to change their orientation from the coronal to the sagittal plane.[11]

In the lumbar spine the space available for the neural structures increases significantly as the canal progresses caudally. For a given degree of displacement, neural injury is often less severe and there is greater potential for recovery than at other levels. This is true because of the increased space available for neural structures, and because the spinal cord ends in the vicinity of L2 and the peripheral nerves of the cauda equina have a greater capacity to resist injury and recover from injury more readily than the spinal cord. As a result there is poor correlation between the degree of canal compromise as measured by CT scanning and the resulting neurologic deficit.[12-17]

Contiguous and Noncontiguous Spinal Injury

A major error in early patient evaluation is failure to demonstrate other coexisting spinal injuries.[18] Four to 17% of patients with spine fractures have noncontiguous fractures, of which approximately 20% will be potentially unstable.[1,19-22] The majority of noncontiguous injuries are at the extremes of the spine, especially at C1-C2 and L4-L5.[19,23] As soon as a fracture at any level has been identified, screening x-rays of the entire spine should be taken, and special attention should be paid to the craniocervical and lumbosacral junctions.[11,19,23,24] Contiguous injuries are most frequently compression fractures occurring either above or below a severe burst fracture in the thoracolumbar spine.

Classification of Thoracic and Lumbar Injuries

Early Classification Schemes

Nicoll was the first to differentiate between stable and unstable injuries in a study of injuries sustained by coal miners.[25] Holdsworth and Hardy modified the Nicoll classification in 1953.[26] This classification led to a better understanding of the mechanisms of injury and clarified the indications for operative and nonoperative treatment. It was recognized that the thoracic and lumbar spine may be subjected to (1) flexion injuries in which the posterior ligaments do not rupture, (2) flexion forces with a rotatory component which may cause rupture of the posterior ligamentous complex, (3) hyperextension causing injury to the posterior elements with the potential for dislocation, and (4) axial compression forces.

Each individual or coupled force could result in specific fracture patterns identifiable on radiographs. Holdsworth insisted that rupture of the posterior column alone was sufficient to create instability of the spine. Wedge compression fractures and burst compression fractures were considered stable, while all dislocations, extension fracture dislocations, and rotational fracture dislocations were considered unstable.

Although the Holdsworth classification has remained the cornerstone of all subsequent classification schemes, this classification is no longer considered wholly accurate. Many burst compression fractures that Holdsworth considered stable are now classified as unstable.

Two and Three Column Concepts

The two-column concept (anterior and posterior) of the anatomy of the spine was first introduced by Kelly and Whitesides.[27] The vertebral body and its ligamentous attachments represent the anterior column. Everything posterior to and including the pedicles was considered the posterior column. However, the descriptive two-column classifications rapidly yielded to a three-column theory with the advent of computerized tomography.[5,13] Denis introduced the concept of the middle column, an osteoligamentous column whose integrity is critical to the stability of the spine. Spinal stability also was realized to be dependent on the status of the middle spinal column and not solely the posterior ligamentous complex.

One or more of the three columns predictably fails in axial compression, axial distraction, or translation from combinations of forces in different planes.[13] With compression alone, the middle column can remain intact and will act as a hinge, resulting in anterior or lateral wedge fractures. For example, "Chance" fractures involve failure of the posterior and middle columns due to flexion and distraction. Burst fractures represent disruptions of the anterior and middle columns from axial loading.

Mechanistic Classifications

Further development of the mechanism of injury as a method of classification led to the mechanistic classification of thoracic and lumbar injuries. Ferguson and Allen[28] describe seven major groups of injuries: compressive flexion, distractive flexion, lateral flexion, translational injuries, torsional flexion, vertical compression, and distractive extension injuries.

Nonoperative Treatment

The mainstays of nonoperative treatment in the past were postural reduction and prolonged recumbency.[29-32] If a patient were kept at bed rest long enough, it was believed, osseous stability could be achieved.

Historically, "conservative treatment" meant postural reduction for 6 to 12 weeks. Pillows were used to maintain lordosis of the lumbar spine, and this posture had to be maintained continually for two to three weeks to prevent redisplacement, even while the patient was turned frequently to prevent decubiti.[30,33,34] Injudicious handling during the early postinjury period could result in redisplacement of unstable fractures, loss of reduction, and further injury to nerve roots that might otherwise have had the capacity to recover.[35] Bed rest was followed by mobilization in a cast or orthosis [8,30,33,36] for a prolonged period.

Operative reduction allows earlier ambulation and anatomic fracture reduction. The choice between surgical and conservative treatment is made after examination of fracture morphology on plain radiographs and CT scans. An assessment of initial fracture instability, kyphosis, age at the time of injury, and degree of canal compromise is necessary to choose the best possible candidates for conservative management.[37] Considerations in this decision include the patient's neurologic status, the fracture morphology, the medical condition of the patient, the presence of associated injuries, and the desires of the patient.

CT scans must be carefully examined for evidence of occult posterior element injury which tips the decision-making balance away from conservative management.[37] The presence of canal compromise secondary to retropulsed bone fragments is not by itself an indication for surgical decompression. The presence of canal occlusion at the time of injury does not guarantee that it will remain occluded. Resorption of bone fragments causing canal compromise does occur, especially in those patients with less than 50% canal occlusion. Krompinger et al demonstrated that canal occlusion of greater than 25% decreased in over 75% of the patients and canal compromise of 25% or less resolved completely in 50%.[37] Patients with canal compromise of up to 60% have been managed nonoperatively in the absence of neurologic deficit without neurologic deterioration.[37,38]

Certain fracture patterns are unsuitable for nonoperative management. These include (1) all translational and flexion/rotation fracture-dislocations, (2) the majority of three-column fractures, and (3) distraction injuries with posterior ligamentous disruption and kyphotic deformities of greater than 30°.

Neurologically intact patients treated conservatively can suffer residual kyphosis, spinal stenosis, late instability, or radiculopathy which interferes with a good functional result. Back pain in these patients may result from instability, kyphosis, retained fragments, or foraminal stenosis which might have been corrected at the time of injury with anatomic reduction and rigid fixation.[34,37] In one report approximately 20% of neurologically intact patients with burst fractures developed either frank neurological symptoms[39] or severe leg pain[37] when treated nonoperatively.

Nonoperative management can lead to progressive kyphotic deformity of 10° or more in at least 20% of patients. Patients with initial kyphosis of 10° or less do not progress more than 10° (Figure 1).[37,40] Progression occurs most frequently at the thoracolumbar junction in patients with initial kyphosis greater than 15° or 50% canal occlusion. Late back pain is not uncommon in patients with more than 20° of residual posttraumatic kyphosis.[41] Correction of this late posttraumatic kyphosis may require combined anterior and posterior fusion or anterior osteotomy, instrumentation, and fusion.[42-44]

Operative Treatment: General Considerations

Good evidence exists that stabilization of unstable thoracic and lumbar spine fractures promotes more rapid mobilization, faster rehabilitation, more rapid ambulation and wheelchair use, and easier nursing care with fewer complications. Operative therapy is associated with less residual deformity and prevents progression of deformity. Operative therapy minimizes the high expense and complications associated with recumbent management and decreases hospitalization in patients with minimal or no neurologic deficit, permitting mobilization in days rather than months.[12,28,36,40,41,45-60,196,201]

Indications

The strongest indication for surgical stabilization occurs in those patients who have sustained injuries that are mechanically unstable.[61] The determination of stability is not always an easy task. Stability is a relative term that depends on the severity and anatomy of the injury and the potential stresses which will be applied to a spinal motion segment prior to and after successful healing.[51,62]

A reasonable integration of knowledge to date suggests the following definitions:

1. A "stable fracture" is one where only a few days of bed rest are required to ameliorate the acute effects of the fracture. The patient may then be mobilized upright walking either with or without immobilization.

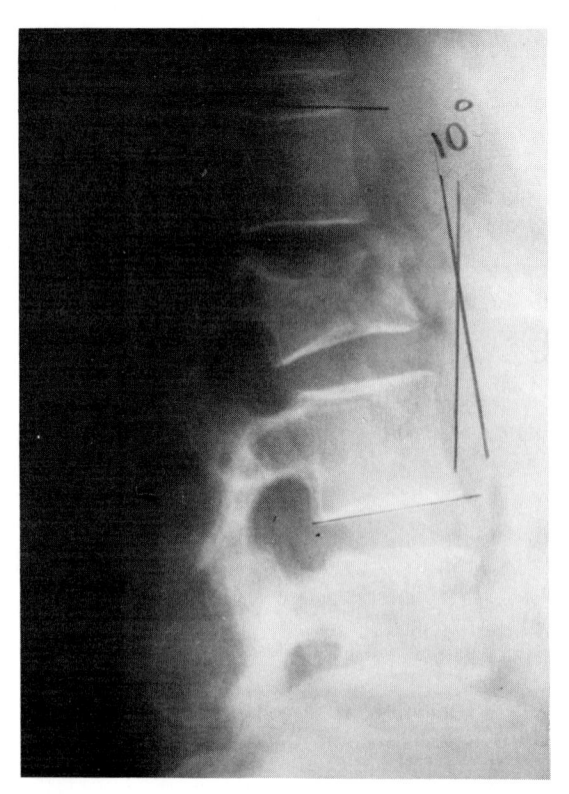

Figure 1. Note burst fracture of L2 with 10° of kyphosis as measured from the top of L1 to the bottom of L3.

2. An "unstable fracture" can then be defined as one where early mobilization in a cast or brace leads to an unacceptable risk of fracture fragment migration, subluxation, or frank dislocation which may lead to a long-term deleterious effect manifested by pain, loss of neurologic function, or spinal deformity.

Conservative management of an "unstable fracture" is possible: a period of bed rest or postural reduction allows enough healing to occur over 6 to 12 weeks to permit mobilization in a cast or brace. Some late deleterious effects may occur, but they are thought by proponents of nonoperative management to be acceptable.

"Highly unstable" fractures represent a subcategory of unstable fractures. These are fractures in which reduction is difficult to maintain even with prolonged bed rest followed by external immobilization. These fractures include the fracture/dislocations, especially those with translation, and burst fractures with posterior element damage. All such fractures must be treated with operative stabilization.

The Role of Decompression

Decompression is carried out only in patients with *incomplete* neurologic deficit in whom there is evidence of canal compromise by bone or disc. Single nerve root lesions are probably not an indication for decompression, as this problem usually improves spontaneously. Patients with complete loss of sensory and motor function do not require any decompressive procedure[5,7] because meaningful neurological improvement from decompression of neural elements is extremely unlikely.

The effects of decompression on neural functioning have been difficult to document. Operation on patients with total neurological deficit is unlikely to result in improvement of function.[45,48,53,55,62,63] Because incomplete lesions tend to improve with time and nonoperative therapy, it has been difficult to demonstrate that surgical decompression has any positive effects.[32,53,62,64]

Restoration of Alignment

Restoration of normal spinal alignment may lead to adequate decompression if the canal is restored to normal dimensions early, if there are no comminuted fragments in the canal, and the posterior longitudinal ligament is intact.[14,45,50,51,62,65] Restoration of the neural foramina and spinal canal is maximized by the correction of vertebral height, alignment, and displacement.[66]

However, even a technically acceptable reduction, using posterior instrumentation to reduce and stabilize a thoracolumbar fracture, does not necessarily alleviate continued compression from fragments of bone or disc within the spinal canal (Figure 2).[67-70] Dickson[48,49] and Flesch[50] both described iatrogenic progressive neurologic deficit and transient paresthesias in several patients after Harrington rod instrumentation without anterior decompression. Fountain used intraoperative myelography to demonstrate that

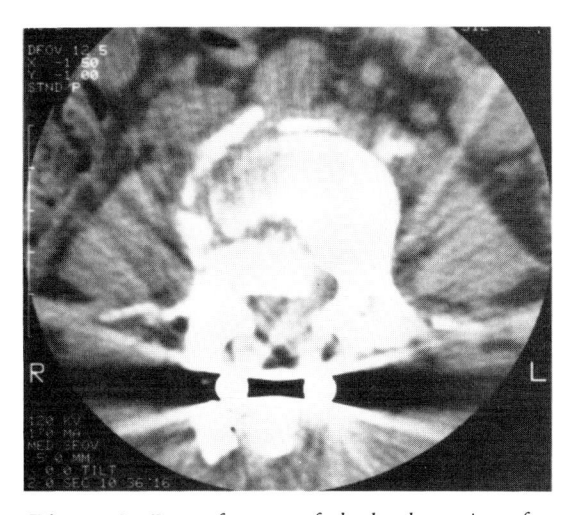

Figure 2. Burst fracture of the lumbar spine after "reduction" with dual Harrington rods. Despite the scatter artifact noted on the CT scan the residual bone fragments within the spinal canal are obvious.

dual Harrington distraction rods frequently do not decompress the spinal canal.[71] Dual posterior Harrington instrumentation with or without posterolateral decompression often leaves persistent anterior impingement.[68,72,73]

In patients with incomplete neurologic injury, who have radiographically demonstrable residual neural compression by bone or disc fragments, anterior decompression is the most common secondary surgical procedure after posterior stabilization.[69,70,73-75]

Laminectomy

Which type of decompressive operation is most effective remains a controversial subject. Holdsworth and Hardy were the first to demonstrate the deleterious effects of laminectomy on spinal stability and neurological functioning.[5,8,26,50,76-79,198] Laminectomy will not produce dural decompression from anteriorly placed bone or soft tissue, rarely results in neurologic improvement,[45,50,80,81,199,200] and will not relieve myelographic block[53,82] or pressure on the dura secondary to anteriorly placed lesions. Laminectomy has no decompressive effect with up to 35% occlusion of the canal.

Moreover, laminectomy increases operative time, blood loss, postoperative pain, subsequent instrument failure,[55,81,83] and early and late instability. The most significant postinjury kyphosis occurs in patients in whom laminectomy has been performed. Laminectomies spanning more than 1.5 segments will complicate stabilization by necessitating fusion over a greater length than the injury would have called for otherwise.[1,18,48-50,61,81,84-86] The presence of a dural tear on CT-myelography is not an indication for laminectomy and repair as traumatic dural tears are frequently on the anterior surface of the dura and cannot be repaired by means of a laminectomy.[18]

In short, no operative procedure other than removal of an anterior mass is beneficial when there is anterior compression of the dural tube. Although laminectomy has been condemned frequently in the past, this point deserves to be reemphasized. Thirty percent of fractures recently reported to a Regional Spinal Cord Injury Center are still being treated with laminectomy.[87] The only rare indication for laminectomy is significant posterior impingement by fragments of the neural arch.[18,66]

Posterolateral Decompression

Unilateral or bilateral posterolateral decompression has been proposed as a method of decompressing the anterior surface of the spinal canal.[50,52,67,70,84,88] This approach has the advantage of allowing concomitant posterior stabilization to be performed without changing the patient's position on the operating table.[50,67,70,83,84,89] Intraoperative sonography can confirm the adequacy of decompression when posterior reduction and posterolateral decompression of burst fragments in the canal are attempted.[12,90,91]

Considerable morbidity is added to the stabilization procedure by this method of decompression. It requires retraction of the dura, and adjacent nerve roots, with the potential for spinal cord injury[12,74,92-94] when decompression is performed at the L2 level and above. In addition, in old injuries retraction may be made difficult by the presence of tethering and scarring at the fracture site.[94] The posterolateral approach frequently does not offer adequate visualization across the entire width of the canal.[69,74,92,93,95] It can lead to excessive hemorrhage,[12] and pneumothorax occurs frequently.[70] Removal of a pedicle can add significant instability to the already injured spine.[50,73] The results of posterolateral decompression are in large part dependent upon the skill of the surgeon, and are not uniformly good. CT frequently demonstrates inadequate decompression after posterior procedures.[67,86,96]

Anterior Decompression

In this author's opinion, anterior decompression is the most effective means of

Thoracolumbar Spine Injuries

treating ventral masses compressing the dura. This approach allows direct visualization and relief of the compression with minimal manipulation of the dural tube, and results in the optimum environment for the recovery of incomplete neural deficits.[3,5,7,35,45,64,69,80,92,93,97-101]

Anterior decompression can bring about complete recovery of neurological deficit in some patients, and the majority with preserved neurological function will improve at least one Frankel grade.[69,102-104] Progressive deficits are halted after anterior decompression.[74] Bradford and McBride demonstrated greater neurologic improvement after anterior spinal decompression than after posterior or posterolateral decompression procedures. The return of bowel and bladder function was more frequent after anterior decompression than after posterior or posterolateral procedures. Only 17% of those approached anteriorly failed to improve, compared with 60% after posterior procedures. The inferior results after the posterior procedures were correlated with residual bony stenosis on CT. Following posterior procedures the average area found to be occupied by bony fragments was approximately 25% of the canal area. After anterior procedures, less than 1% stenosis remained (Figures 3a,b).[47,73]

Specific Injuries and Their Management

Compressive Flexion

Axial loading of the spine in the flexed position causes compressive stress to pass through and damage the anterior elements. The three patterns of injury in this group depend upon whether the posterior and/or middle elements fail in tension.[5,13,28]

Anterior Wedge Compression Fractures

The first pattern is the simple anterior wedge compression fracture. The anterior ele-

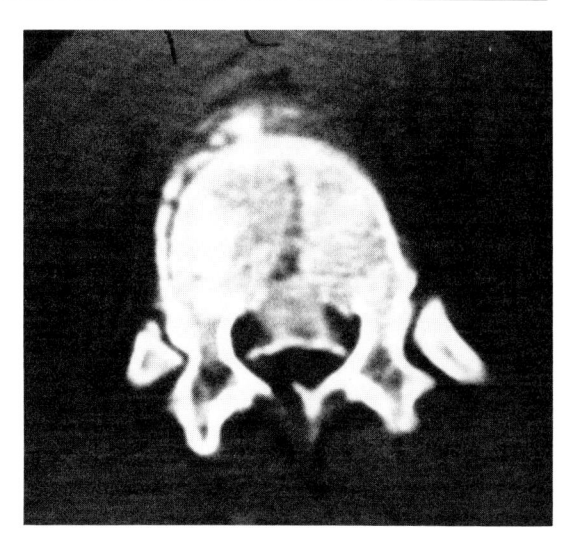

Figure 3a. Burst fracture of T12 with marked canal compromise in a patient with incomplete paraplegia.

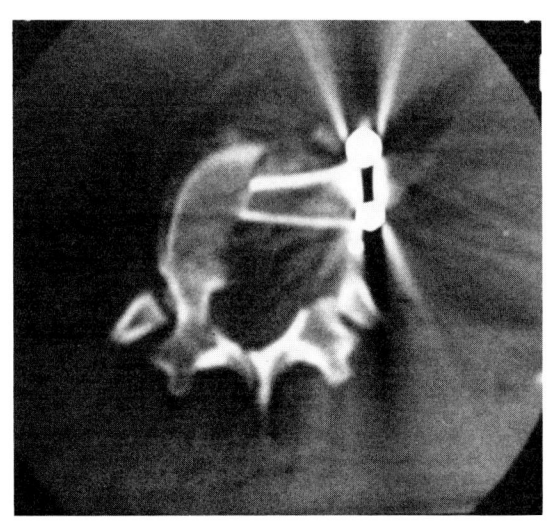

Figure 3b. After anterior decompression, bone grafting, and instrumentation there was complete decompression of the spinal canal. The patient recovered to full walking ability.

ments fail in compression and the posterior and middle elements remain intact.[13,28,34,105,106] Due to the stabilizing effect of the rib cage, simple wedge compression fractures are most commonly seen in the thoracic spine.[106] Less than 50% of the vertebral body height usually is lost. If anterior compression is limited to less than 50%, sufficient posterior ligamentous integrity remains and the fracture is stable.[13,28,105,107]

The radiographic hallmark of this fracture is a decreased anterior vertebral height while the posterior height is unchanged (Figure 4).[12,13,105] The posterior vertebral cortex is intact, so the middle column has not been disturbed. CT scanning demonstrates an irregular arc of anterior bony density displaced circumferentially from the vertebral body, confirming that the neural elements are not disrupted and that the canal has not been transgressed.[13,16,105] If less than 50% of the body height is lost and the CT scan confirms the absence of posterior column disruption, these fractures may be safely treated with early bracing and ambulation.

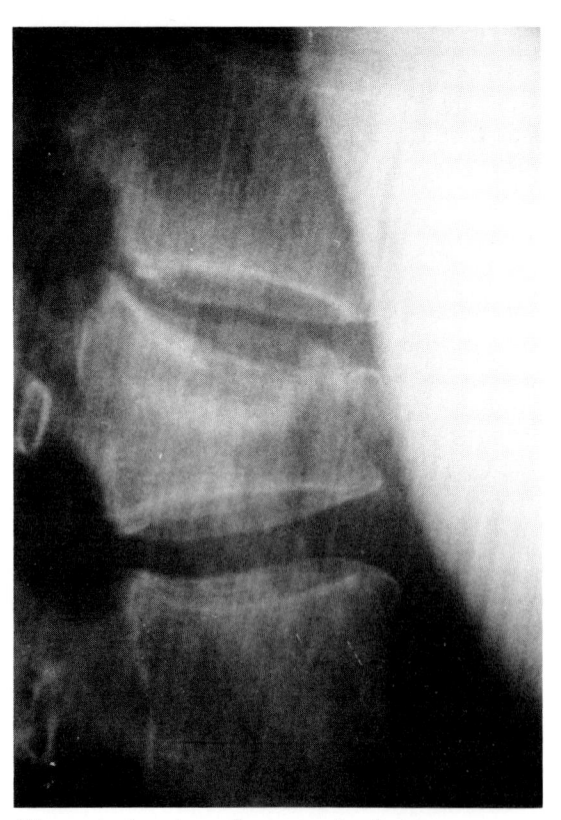

Figure 4. Anterior wedge compression fracture.

Anterior Wedge Compression Fracture and Posterior Element Disruption

Posterior element disruption in association with an anterior wedge fracture is the second stage of injury, and is the most common injury in the lumbar spine.[53] Greater than 50% compression of the anterior vertebral body is usually combined with tension failure and severe disruption of the posterior ligamentous complex.[1,5,28,34,108] Progression of deformity is more likely in this injury than in isolated wedge compression fracture due to tension failure of the posterior elements. Neurologic injury is also more likely. The middle column remains intact, acts as a hinge around which the vertebral body rotates, prevents subluxation, and protects the neural elements.[13,105] The posterior injury is demonstrated on lateral x-ray with an increase of the interspinous distance and adjacent pedicles.[12,105] The articular processes are usually subluxed or dislocated.[13,28,105,107,109] Failure to stabilize this injury may result in an unacceptable, late, painful deformity.[7] These fractures are "unstable" and are best treated with operative stabilization.

Three-Column Injury

The third pattern is the most severe. It is a combined injury of middle element failure along with two other columns. Failure of the middle column to bear load creates a high probability of progression and neurologic injury. It must be recognized and properly treated.[28] The lateral x-ray shows that the posterior vertebral wall height is equal to or increased when compared with the adjacent, inferior vertebral body. In contradistinction to burst fractures, the pedicles remain in continuity with the vertebral body and are not splayed apart.[34] The middle column fails in tension and the posterior wall of the vertebral body is not shortened.[28,108] This injury has a high association with neurologic deficit and progressive spinal deformity. Operative stabilization is essential.

Treatment

Wedge compression fractures with anterior failure alone have no propensity for further progression of spinal deformity or neurologic injury, even with early ambulation.[107,110] Patients are most appropriately treated in a Jewett or other hyperextension brace.[27,34,86,101,111,112]

When the anterior and posterior elements have failed and the middle column remains intact, operative stabilization is required to prevent further deformity. Most authors prefer Harrington instrumentation, and many variations of this technique have been used. Harrington instrumentation with bilateral distraction will restore vertebral body height (Figure 5).[57,66,78,86,113,114] Combined distraction and compression instrumentation with an additional midline compression rod will also serve to preserve lumbar lordosis.[115] Locking hook and spinal rod devices,[116,117] segmental interspinous process wiring,[118] and sublaminar wires[119,120-122] have been used to increase the stability of the construct in an attempt to preserve lordosis. Sublaminar wires may further decrease the incidence of pseudoarthrosis and obviate the need for external immobilization, speeding rehabilitation.[120,122]

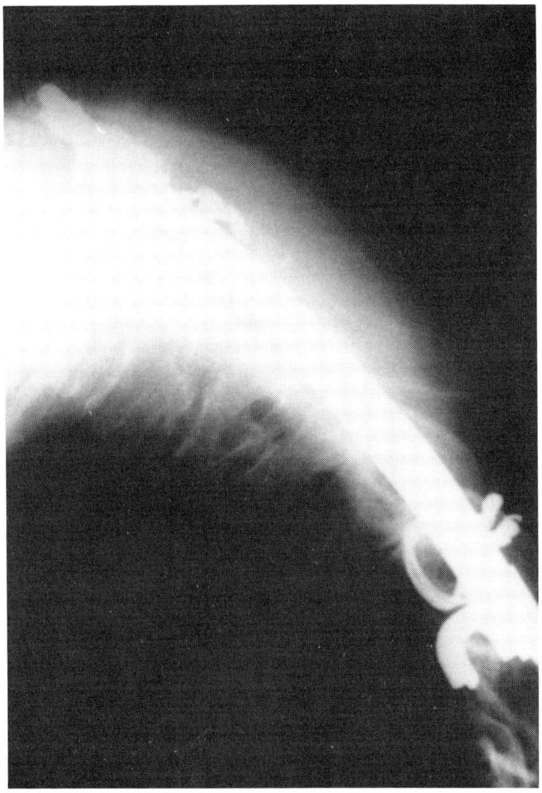

When bone fragments are in the canal or subluxation is present, a distraction apparatus may be chosen.[28,50,60,123] Partial indirect decompression of the retropulsed fragment is sometimes possible when the posterior longitudinal ligament remains attached to this fragment. When sufficient lordosis is restored to the spinal segment, the fragment may be reduced back into position with the ligament. This phenomenon is known as ligamentataxis.[34] Although several authors advocate their use,[124,125] L-rod instrumentation is not appropriate for compression fractures of the thoracolumbar spine. This type of segmental instrumentation does not produce the distracting forces necessary to reduce compression fractures.

Flexion-Distraction

This injury occurs as a result of tension failure of all three columns. The original fracture that Chance described in 1948[126] is a purely bony injury with horizontal splitting of the spinous process and the neural arch. With the flexion component the axis of rotation is anterior to the anterior longitudinal ligament and lies at the level of the abdominal wall.[5,28,127] This is why the injury is frequently associated with lap belt wear.[56,86,127-131] The seat belt acts as a fulcrum around which hyperflexion occurs.

Distraction is an important component of the disruptive force.[13,86,130,131] These injuries are especially likely to occur if the victim is wearing a high-riding or otherwise malpositioned seat belt[132,133] or has slipped under the belt after impact.[130] The resultant flexion-distraction injuries are usually located in the upper lumbar spine, occasionally as high as T12,[127] rarely below L3.[13,53,54,129,130,133]

Concomitant intraabdominal injury is common with this fracture, and may be difficult to diagnose in patients with neurologic

Figure 5. Bilateral Harrington distraction rods used in conjunction with sublaminar wiring in the upper thoracic spine.

deficit. It is thus essential that such patients undergo minilaparotomy and paracentesis after spinal injury.[129,130,133-135] Associated rib, sternal, and long-bone fractures are common.[127,130-133,135,136] Craniofacial trauma is frequently seen as a result of the victim's face and head striking the dash or seat in front of him as he is thrown forward around the belt.

The distractive flexion injuries have been subdivided by Denis, depending on the direction and the type of tissue through which the injury has progressed in a posterior to anterior direction.[13] Type A are fractures which occur at one level—the classic Chance fracture. Type B fractures are also a one-level injury, a flexion-distraction dislocation that is purely ligamentous in nature. Type C fractures are two-level injuries through bone at the level of the middle column. Type D is a two-level injury, passing through ligamentous tissue at the level of the middle column (Figure 6). Gumley et al[130] demonstrated that injury to the posterior elements may occur through the middle or base of the spinous processes, or there may be an asymmetric injury of the posterior elements due to rotatory forces.

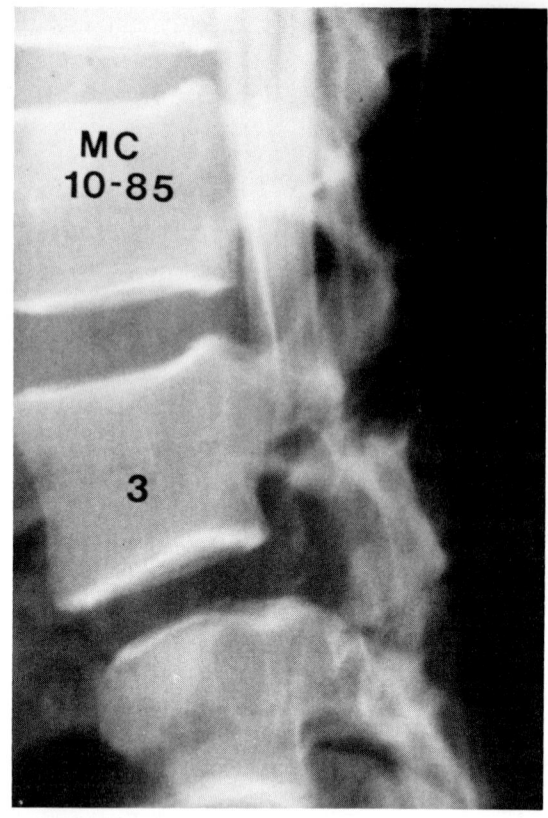

Figure 6. Distractive flexion injury. The injury passes through the posterior bony elements of L3 and disrupts the L3-L4 disc space. Note the myelographic block at the injury site.

Treatment

The true Chance fracture, Denis type A, is fairly uncommon. Union of the vertebral cancellous surfaces occurs with regularity if the fracture is reduced and there is coaptation of the cancellous surfaces[130] while the patient is immobilized in a hyperextension cast or brace. Surgical reduction and bracing is also an acceptable option for more immediate mobilization.[83,86,111]

Operative treatment is necessary for the majority of flexion-distraction injuries, which occur through ligamentous tissue. Although they are stable initially, late instability may occur.[7,130] Because the posterior anatomic hinge has been disrupted, the treatment of choice is bilateral compression instrumentation to counter the tension failure of the posterior elements.[1,12,28,52,60,62,66,86,114] If there is moderate to severe anterior compression of the vertebral body, distraction rods[129] or a combination of distraction and compression instrumentation may be necessary.[1]

Compression instrumentation acts as a hinge, creating a posterior tension banding system,[12,60,66,85,108,114] providing superior stability and better restoration of anatomy than other types of instrumentation (Figure 7).[85,135] Distraction instrumentation may be used but requires fusion over a longer distance, requiring an average of 5.5 segments as compared to the two segments needed for compression instrumentation.[66,108,135,137]

Lateral Flexion

Lateral flexion injuries occur from eccentric axial loading forces that cause lateral bending of the spine.[28] Compression failure

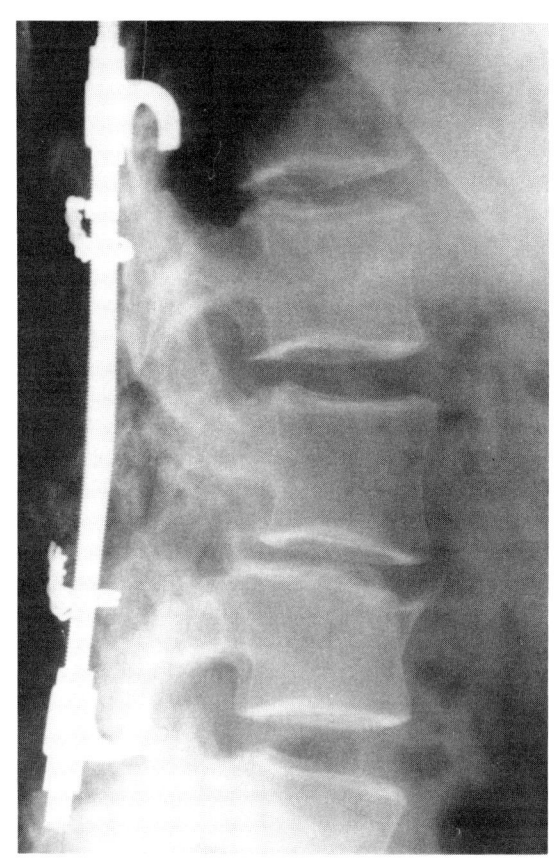

Figure 7. Lateral x-ray after reduction and fusion of a Chance fracture with bilateral Harrington compression rods.

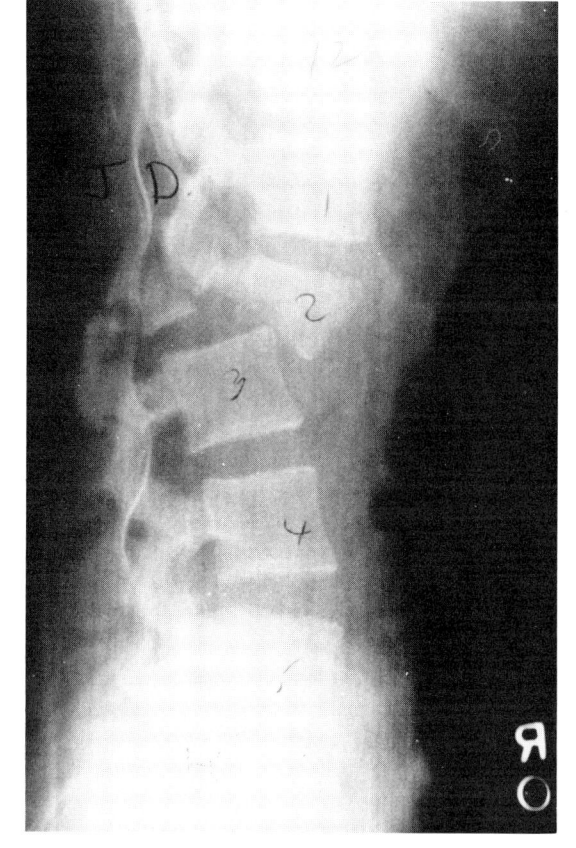

Figure 8. Posterior-anterior shear injury with resultant dislocation of L2 on L3.

occurs on the concave side of the spine while tension failure of the bony and ligamentous structures occurs on the convex side, with the fulcrum located within the vertebral body (Figure 8).

If only the middle and anterior columns are involved, the deformity is unlikely to progress. If the posterior elements also fail, the incidence of late pain due to continued deformity increases. Neurologic injury may occur if the middle column element encroaches on the neural canal.[27,28] Patients with neurologic deficit after this fracture show the best overall improvement with the least profound deficits when compared to patients with other types of injuries.[61]

Several techniques are available to treat this fracture pattern. Harrington distraction instrumentation or segmental spinal instrumentation has been applied successfully.[28,108] Harrington distraction rods are used on the concave side of the deformity combined with compression rods on the convex side.[61] If middle-element failure has caused spinal canal impingement, Harrington distraction instrumentation is the procedure of choice to prevent axial loading and possible further encroachment on the neural canal by the middle element. The necessity for anterior decompression is dictated by the severity of neural compression and deficit.[28]

Translational or Shear Type Fracture/Dislocation

Fracture dislocations secondary to shear are caused by forces of injury which displace the vertebral body anteriorly, posteriorly, or laterally.[5,13,28,105] Shearing forces are most commonly the result of massive blows to the back.[11,138] Gross displacement of the vertebral bodies is associated with fractures of the articular processes and ligamentous rupture. Significant neurologic deficit is common.[11]

Shear occurs for the most part in the sagittal plane. Posteroanterior shear, when the segment above shears forward off the segment below, is seen when injury occurs with the patient in an extended position. There is no loss of vertebral height.[13] The posterior arch of the vertebral segment is fractured as it rides forward through the posterior elements of the level below, leading to free-floating laminae, fractures of several spinous processes, fracture of the superior facet of the inferior vertebra, and disruption of the anterior longitudinal ligament.[11,13,58]

With displacements of 25% or more, the articular processes and all ligamentous structures, including the anterior longitudinal ligaments, are ruptured. If the articular processes are also fractured, there are few, if any, elements providing spinal stability. Acute and chronic deformities may result. These are highly unstable lesions which require operative stabilization.[5,7,11,13,58,105]

Shear is frequently associated with other injury mechanisms and rarely occurs in a pure form. Associated injuries usually include rib fractures, and lung contusions, sternal fractures, and most frequently, pneumothorax, hemothorax, or both.[50,58,95]

Due to the extreme degree of canal compromise, 80% or more of patients with injuries at the thoracolumbar junction and above sustain complete paraplegia. Discontinuity of the spinal canal is nearly complete.[13,34,86] There are isolated reports of patients who have sustained significant bony injuries without neurologic compromise, when multiple pedicular fractures dissociate the anterior elements from the posterior elements. This traumatic spondylolysis causes widening of the spinal canal, leaving the neural elements intact.[58,139-142,195] In the lumbar spine, there is a large area for the conus medullaris or cauda equina, and few patients sustain significant neural injury after this fracture.[34,138]

Treatment

Reduction of these dislocations can be difficult,[138] especially when there is dissociation of the body from the spinous processes. Operative treatment in the past used Harrington distraction.[49,57,78] The posterior longitudinal ligament is usually completely transected. If the body is displaced more than 25%, the anterior longitudinal ligament may also be ruptured, allowing overdistraction to occur.[28,75] To minimize overdistraction, the posterior elements of the injured vertebra may be wired together before distraction,[115] and a short midline compression rod across the injured vertebral segments may counteract the distraction.[85,143]

A significant failure rate accompanies the use of Harrington rods to treat this injury. Pseudarthrosis is most likely to occur after distraction instrumentation of translational injuries, and is associated with hook dislodgement.[55,61,75] The use of Harrington distraction rods supplemented by sublaminar wires improves resistance to axial loads, lateral bending, and forward flexion, but the greatest improvement is in resistance to rotatory stresses. Sublaminar wiring will decrease the pseudoarthrosis rate and the incidence of hook cutout.[111,119,120,122]

The use of L-rods and sublaminar wiring produces very rigid fixation, especially with respect to rotation.[114,144] Luque instrumentation is best reserved for complete neural injuries[83,114,119,121,145,146] as external immobilization is no longer necessary when the segmental fixation is employed.[121] Segmental fixation with either Harrington distraction rods supplemented by sublaminar,[119,120-122,146] interspinous wires,[118] or Luque rods may be used.[28] Since Luque rods require no stability from the anterior longitudinal ligament, overdistraction cannot occur. These rods afford an excellent means of stabilizing translational injuries.[28] Roy-Camille plates and pedicular fixation have also been used for this injury[147,148,149,150] as has the internal fixator of Dick.[65]

Torsional Flexion or Rotation/ Flexion Dislocation

The most unstable fracture of the thoracolumbar spine is the rotatory fracture dislocation.[11,13,28,101] These unstable flexion/rotation dislocations are frequently located at the thoracolumbar junction (Figure 9). This injury occurs from torsion and compression of the anterior elements and simultaneous tension and torsion of the posterior elements.[13,28,105,106] The articular processes are usually fractured and dislocated as a result of the rotatory forces which produce the injury.[11,13,105] Middle-column injuries are frequently present and occur through either the vertebral body or disc along with wedging of the inferior vertebral body.[13] Usually, a slice of the inferior vertebral body attached to the annulus is fractured in the sagittal plane and translated anteriorly or laterally.[5,11,13,94,106] The anterior longitudinal ligament is usually stripped from the anterior border of the involved vertebra.[5,13,28]

This lesion is most common in the thoracic spine, and the majority of patients sustain complete neurologic injury. The most unstable patients are those with anterior subluxation. Roberts and Curtiss[123] were able to demonstrate only a very low incidence of spontaneous fusion with progressive deformity in most patients. Fractures occurring above T8-T9 have little further progression of the deformity due to the stabilizing influences of the rib cage. Although Denis noted no neurologic injury in 25% of his fracture/dislocations, more than 50% of patients had complete neurologic injury.[13]

Other authors have also documented profound neurologic deficit from this injury. Sixty to 70% of patients will have complete injuries, and the remainder significant though incomplete injury.[50,61] Neural recovery after decompression of flexion/rotation injuries is not as complete as that obtained after decompression of burst fractures.[151]

Treatment

Patients with complete spinal cord injury and grossly unstable rotatory fracture-dislocation will require posterior open reduction and internal fixation with posterior arthrodesis. These torsional flexion injuries may be treated with Harrington instrumentation.[5,28,49,57,61,62,71,78] Bilateral Harrington rod instrumentation acts like a beam lying between the spinous processes and facets to prevent rotation.[52,152,153] However, Harrington rods are relatively weak in preventing rotation,[65] and supplementation with either a short compression rod to resist tensile forces or with sublaminar wiring is recommended.[83,143,146] Segmental spinal instrumentation with L-rods has been recommended for this injury[28,119,146] and is best for preventing rotation.[65] Roy-Camille also describes his experience with pedicular screw plating for this fracture.[147-150] Patients who

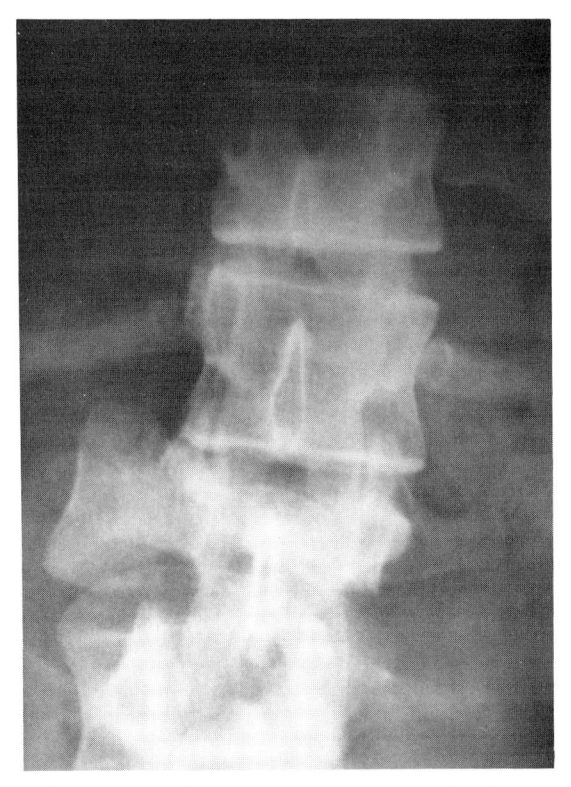

Figure 9. Flexion/rotation dislocation of the thoracolumbar junction.

have sustained complete neurologic injury are probably best treated by compression instrumentation; a shorter length of spine needs to be instrumented and fixation is stronger.[52]

Burst Fracture

The burst compression fracture of the thoracolumbar spine is the most common major spine injury. Holdsworth[26] believed that this injury occurred when the entire spine was placed in a relatively straight position with axial compression applied to the body in a nearly symmetric fashion, causing the vertebral body to explode. The height of the vertebral body diminishes as the anterior, posterior, and lateral walls of the vertebral body are disrupted. The longitudinally oriented anterior and posterior longitudinal ligaments are vertically shortened and bowed out around the expanded bone. As the cephalic half of the vertebral body is crushed, the rim of cortical bone is broken into a number of fragments which are displaced outward from the vertebral body in a circumferential fashion (Figure 10).[5,11,28,34,105,154]

The majority of burst fractures occur between T10 and L2.[13,38,39,48,89,101,151,155]

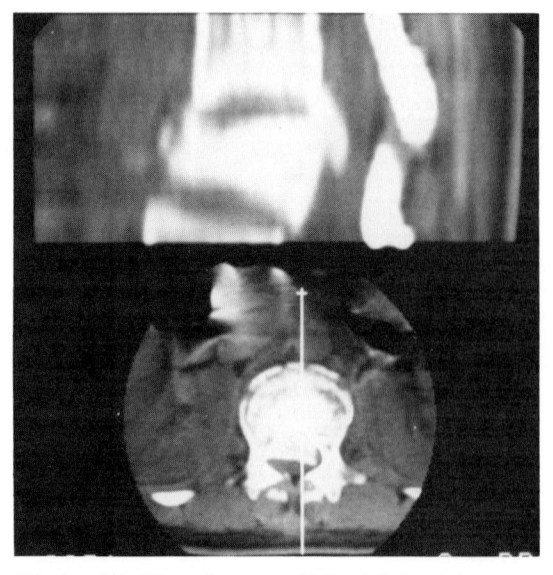

Figure 10. Burst fracture of L2 with bone fragments circumferentially displaced outward from the body and retropulsed into the spinal canal.

Severe burst fractures are frequently accompanied by compression fractures above or below the fractured level.[11,156] These injuries may be associated with posterior dural tears, allowing posterior interlaminar herniation of the cauda equina and entrapment or amputation of nerve roots.[157] A significant association is seen between fracture of the os calcis and long bones as well as between ligamentous injuries to the knee and intraabdominal injuries.[39]

The radiographic hallmark of these fractures on plain x-ray is widening of both the AP and transverse diameters of the vertebral body. On the AP film there is widening of the interpedicular distance.[7,13,28,156] On the lateral x-ray, posterior height is lost and there is spreading of the vertebral body, representing failure of the middle column.[7,12,13,105]

Axial CT scanning is essential in the evaluation of burst fractures, and is especially helpful in assessing the degree of compromise of the spinal canal (Figure 11).[1,2,7,11,12,14,16,24,39,86,89,156,158-165] CT scanning also offers the best assessment of facet congruity,[86] the degree of foraminal compromise,[155] the extent of disruption of the anterior and posterior borders of the vertebral body, and comminution of the vertebral bodies.[13,86]

Sagittally oriented fractures are usually noted in the lower third of the vertebral body.[16,166] Vertebral body fragments are distributed in a centripetally oriented array, in-

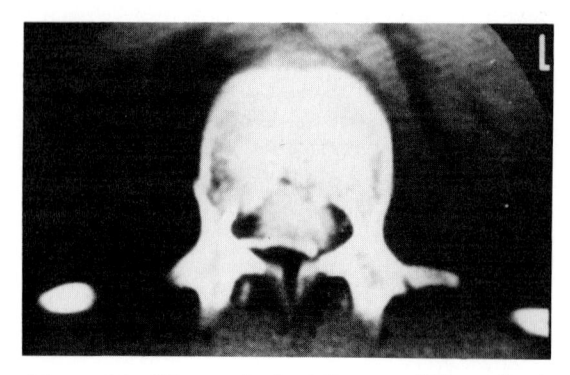

Figure 11. CT scan of a burst fracture which reveals almost complete obliteration of the spinal canal.

dicating that the longitudinal ligaments are intact.[154,156,166] Although this is the usual case,[75,167] the fragments do not always remain attached to the longitudinal ligaments.[168]

The hallmark of axial compression is retropulsion of the vertebral body into the spinal canal. The fragment may pivot so that the cortical surface normally facing the spinal canal no longer is vertical but projects into the canal. The fragment is displaced 2-4 mm or more posteriorly so that it is posterior to the lower corner of the adjacent vertebral body[9,16,94] rather than directly below it.

Holdsworth considered all burst fractures to be stable, and treated them with a body cast or an orthosis.[83,86] However, subsequent experience has shown that ambulation of a patient with a disrupted middle column may cause further axial loading of the spine and progression of neurologic deficit.[108,162] These fractures are now considered to be unstable. Within this subgroup of unstable fractures there are injuries with a greater relative inherent stability ("stable" burst fractures) and those which are highly unstable. Burst fractures have been considered "stable" if the posterior column remains intact. A burst fracture is unstable if there is subluxation of one or more facet joints, a displaced fracture of the neural arch, posterior ligamentous injuries, or gross displacement of neural elements.[86,89,101,108,109,156]

Neurologic deficit sustained after burst fractures is usually incomplete.[13,73] Unstable burst fractures are associated with the most severe neurologic deficits, although there are instances where the canal can be occluded up to 90% in "stable" burst fractures.[69,86] Denis found few neurologic injuries where the canal was compromised 50% or less and few injuries of Frankel grade B or C were sustained with canal occlusions 75% or greater.[13] Most authors have found no direct correlation between the amount of canal encroachment and associated neurologic injury.[13-17,61,86,89]

Many authors feel that conservative treatment of burst fractures carries an unacceptably high percentage of unsatisfactory results. Nonoperative treatment of burst fractures may be associated with progressive neurologic deficit and posttraumatic spinal stenosis. Posttraumatic kyphosis has been reported to increase in at least 20% of patients treated without operation. Paraparesis and radicular symptoms were demonstrated in 17% of patients treated nonoperatively in one study,[39] although neurological deterioration does not always occur in patients with canal compromise.[37,38] Resolution of small bony fragments and adaptive changes in canal morphology by bony remodeling may occur. These changes are age related, presenting more frequently in younger patients.[37]

Treatment

Prophylactic stabilization and fixation of so-called "stable" burst fractures in intact patients prevents neurologic deficits, allows early, safe mobilization, prevents late kyphosis and degenerative changes, and decreases postoperative pain.[37,39,152,153] However, operative risks include failure of fixation, pseudarthrosis, neurologic damage, and failure to decompress the neural elements adequately.[37]

Bilateral Harrington distraction instrumentation has been used most frequently in posterior stabilization. It has been the most effective instrumentation in restoring vertebral height. Harrington instrumentation may partially reduce the retropulsed posterior wall of the vertebral body. Angulation is resisted by the beam effect on the intact lamina.[1,5,12,28,57,66,78,85,86,96,102,114,169]

Harrington instrumentation has weaknesses that limit its effectiveness in treating burst fractures. While distraction does tend to lengthen the middle column, it depends upon distraction to keep the hooks under the lamina. Harrington rods have very limited firm skeletal purchase.[111,170] A burst fracture may settle even after Harrington instrumentation and may recur if straight Harrington rods are used.[41]

Several adaptations of posterior instrumentation have been used to correct these shortcomings. Harrington and "universal" rods have been supplemented by the application of variously sized rod sleeves. These allow shorter fusions and application of an anteriorly directed force while preserving lordosis. Rod sleeves allow the use of noncontoured rods and make it easier to insert hooks.[66,154] The locking rods of Jacobs can also be used, with contouring of the rods to preserve lordosis and maintain the tension on the anterior structures.[116,117]

Wired Harrington rods provide improved axial stability and are best at resisting compressive loads. Many authors advocate their use in treating unstable burst fractures.[65,83,108,111,119,121,167] The addition of the sublaminar wires prevents progression of kyphosis[154] and decreases the need for external immobilization.[83,119,145,146] The use of segmental spinal fixation with sublaminar wires must be carefully considered in light of its risk in intact patients[114] and should be avoided at and adjacent to the site of injury.

Cotrel-Dubousset instrumentation is used with increasing frequency in the treatment of burst fractures and other spinal fractures (Figure 12a,b). The technique accomplishes

Figure 12a. An L1 burst fracture in an incomplete paraplegic treated with posterior Cotrel-Dubousset instrumentation and fusion.

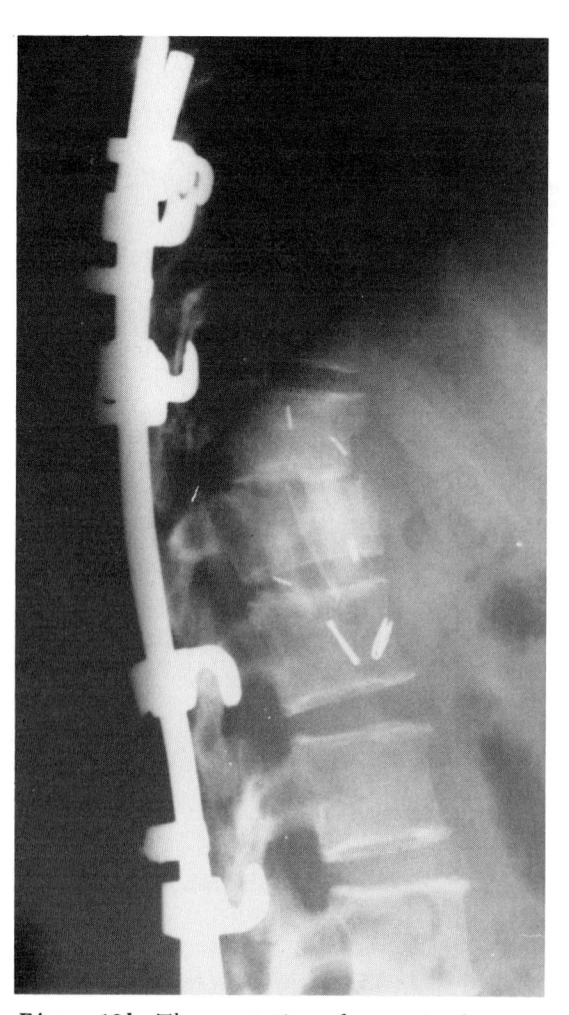

Figure 12b. The same patient after anterior decompression and strut grafting with iliac crest bone grafts.

three-point bending as does the classic Harrington system. It is rigidly attached to the uppermost vertebra so that overdistraction is not necessary to maintain the superior hook in position. Segmental fixation is accomplished without the need for sublaminar wires. Rotational stability can be improved by the use of the DTT between the two rods.[154,171,172]

The pedicle is considered by some to be ideal for fixation in these injuries.[173] Pedicle screw plates have been used[149,150] and an internal spinal skeletal fixator has been designed by Dick et al.[174] The major advantage of the "internal fixator" is that it is only applied to the vertebrae immediately adjacent to the fracture, thereby decreasing the extent of surgical fusion and preserving lordosis. Strong fixation allows rapid mobilization with good restoration of vertebral anatomy and indirect decompression of the neural canal without the need for further anterior decompression.[65,173-177]

Because of the mechanical defect still present in the anterior and middle columns, anterior bone grafting through the pedicle or via an anterior approach to reduce the incidence of fatigue failure of the internal fixator has been suggested.[65,174,176,177] The internal fixator can be used in any type of lesion; it does not require the presence of intact longitudinal ligaments, nor does it depend upon intact posterior elements or the posterior wall of the vertebral body.[65,174]

Luque instrumentation has no role in the treatment of burst fractures as it cannot be used to produce axial distraction.[125] The use of Luque rods in patients with burst fractures is associated with the highest percentage of reoperation of any form of instrumentation.[45]

Although favored in the past, Harrington rods have been less than ideal in the treatment of burst fractures, and should not be the primary treatment in patients with incomplete neurologic deficit.[64,168] Although the vertebral body fragments within the canal can be successfully reduced with distraction in some cases, ligamentaxis may not always be successful in reducing the fragment.[12,14,68,161] Many authors have found that better results can be obtained with removal of the anterior vertebral body.[5,14,28,34,48,68,96,103,154,168] Dickson[48] and Flesch[50] both documented progressive neurologic deficit after Harrington rod instrumentation in patients who did not undergo anterior decompression.

Considerable controversy exists regarding the timing of anterior decompression, and whether anterior or posterior instrumentation should be employed. Some authors have suggested that it is unnecessary to perform anterior surgery soon after injury, treating only those who develop new neurologic deficit or whose recovery plateaus with later anterior surgical decompression.[51,80,98] Whitesides and Shah were the first to advocate a two-stage approach: posterior spinal fusion followed by anterior decompression.[69,89,99,101] A number of authors believe that a posterolateral approach used with posterior instrumentation affords sufficient decompression.[50,83,84,89]

Numerous attempts have been made to carry out anterior decompression and instrumentation. Anterior fusion without instrumentation was associated with progressive kyphosis, although no greater than that allowed by posterior Harrington instrumentation.[35] Zielke instrumentation has been used, but was not biomechanically suited for fracture management.[99] AO broad plates were used for anterior fixation after Harrington instrumentation was used for distraction[58] but these plates were associated with nonunion,[168] and the Dunn instrumentation device[93] has been withdrawn from the market because of a small incidence of vascular injuries occurring after long-term implantation.[154]

Kostuik reported on anterior decompression along with anterior fixation for burst fractures in patients with and without incomplete neurologic injuries.[103,168] There is no need for posterior fusion and instrumentation when using the Kostuik/Harrington distraction rods and compression system. This combination is sufficiently rigid to allow early rehabilitation and ambulation with an orthosis. The anterior decompression is performed and the defect is filled by iliac crest grafting.[168]

The indications for this approach include the following: (1) acute burst fractures involving the anterior and middle columns with retropulsion of bone into the canal in patients with neurologic deficit, (2) late burst injuries (those that are treated 10 or more days after injury) that are difficult to reduce posteriorly, (3) painful and/or progressive kyphosis with or without neurologic deficit. Kostuik also believes that anterior surgery serves to preserve motion segments if there is no injury at the lower lumbar spine.[7,93,162] Stabilization is limited to one vertebral body above and below the fracture.[154,162] Lordosis can be preserved with this approach, and kyphosis is eliminated (Figures 13a,b).

Classification of Burst Fractures

Opinion regarding the treatment of burst fractures remains fragmented.[69,89,93,99,101] In order to select a treatment it is necessary to distinguish among upper burst fractures (T12-L1), middle burst fractures (L2-L3), and lower burst fractures (L4-L5). Each of these areas demands special consideration because of unique anatomy. In each category the differentiation between a stable burst injury and an unstable burst injury must be made.

Decision Making in Upper Burst Injuries

The upper burst fracture is anatomically unique from the other two because the canal still contains the spinal cord or conus medullaris. Of considerable importance as well is the availability of at least four or five interspaces below the fracture, depending upon the exact level of injury and the presence or absence of lumbosacral anaomalies. Each of these factors will weigh in the decision making.

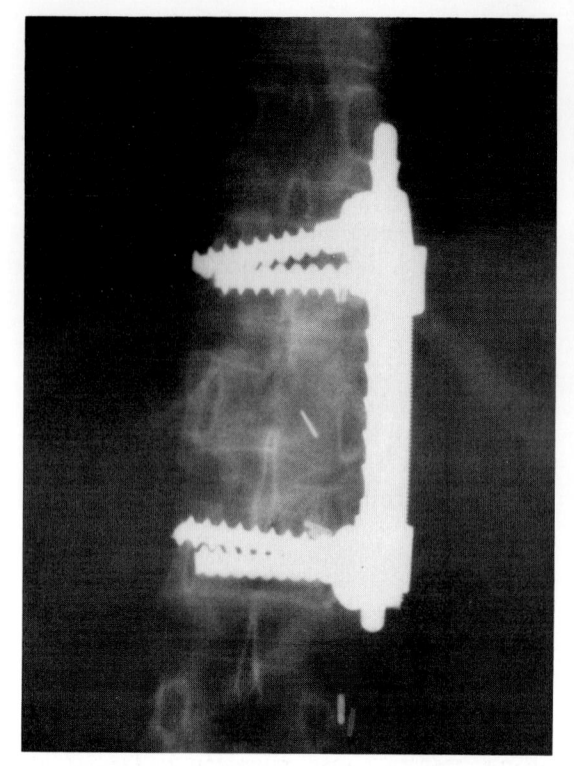

Figure 13a. AP view of anterior Kostuik-Harrington instrumentation and fusion.

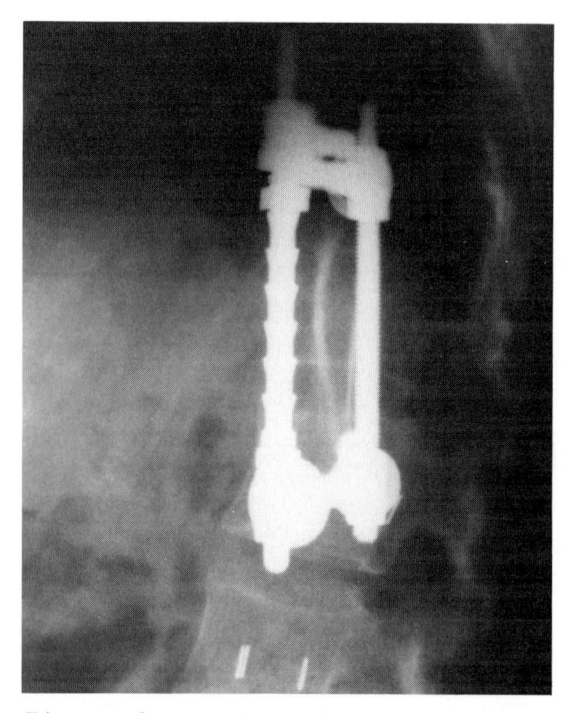

Figure 13b. Lateral view of anterior Kostuik-Harrington instrumentation and fusion.

Thoracolumbar Spine Injuries

The presence or absence of neurologic deficit is the single most important factor in decision making. The presence of profound but incomplete neural deficit in association with canal compromise represents an urgent indication for surgical decompression. Three methods of decompression are available, two direct and one indirect.

Indirect decompression is accomplished by a variety of posterior instrumentation procedures, relying upon correction of kyphosis and ligamentaxis to achieve canal clearance. As mentioned previously, this is not without risk of iatrogenic neural injury and at best produces incomplete canal decompression. This technique is the most dangerous at the upper level where the spinal cord and conus medullaris are present.

Direct decompression may be achieved through a posterolateral or anterior approach. Posterolateral decompression may be performed after partial indirect decompression using posterior instrumentation. Posterolateral decompression usually entails unilateral pedicle resection, which has the disadvantage of exacerbating preexisting instability. However, the far side of the spinal canal is difficult to decompress with unilateral posterolateral decompression, even in experienced hands. Bilateral posterolateral decompression obviates this disadvantage but further enhances instability.

The remaining choice involves direct anterior decompression, either combined with anterior stabilization or following a posterior instrumentation and decompression. The risk of iatrogenic neurologic injury is lowest with this procedure given the proximity of the cord and conus, and it is the most effective means of decompressing the spinal canal.[103,168]

No firm criteria have yet been established for the neurologically intact patient regarding the need for and the extent to which canal decompression must be performed. A partial decompression in the neurologically intact patient combined with reduction of the kyphus and a stable fusion may well suffice. The answer to this can only be determined after long-term follow-up.

There is no one overwhelming choice of instrumentation systems to suggest to the reader. In treating these patients the surgeon has great latitude in selecting surgical techniques (Figures 14a,b). Each surgeon should select a technique with which he is familiar

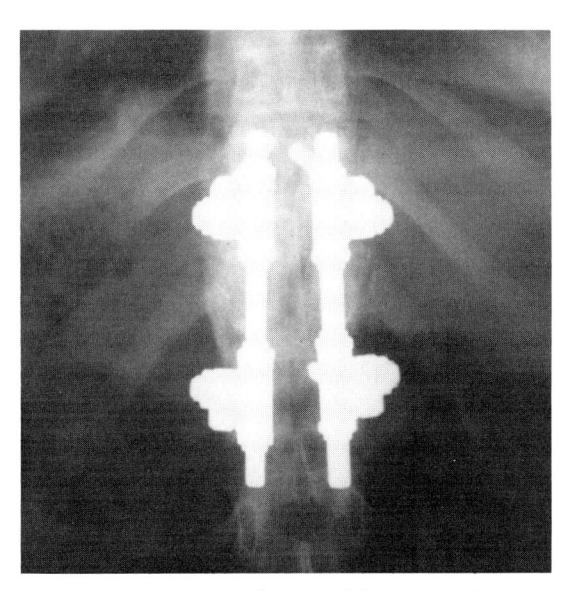

Figure 14a. AP view of "internal fixator" used to treat a T12 burst fracture.

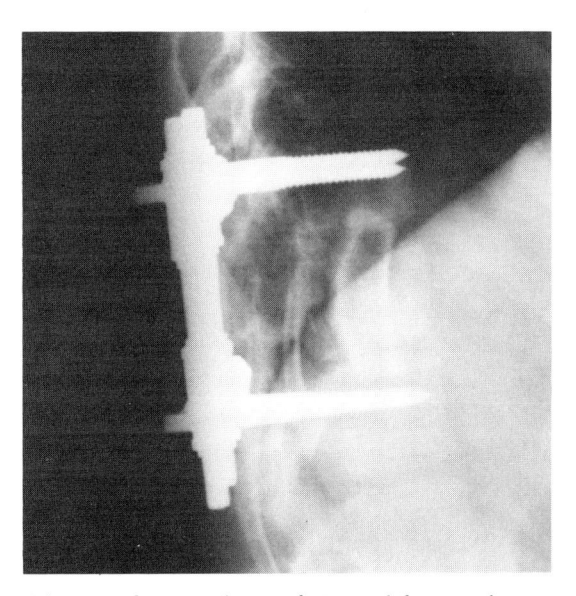

Figure 14b. Lateral view of "internal fixator" showing instrumentation and decompression and strut grafting of T12.

and knows is well within his surgical capabilities. The incomplete lesion of the upper lumbar spine is not the place to use a technique with which the surgeon is still on his "learning curve." However, because of the availability of multiple open segments below the injury level, standard techniques more familiar to surgeons as well as the newer techniques including pedicular fixation techniques may be selected.

In this author's opinion, patients with neurologic deficits and bony injury in this region should be treated with anterior decompression and internal fixation (Figures 15a,b). "Highly unstable" burst fractures should have supplemental posterior fixation. Neurologically normal patients may be treated either anteriorly or posteriorly, depending on the patient's medical condition, age, degree of canal compromise, and stability.

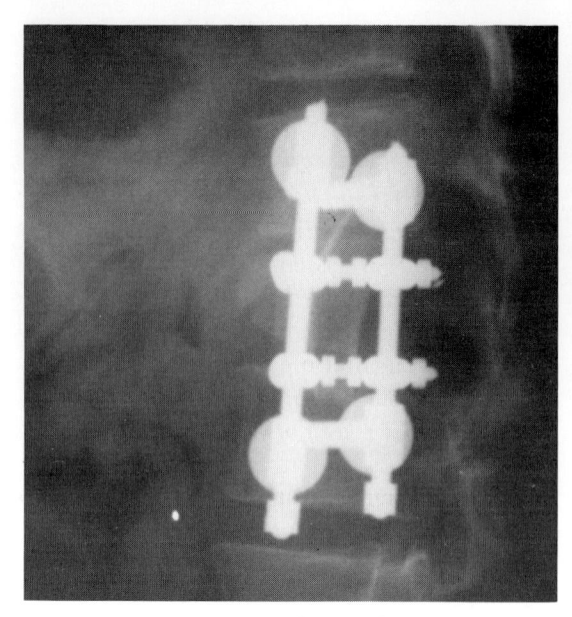

Figure 15b. Lateral view showing the dual compression rods linked by two "DTT" devices.

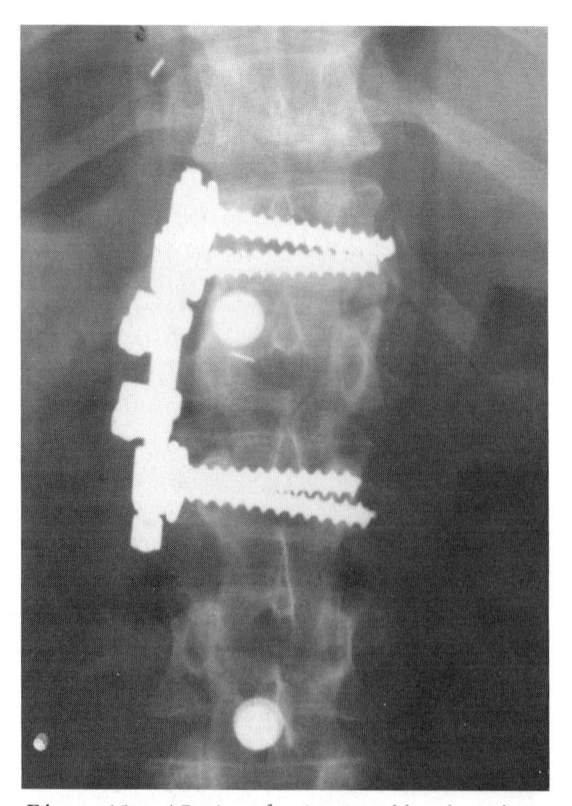

Figure 15a. AP view of a 31-year-old male with L1 burst fracture and incomplete paraplegia treated with primary anterior decompression, fusion, and anterior Kostuik-Harrington instrumentation.

Decision Making in Middle Burst Injuries without Neurologic Injury

Injuries to the L2-L3 vertebral levels are relatively common. In this area, the conus medullaris gives way to the cauda equina. The increased size of the spinal canal and the presence of peripheral nerve rather than spinal cord accounts for the number of patients who are neurologically normal despite a significant degree of canal compromise.

The choices for decompression of middle burst fractures are the same as with upper burst fractures. Once again, indirect decompression and posterolateral decompression may be used. Improved decompression can be achieved if reduction is performed soon after injury. Iatrogenic injury is less likely to occur at this level because the spinal cord and conus are no longer present. Anterior decompression is more complete; however, this must be balanced by the unknown factor of how much decompression is necessary below the level of the conus to restore function of the cauda equina.

The selection of instrumentation in middle burst fractures is more crucial than in upper lumbar injuries. Instrumentation which permits fixation of only one level below the fracture will help preserve needed lumbar mobility. The injury to the anterior and middle column will put significant stress on posterior instrumentation. Significant posterior column involvement will produce three-column instability, which will significantly stress any instrumentation system. For this reason, serious consideration should be given to anterior grafting procedures, with or without anterior instrumentation, to provide additional stability in cases where excellent anatomic reduction of fragments has not been achieved.

Anterior grafting may be performed with a bone strut of iliac crest, fibula, or bone allograft. A form of anterior grafting for body reinforcement may also be accomplished by adding morselized bone via the transpedicular route prior to pedicular fixation.[65,174] Anterior strut grafting may be performed as the primary procedure and followed by posterior instrumentation or may be done after posterior stabilization is accomplished.

When a primary anterior decompression, instrumentation and bony fusion has been selected, a posterior approach can often be avoided. The exception to this would be the highly unstable burst fracture with complete disruption of one or more facets posteriorly. Translation on the AP x-ray or documentation of posterior element destruction on the CT scan is also a sign of a highly unstable injury, and requires posterior stabilization after anterior decompression and stabilization. Failure to perform posterior stabilization will result in instrument failure, progressive deformity, or neurologic injury.

The surgeon's choices are much more restricted here than in upper lumbar lesions. However, neurologic impairment is less common in these lesions and the indications for operative decompression fewer. The primary decision making on instrumentation techniques should be determined by the surgeon's decision not to fuse lower than L3 or L4. Conservative management is a far better solution with greater future options open to the patient than a long fused lumbar spine with loss of lordosis and only the L5-S1 disc preserved.

The middle burst injury is best treated by either anterior or posterior instrumentation one level above or below the injury. There is no role for "long" instrumentation techniques, or distraction at this level in the lumbar spine.

Decision Making in Lower Burst Injuries

Although burst compression fractures of L4 and L5 are uncommon injuries[155,178,192] they deserve special comment (Figures 16a,b). Several authors have shown that residual bony deformity after conservative care in a cast or brace causes less morbidity than reduction with Harrington rods or Luque instrumentation.[7,155,178] Although loss of lordosis occurs in all patients with fractures at this level, whether they are treated conser-

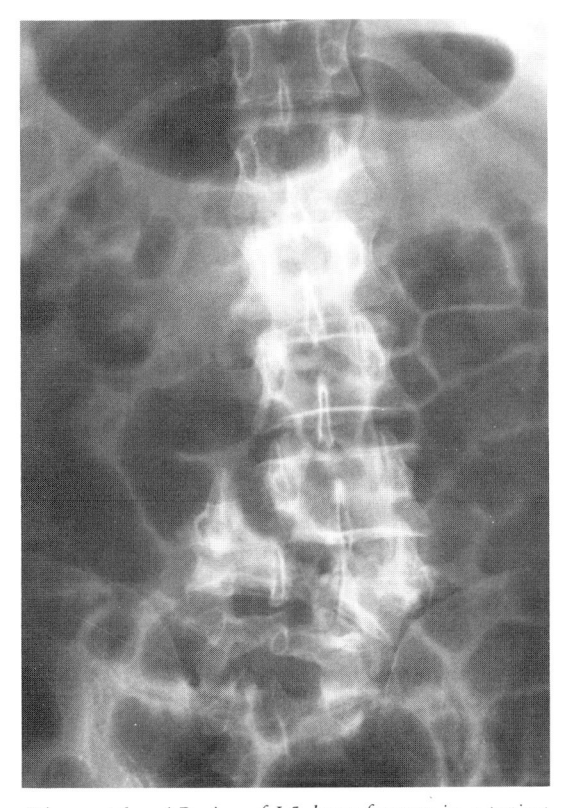

Figure 16a. AP view of L5 burst fracture in a patient with six lumbar vertebrae.

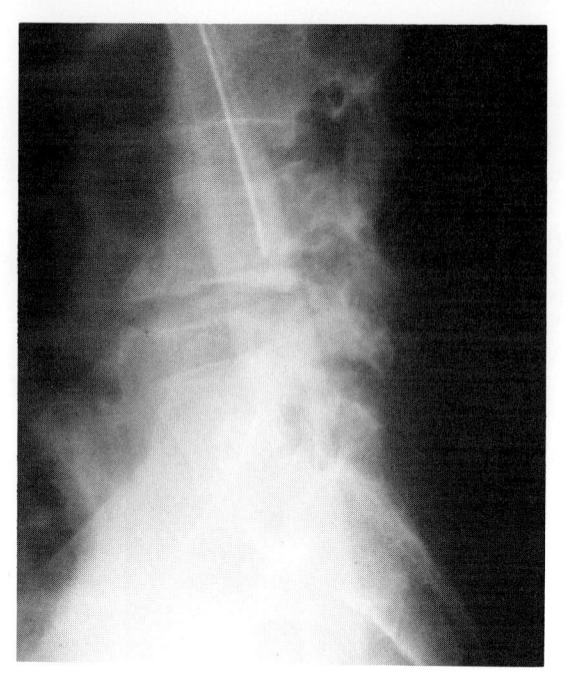

Figure 16b. Lateral view of severe burst injury of L5.

vatively or with instrumentation, the loss of lordosis in patients treated with Harrington distraction instrumentation is greater than in patients treated conservatively.[178]

Several authors reported better results using posterior instrumentation. Byrd reports solid fusion and preservation of lordosis after decompression, posterolateral fusion, and Steffee plating. Edwards advocates use of the rod-sleeve instrumentation with pedicular fixation in the middle segment for burst fractures of L4-L5. This system restricts fusion to two levels, and preserves lordosis.[179]

Neurologic deficit is usually minor after burst fractures of L4 or L5, despite significant neural encroachment.[178] If there is progressive neurologic deficit and radiologic evidence of bony enroachment on the spinal canal or foramina, the patient should be treated operatively with posterior decompression and fusion.[155] Decompression also may be performed via a transabdominal approach, but there are hazards in leaving metallic fixation near vascular structures. At these lower levels of the lumbar spine, laminectomy may be sufficient for posterior decompression. There is room for access to the anterior fragments of bone, and the dural tube containing the cauda equina can be retracted out of the way more safely than the conus medullaris.[5,89] These fractures may also be appropriately treated using posterior pedicular systems that will allow for decompression as necessary.

Distractive Extension Injuries

Distractive extension fractures are uncommon. These injuries occur when the major compressive forces are applied to the posterior elements, resulting in a fracture of the lamina or pars interarticularis in the low lumbar region.[106] They are very rare in the thoracolumbar spine[61,106] and are considered to have no propensity for progression of deformity or neurologic injury.[28,107] Since the injuries are stable in flexion, they can be treated in an orthosis.[106] If operative therapy becomes necessary for other reasons, patients can be treated successfully with bilateral Harrington distraction rods.[61] Other types of posterior instrumentation used in a distraction or stabilization mode might be equally successful. In the low lumbar region, pedicular systems will allow the surgeon to limit the fusion levels and preserve mobility.

Lumbosacral Dislocation

Lumbosacral dislocation is a rare injury resulting from combined flexion, rotation, and compression forces. It is not a simple flexion-distraction injury and does not fit simply into the Ferguson and Allen classification. Patients who sustain this injury are either crushed in a stooped position[180] or have had heavy weights land on them. The bony injury that they sustain is either a pure dislocation or dislocation with facet fracture.[181] It can be unilateral[182-185] or bilateral. The application of this force to the lumbosacral junction results in a traumatic anterior spondylolisthesis.

The pathognomonic feature of this injury is the presence of multiple transverse process fractures above the dislocation[180,181,183-190] and is an important finding in the early diagnosis of lumbosacral fracture dislocations.[187] CT scanning is diagnostic and will demonstrate the absence of articulation between the lumbar and sacral facets.[181]

Many patients demonstrate neurologic deficit as a result of injury to the cauda equina. Reduction is usually associated with at least a partial return of neurologic function.[132,180,181,186,188]

This ligamentous injury requires operative intervention.[26] Conservative treatment has been only partially successful[182,185,186,189] and the dislocation often cannot be reduced by closed methods. Partial facetectomy may facilitate reduction and may be required to reduce the dislocation.[180,181,186,188,190] Laminectomy is required only if the dislocation is irreducible[186] or if there is bone or soft tissue within the spinal canal causing neural compromise.[188] Decompression and reduction should be followed by pedicular fixation and posterolateral fusion. In the past, fixation was obtained by wiring the bases of the spinous processes together[180,181,183,184] or with the use of Harrington instrumentation.[188]

Conclusion

In this chapter we have attempted to give an overview of the different types of injuries that affect the thoracolumbar spine. Vigilance and a high degree of suspicion are essential for their detection. Associated injuries must be discovered and treated. Careful, systematic examination of x-rays will lead to the correct diagnosis. Treatment should then be based on the mechanism of injury.

There is often no one best treatment plan for any specific injury. The most appropriate treatment for each patient and injury is determined both by the nature of the injury and the surgeon's familiarity with each of the instrumentation techniques. While we all wish to offer patients the rapid mobilization afforded by surgical techniques, nonoperative management can yield better results than a poorly performed sophisticated technique.[191-200]

References

1. Keene JS. Thoracolumbar fractures in winter sports. *Clin Orthop*. 1987;216:39-49.
2. White RR, Newberg A, Seligson D. Computerized tomographic assessment of the traumatized dorsolumbar spine before and after Harrington instrumentation. *Clin Orthop*. 1980;146:150-156.
3. Riska EB. Antero-lateral decompression as a treatment of paraplegia following vertebral fracture in the thoracolumbar spine. *Int Orthop*. 1977;1:22-32.
4. Zwimpfer TJ, Gertzbein SG. Ultralight aircraft crashes: their increasing incidence and associated fractures of the thoracolumbar spine. *J Trauma*. 1987;27:431-436.
5. Bohlman HH. Treatment of fractures and dislocations of the thoracic and lumbar spine. *J Bone Joint Surg Am*. 1985;67A:165-169. Current Concepts Review.
6. Dommisse GF. The blood supply of the spinal cord: a critical vascular zone in spinal surgery. *J Bone Joint Surg Br*. 1974;56B:225-235.
7. King AG. Spinal column trauma. In: Anderson LD, ed. *Instructional Course Lectures*. St. Louis, Mo; CV Mosby Co; 1986;35:40-51.
8. Waters RL, Morris JM. Effect of spinal supports on the electrical activity of muscles of the trunk. *J Bone Joint Surg Am*. 1970;52A:51-60.
9. Bedbrook GM, Clark WB. Thoracic spine injuries with spinal cord damage. *J R Coll Surg Edinb*. 1981;26:264-271.
10. White AA, Panjabi MM. *Clinical Biomechanics of the Spine*. Philadelphia, Pa: JB Lippincott Co; 1978.
11. Angtuaco EJ, Binet EF. Radiology of thoracic and lumbar fractures. *Clin Orthop*. 1984;189:43-57.
12. Casey MP, Asher MA, Jacobs RR, Orrick JM. The effect of Harrington rod contouring on lumbar lordosis. *Spine*. 1987;12:750-753.
13. Denis F. The three column spine and its significance in the classification of acute thoracolumbar spinal injuries. *Spine*. 1983;8:817-831.
14. Durward QJ, Schweigel JF, Harrison P. Management of fractures of the thoracolumbar and lumbar spine. *Neurosurgery*. 1981;8:555-561.
15. Gertzbein SD, Court-Brown CM, Marks P, Martin C, Fazl M, Schwartz M, et al. The neurological outcome following surgery for spinal fractures. *Spine*. 1988;13:641-644.
16. Kilcoyne RF, Mack LA, King HA, Ratcliffe SS, Loop JW. Thoracolumbar spine injuries associated with vertical plunges: reappraisal with computed tomography. *Radiology*. 1983;146:137-140.
17. Shuman WP, Rogers JV, Sickler ME, Hanson JA, Crutcher JP, King HA, et al. Thoracolumbar burst fractures: CT dimensions of the spinal canal relative to postsurgical improvement. *AJR*. 1985;145:337-341.
18. Levine A, Edwards CC. Complications in the treat-

ment of acute spinal injury. *Orthop Clin North Am.* 1986;17:183-203.
19. Calenoff L, Chessare JW, Rogers LF, Toerge J, Rosen JS. Multiple level spinal injuries: importance of early recognition. *AJR.* 1978;130:665-669.
20. Kewalrami LS, Taylor RG. Multiple non-contiguous injuries to the spine. *Acta Orthop Scand.* 1976;47:52-58.
21. Scher AT. Double fractures of the spine: an indication for routine radiographic examination of the entire spine after injury. *S Afr Med J.* 1978;53:411-413.
22. Tearse DS, Keene JS, Drummond DS. Management of non-contiguous vertebral fractures. *Paraplegia.* 1987;25:100-105.
23. Bentley G, McSweeney T. Multiple spinal injuries. *Br J Surg.* 1968;55:565-570.
24. Keene JS. Radiographic evaluation of thoracolumbar fractures. *Clin Orthop.* 1984;189:58-64.
25. Nicoll EA. Fractures of the dorso-lumbar spine. *J Bone Joint Surg Br.* 1949;31B:376-394.
26. Holdsworth FW, Hardy A. Early treatment of paraplegia from fractures of the thoraco-lumbar spine. *J Bone Joint Surg Br.* 1953;35B:540-550.
27. Kelly RP, Whitesides TE Jr. Treatment of lumbodorsal fracture-dislocations. *Ann Surg.* 1968;167:705-717.
28. Ferguson RL, Allen BL Jr. A mechanistic classification of thoracolumbar spine fractures. *Clin Orthop.* 1984;189:77-88.
29. Bedbrook GM. Spinal injuries with tetraplegia and paraplegia. *J Bone Joint Surg Br.* 1979;61B:267-284.
30. Bedbrook GM: Treatment of thoracolumbar dislocation and fractures with paraplegia. *Clin Orthop.* 1975;112:27-43.
31. Bedbrook GM. Fracture dislocations of the spine with and without paralysis: the case for conservatism and against operative techniques. In: Leach RE, Hoaglund FT, Riseborough EJ, eds. *Controversies in Orthopedic Surgery.* Philadelphia, Pa: WB Saunders Co; 1982.
32. Frankel HL, Hancock DO, Hyslop G, Melzak J, Michaels LS, Ungar GH, et al. The value of postural reduction in the initial management of closed injuries of the spine with paraplegia and tetraplegia: part 1. *Paraplegia.* 1969;7:179-192.
33. Burke DC, Murray DD. The management of thoracic and thoraco-lumbar injuries of the spine with neurological involvement. *J Bone Joint Surg Br.* 1976;58B:72-78.
34. Levine A, Edwards CC. Lumbar spine trauma. In: Camins MB, O'Leary PF, eds. *The Lumbar Spine.* New York, NY: Raven Press; 1987:183-212.
35. Young B, Brooks WH, Tibbs PA. Anterior decompression and fusion for thoracolumbar fractures with neurological deficits. *Acta Neurochir.* 1981;57:287-298.
36. Bohler J. Operative treatment of fractures of the dorsal and lumbar spine. *J Trauma.* 1970;10:1119-1122.
37. Krompinger WJ, Fredrickson BE, Mino DE, Yuan HA. Conservative treatment of fractures of the thoracic and lumbar spine. *Orthop Clin North Am.* 1986;17:161-170.
38. Weinstein JN, Collalto P, Lehmann TR. Thoracolumbar "burst" fractures treated conservatively: a long-term follow-up. *Spine.* 1988;13:33-38.
39. Denis F, Armstrong GWD, Searls K, Matta L. Acute thoracolumbar burst fractures in the absence of neurologic deficit: a comparison between operative and nonoperative treatment. *Clin Orthop.* 1984;189:142-149.
40. Willen J, Lindahl S, Nordwall A. Unstable thoracolumbar fractures: a comparative clinical study of conservative treatment and Harrington instrumentation. *Spine.* 1985;10:111-122.
41. Gertzbein SD, Macmichael D, Tile M. Harrington instrumentation as a method of fixation in fractures of the spine. a critical analysis of deficiencies. *J Bone Joint Surg Br.* 1982;64B:526-529.
42. Kostuik JP, Errico TJ, Gleason TF. Techniques of internal fixation for degenerative conditions of the lumbar spine. *Clin Orthop.* 1986;203:219-231.
43. Malcolm BW, Bradford DS, Winter RB, Chou SN. Post-traumatic kyphosis: a review of forty-eight surgically treated patients. *J Bone Joint Surg Am.* 1981;63A:891-899.
44. McBride GG, Bradford DS. Vertebral body replacement with femoral neck allograft and vascularized rib strut graft: a technique for treating post-traumatic kyphosis with neurologic deficit. *Spine.* 1983;8:406-415.
45. Aebi M, Mohler J, Zack G, Morscher E. Analysis of 75 operated thoracolumbar fractures and fracture dislocations with and without neurological deficit. *Arch Orthop Trauma Surg.* 1986;105:100-112.
46. Braakman R. The value of more aggressive management in traumatic paraplegia. *Neurosurg Rev.* 1986;9:141-147.
47. Bradford DS, Thompson RC. Fractures and dislocations of the spine: indications for surgical intervention. *Minn Med.* 1976;59:711-720.
48. Dickson JH, Harrington PR, Erwin WD. Results of reduction and stabilization of the severely fractured thoracic and lumbar spine. *J Bone Joint Surg Am.* 1978;60A:799-805.
49. Dickson JH, Harrington PR, Erwin WD. Harrington instrumentation in the fractured, unstable thoracic and lumbar spine. *Tex Med.* September 1973;69:91-98.
50. Flesch JR, Leider LL, Erickson DL, Chou SN, Bradford DS. Harrington instrumentation and spine fusion for unstable fractures and fracture-dislocations of the thoracic and lumbar spine. *J Bone Joint Surg Am.* 1977;59A:143-153.
51. Gaines RW, Humphreys WG. A plea for judgement in management of thoracolumbar fractures and fracture-dislocations: reassessment of surgical indications. *Clin Orthop.* 1984;189:36-42.
52. Jacobs RR, Asher MA, Snider RK. Thoracolumbar spinal injuries: a comparative study of recumbency and operative treatment in 100 patients. *Spine.* 1980;5:463-477.
53. Kaufer H, Hayes JT. Lumbar fracture dislocation: a study of 21 cases. *J Bone Joint Surg Am.* 1966;48A:712-730.
54. Lewis J, McKibbin B. The treatment of unstable fracture-dislocations of the thoracolumbar spine accompanied by paraplegia. *J Bone Joint Surg Br.* 1974;56B:603-612.
55. Osebold WR, Weinstein SL, Sprague BL. Thor-

acolumbar spine fractures: results of treatment. *Spine*. 1981;6:13-34.
56. Soreff J, Axdorph G, Bylund P, Odeen I, Olerud S. Treatment of patients with unstable fractures of the thoracic and lumbar spine: a follow-up study of surgical and conservative treatment. *Acta Orthop Scand*. 1982;53:369-381.
57. Svensson O, Aaro S, Ohlen G. Harrington instrumentation for thoracic and lumbar vertebral fractures. *Acta Orthop. Scand*. 1984;55:38-47.
58. Weber SC, Sutherland GH. An unusual rotational fracture-dislocation of the thoracic spine without neurologic sequelae internally fixed with a combined anterior and posterior approach. *J Trauma*. 1986;26:474-479.
59. Yocum TD, Leatherman KD, Brower TD. The early rod fixation in treatment of fracture-dislocations of the spine. *J Bone Joint Surg Am*. 1970;52A:1257. Proceedings of The American Academy of Orthopaedic Surgeons.
60. Yosipovitch Z, Robin GC, Makin M. Open reduction of unstable thoracolumbar spinal injuries and fixation with Harrington rods. *J Bone Joint Surg Am*. 1977;59A:1003-1015.
61. Cotler JM, Vernace JV, Michalski JA. The use of Harrington rods in thoracolumbar fractures. *Orthop Clin North Am*. 1986;17:87-103.
62. Bradford DS, Akbarnia BA, Winter RB, Seljeskog EL. Surgical stabilization of fracture and fracture dislocations of the thoracic spine. *Spine*. 1977;2:185-196.
63. Davies WE, Morris JH, Hill V. An analysis of conservative (non-surgical) management of thoracolumbar fractures and fracture-dislocations with neural damage. *J Bone Joint Surg Am*. 1980;62A:1324-1328.
64. Bohlman HH. Traumatic fractures of the upper thoracic spine with paralysis. *J Bone Joint Surg Am*. 1974;56A:1299. Proceedings of The American Academy of Orthopaedic Surgeons.
65. McAfee PC, Werner FW, Glisson RR. A biomechanical analysis of spinal instrumentation systems in thoracolumbar fractures: comparison of traditional Harrington distraction instrumentation with segmental spinal instrumentation. *Spine*. 1985;10:204-217.
66. Edwards CC, Levine AM. Early rod-sleeve stabilization of the injured thoracic and lumbar spine. *Orthop Clin North Am*. 1986;17:121-145.
67. Garfin SR, Mowery CA, Guerra J Jr, Marshall LF. Confirmation of the posterolateral technique to decompress and fuse thoracolumbar spine burst fractures. *Spine*. 1985;10:218-223.
68. Lifeso RM, Arabie KM, Kadhi SKM. Fractures of the thoracolumbar spine. *Paraplegia*. 1985;23:207-224.
69. McAfee PC, Bohlman HH, Yuan HA. Anterior decompression of traumatic thoracolumbar fractures with incomplete neurological deficit using a retroperitoneal approach. *J Bone Joint Surg Am*. 1985;67A:89-104.
70. Maiman DJ, Larson SJ, Benzel EC. Neurological improvement associated with late decompression of the thoracolumbar spinal cord. *Neurosurgery*. 1984;14:302-307.
71. Fountain SS. A single-stage combined surgical approach for vertebral resections. *J Bone Joint Surg Am*. 1979;61A:1011-1017.
72. Bradford DS, McBride G. Thoracic/lumbar spine fractures with incomplete neurologic deficit: a correlative study on the adequacy of decompression vs. neurologic return. *Orthop Trans*. 1984;8:159-160.
73. Bradford DS, McBride GG. Surgical management of thoracolumbar spine fractures with incomplete neurologic deficits. *Clin Orthop*. 1987;218:201-216.
74. Johnson JR, Leatherman KD, Holt RT. Anterior decompression of the spinal cord for neurological deficit. *Spine*. 1983;8:396-405.
75. McAfee PC, Bohlman HH. Complications following Harrington instrumentation for fractures of the thoracolumbar spine. *J Bone Joint Surg Am*. 1985;67A:672-686.
76. Guttmann L. Surgical aspects of the treatment of traumatic paraplegia. *J Bone Joint Surg Br*. 1949;31B:399-403.
77. Guttmann L. Spinal deformities in traumatic paraplegics and tetraplegics following surgical procedures. *Paraplegia*. 1969;7:38-58.
78. Hannon KM. Harrington instrumentation in fractures and dislocations of the thoracic and lumbar spine. *South Med J*. 1976;69:1269-1273.
79. Stauffer ES. Internal fixation of fractures of the thoracolumbar spine. *J Bone Joint Surg Am*. 1984;66A:1136-1138. Current Concepts Review.
80. Bohlman HH, Freehafer A, Dejak J. The results of treatment of acute injuries of the upper thoracic spine with paralysis. *J Bone Joint Surg Am*. 1985;67A:360-369.
81. Jodoin A, Dupuis P, Fraser M, Beaumont P. Unstable fractures of the thoracolumbar spine: a 10-year experience at Sacre-Coeur Hospital. *J Trauma*. 1985;25:197-202.
82. Pierce DS. Long-term management of thoracolumbar fractures and fracture dislocations. In: American Academy of Orthopedic Surgeons, ed. *Instructional Course Lectures*. St. Louis, Mo: CV Mosby Co; 1972;21:102-107.
83. Sullivan JA. Sublaminar wiring of Harrington distraction rods for unstable thoracolumbar spine fractures. *Clin Orthop*. 1984;189:178-185.
84. Erickson DL, Leider LL, Brown WE. One-stage decompression-stabilization for thoracolumbar fractures. *Spine*. 1977;2:53-56.
85. Keene JS, Wackwitz DL, Drummond DS, Breed AL. Compression-distraction instrumentation of unstable thoracolumbar fractures: anatomic results obtained with each type of injury and method of instrumentation. *Spine*. 1986;11:895-902.
86. McAfee PC, Yuan HA, Fredrickson BE, Lubicky JP. The value of computed tomography in thoracolumbar fractures: an analysis of one hundred consecutive cases and a new classification. *J Bone Joint Surg Am*. 1983;65A:461-473.
87. Allen BL Jr, Tencer AF, Ferguson RL. The biomechanics of decompressive laminectomy. *Spine*. 1987;12:803-808.
88. Larson SJ, Holst RA, Hemmy DC, Sances A Jr. Lateral extracavitary approach to traumatic lesions of the thoracic and lumbar spine. *J Neurosurg*. 1976;45:628-637.
89. McAfee PC, Yuan HA, Lasda NA. The unstable burst fracture. *Spine*. 1982;7:365-373.
90. McGahan JP, Benson D, Chehrazi B, Walter JP, Wagner FC Jr. Intraoperative sonographic monitor-

ing of reduction of thoracolumbar burst fractures. *AJR*. 1985;145:1229-1232.
91. Vincent KA, Benson DR, McGahan JP. Intraoperative sonography for thoracolumbar burst fractures. Poster Exhibited at 55th Annual Meeting, American Academy of Orthopedic Surgeons, February 1988; Atlanta, Ga.
92. Cook WA. Transthoracic vertebral surgery. *Ann Thorac Surg*. 1971;12:54-68.
93. Dunn HK. Anterior spine stabilization and decompression for thoracolumbar injuries. *Orthop Clin North Am*. 1986;17:113-119.
94. Jelsma RK, Kirsch PT, Rice JF, Jelsma LF. The radiographic description of thoracolumbar fractures. *Surg Neurol*. 1982;18:230-236.
95. Meyer PR. Complications of treatment of fractures and dislocations of the dorsolumbar spine. In: Epps CH, ed. *Complications in Orthopedic Surgery*. Philadelphia, Pa: JB Lippincott Co; 1986.
96. Golimbu C, Firooznia H, Rafii M, Engler G, Delman A. Computed tomography of thoracic and lumbar spine fractures that have been treated with Harrington instrumentation. *Radiology*. 1984; 151:731-733.
97. Benzel EC, Larson SJ. Functional recovery after decompressive operation for thoracic and lumbar spine fractures. *Neurosurgery*. 1986;19:772-778.
98. Bohlman HH, Eismont FJ. Surgical techniques of anterior decompression and fusion for spinal cord injuries. *Clin Orthop*. 1981;154:57-67.
99. Gelderman PW. The operative stabilization and grafting of thoracic and lumbar spinal fractures. *Surg Neurol*. 1985;23:101-120.
100. Paul RL, Michael RH, Dunn JE, Williams JP. Anterior transthoracic surgical decompression of acute spinal cord injuries. *J Neurosurg*. 1975; 43:299-307.
101. Whitesides TE Jr, Shah SGA. On the management of unstable fractures of the thoracolumbar spine: rationale for use of anterior decompression and fusion and posterior stabilization. *Spine*. 1976; 1:99-107.
102. Dunn HK. Neurologic recovery following anterior spinal canal decompression in thoracic and lumbar injuries. *Orthop Trans*. 1984;8:160.
103. Kostuik JP. Anterior spinal cord decompression for lesions of the thoracic and lumbar spine, techniques, new methods of internal fixation results. *Spine*. 1983;8:512-531.
104. O'Laoire SA, Thomas DGT. Surgery in incomplete spinal cord injury. *Surg Neurol*. 1982;17:12-15.
105. Denis F. Spinal instability as defined by the three column spine concept in acute spinal trauma. *Clin Orthop*. 1984;189:65-76.
106. Bucholz RW, Gill K. Classification of injuries to the thoracolumbar spine. *Orthop Clin North Am*. 1986;17:67-73.
107. Weitzman G. Treatment of stable thoracolumbar spine compression fractures by early ambulation. *Clin Orthop*. 1971;76:116-122.
108. Ferguson RL, Allen BL Jr. An algorithm for the treatment of unstable thoracolumbar fractures. *Orthop Clin North Am*. 1986;17:105-112.
109. Nash CL Jr, Schatzinger LH, Brown RH, Brodkey J. The unstable stable thoracic compression fracture: its problems and the use of spinal cord monitoring in the evaluation of treatment. *Spine*. 1977;2:261-265.
110. Dodd CAF, Fergusson CM, Pearcy MJ, Houghton GR. Vertebral motion measured using biplanar radiography before and after Harrington rod removal for unstable thoracolumbar fractures of the spine. *Spine*. 1986;11:452-455.
111. Munson G, Satterlee C, Hammond S, Betten R, Gaines RW. Experimental evaluation of Harrington rod fixation supplemented with sublaminar wires in stabilizing thoracolumbar fracture-dislocations. *Clin Orthop*. 1984;189:97-102.
112. Van Hanswyck EP, Yuan HA, Eckhardt WA. Orthotic management of thoracolumbar spine fractures with a "total contact" TLSO. *Orthotics and Prosthetics*. September 1979;33:10-19.
113. Beerman R, Batt HD, Green BA. Lumbar vertebral reformation after traumatic compression fracture. *AJNR*. 1985;6:455-456.
114. Meyer PR. Posterior stabilization of thoracic, lumbar and sacral injuries. In: Anderson LD, ed. *Instructional Course Lectures*. St. Louis, Mo: CV Mosby Co; 1986;35:401-419.
115. Floman Y, Fast A, Pollack D, Yosipovitch Z, Robin GC. The simultaneous application of an interspinous compressive wire and Harrington distraction rods in the treatment of fracture-dislocation of the thoracic and lumbar spine. *Clin Orthop*. 1986;205:207-215.
116. Jacobs RR, Dahners LE, Gertzbein SD, Nordwall A, Mathys R Jr. A locking hook-spinal rod: current status of development. *Paraplegia*. 1983; 21:197-200.
117. Jacobs RR, Schlaepfer F, Mathys R Jr., Nachemson A, Perren SM. A locking hook-spinal rod system for stabilization of fracture-dislocations and correction of deformities of the dorsolumbar spine: a biomechanical evaluation. *Clin Orthop*. 1984;189:168-177.
118. Drummond D, Guadagni J, Keene JS, Breed A, Narechania R. Interspinous process segmental spinal instrumentation. *J Pediatr Orthop*. 1984;4:397-404.
119. Bryant CE, Sullivan JA. Management of thoracic and lumbar spine fractures with Harrington distraction rods supplemented with segmental wiring. *Spine*. 1983;8:532-537.
120. Gaines RW, Munson G, Satterlee C, Lising A, Betten R. Harrington distraction rods supplemented with sublaminar wires for thoracolumbar fracture dislocations: experimental and clinical investigation. *Orthop Trans*. 1983;7:15.
121. Louw JA. Unstable fractures of the thoracic and lumbar spine treated with Harrington distraction instrumentation and sublaminar wires. *S Afr Med J*. 1987;71:759-762.
122. Sullivan JA, Bryant CE. Management of thoracic and lumbar spine fractures with Harrington rods supplemented with segmental wires. *Orthop Trans*. 1983;7:15.
123. Roberts JB, Curtiss PH Jr. Stability of the thoracic and lumbar spine in traumatic paraplegia following fracture or fracture-dislocation. *J Bone Joint Surg Am*. 1970;52A:1115-1130.
124. Luque ER. Segmental spinal instrumentation in the treatment of fractures of the spine. *Orthop Trans*. 1982;6:22.
125. Luque ER, Cassis N, Ramírez-Wiella G. Segmental spinal instrumentation in the treatment of fractures of the thoracolumbar spine. *Spine*. 1982;7:312-317.

126. Chance CQ. Note on a type of flexion fracture of the spine. *Br J Radiol.* 1948;21:452-453.
127. Cope R, Salmon A, Gaines R. Association of a thoracic distraction fracture and an unusual avulsion fracture: a case report. *Spine.* 1987;12:943-945.
128. Blasier RD, LaMont RL. Chance fracture in a child: a case report with non-operative treatment. *J Pediatr Orthop.* 1985;5:92-93.
129. Gertzbein SD, Court-Brown CM. Flexion-distraction injuries of the lumbar spine: mechanisms of injury and classification. *Clin Orthop.* 1988;227:52-60.
130. Gumley G, Taylor TKF, Ryan MD. Distraction fractures of the lumbar spine. *J Bone Joint Surg Br.* 1982;64B:520-525.
131. Rennie W, Mitchell N. Flexion distraction fractures of the thoracolumbar spine. *J Bone Joint Surg Am.* 1973;55A:386-390.
132. Griffin JB, Sutherland GH. Traumatic posterior fracture-dislocation of the lumbosacral joint. *J Trauma.* 1980;20:426-428.
133. Smith WS, Kaufer H. Patterns and mechanisms of lumbar injuries associated with lap seat belts. *J Bone Joint Surg Am.* 1969;51A:239-254.
134. Carragher AM, Cranley B. Seat-belt stomach transection in association with "Chance" vertebral fracture. *Br J Surg.* 1987;74:397.
135. Levine A, Bosse M, Edwards CC. Bilateral facet dislocations in the thoracolumbar spine. *Spine.* 1988;13:630-640.
136. Huekle DF, Kaufer H. Vertebral column injuries and seat belts. *J Trauma.* 1975;15:304-318.
137. Levine A, Bosse M, Edwards CC. Bilateral facet dislocations in the thoracolumbar spine. *Orthop Trans.* 1988;10:12-13.
138. De Oliveira JC. A new type of fracture-dislocation of the thoracolumbar spine. *J Bone Joint Surg Am.* 1978;60A:481-488.
139. Gertzbein SD, Offierski C. Complete fracture dislocation of the thoracic spine without spinal cord injury. *J Bone Joint Surg Am.* 1979;61A:449-451.
140. Harryman DT. Complete fracture dislocation of the thoracic spine associated with spontaneous neurologic decompression: a case report. *Clin Orthop.* 1986;207:64-69.
141. Sasson A, Mozes G. Complete fracture-dislocation of the thoracic spine without neurologic deficit: a case report. Briefly noted. *Spine.* 1987;12:67-70.
142. Uriarte E, Elguezabal B, Tovio R. Fracture-dislocation of the thoracic spine without neurologic lesion. *Clin Orthop.* 1987;217:261-265.
143. Murphy MJ, Southwick WO, Ogden JA. Treatment of the unstable thoraco-lumbar spine with combination Harrington distraction and compression rods. *Orthop Trans.* 1982;6:9.
144. Fidler MW. Posterior instrumentation of the spine: an experimental comparison of various possible techniques. *Spine.* 1986;11:367-372.
145. Akbarnia BA, Fogarty JP, Tayob AA. Contoured Harrington instrumentation in the treatment of unstable spinal fractures: the effect of supplementary sublaminar wires. *Clin Orthop.* 1984;189:186-194.
146. Gaines RW, Breedlove RF, Munson G. Stabilization of thoracic and thoracolumbar fracture-dislocations with Harrington rods and sublaminar wires. *Clin Orthop.* 1984;189:195-203.
147. Kinnard P, Ghibely A, Gordon D, Tiras A, Basora J. Roy-Camille plates in unstable spinal conditions: a preliminary report. *Spine.* 1986;11:131-135.
148. Roy-Camille R, Saillant G, Berteaux D, Salgado V. Osteosynthesis of thoraco-lumbar spine fractures with metal plates screwed through the vertebral pedicles. *Reconstr Surg Traumatol.* 1976;15:2-16.
149. Roy-Camille R, Saillant G, Mazel CH. Plating of thoracic, thoracolumbar and lumbar injuries with pedicle screw plates. *Orthop Clin North Am.* 1986;17:147-159.
150. Roy-Camille R, Saillant G, Mazel CH. Internal fixation of the lumbar spine with pedicle screw plating. *Clin Orthop.* 1986;203:7-17.
151. Riska EB, Myllynen P, Bostman O. Anterolateral decompression for neural involvement in thoracolumbar fractures: a review of 78 cases. *J Bone Joint Surg Br.* 1987;69B:704-708.
152. Lindahl S, Willen J, Irstam L. Computed tomography of the bone fragments in the spinal canal: an experimental study. *Spine.* 1983;8:181-186.
153. Lindahl S, Willen J, Irstam L. Unstable thoracolumbar fractures: a comparative radiologic study of conservative treatment and Harrington instrumentation. *Acta Radiol Diagnostica.* 1985;26:67-77.
154. King AG. Burst compression fractures of the thoracolumbar spine: pathologic anatomy and surgical management. *Orthopedics.* 1987;10:1711-1719.
155. Frederickson BE, Yuan HA, Miller H. Burst fractures of the fifth lumbar vertebra: a report of four cases. *J Bone Joint Surg Am.* 1982;64A:1088-1094.
156. Atlas SW, Regenbogen V, Rogers LF, Kim KS. The radiographic characterization of burst fractures of the spine. *AJR.* 1986;147:575-582.
157. Miller CA, Dewey RC, Hunt WE. Impaction fracture of the lumbar vertebrae with dural tear. *J Neurosurg.* 1980;53:765-771.
158. Boynton LW, Kalb R. Double lumen sign as demonstrated by computerized tomography in spine dislocation. *Spine.* 1983;8:910-912.
159. Brant-Zawadzki M, Jeffrey RB Jr, Minagi H, Pitts LH. High resolution CT of thoracolumbar fractures. *AJR.* 1982;138:699-704.
160. Brant-Zawadzki M, Miller EM, Federle MP. CT in the evaluation of spine trauma. *AJR.* 1981;136:369-375.
161. Herrlin K, Ekelund L, Sunden G. Radiologic and clinical evaluation of Harrington instrumentation in the injured dorsolumbar spine. *Acta Radiol Diagn.* 1983;24:289-295.
162. Kaneda K, Abumi K, Fujiya M. Burst fractures with neurologic deficits of the thoracolumbar-lumbar spine: results of anterior decompression and stabilization with anterior instrumentation. *Spine.* 1984;9:788-795.
163. Keene JS, Goletz TH, Lilleas F, Alter AJ, Sackett JF. Diagnosis of vertebral fractures: a comparison of conventional radiography, conventional tomography and computed axial tomography. *J Bone Joint Surg Am.* 1982;64A:586-595.
164. Nykamp PW, Levy JM, Christensen F, Dunn R, Hubbard J. Computed tomography for a bursting fracture of the lumbar spine. *J Bone Joint Surg Am.* 1978;60A:1108-1109.
165. Post MJD, Green BA, Quencer RM, Stokes NA, Callahan RA, Eismont FJ. The value of computed

166. Lindahl S, Willen J, Nordwall A, Irstam L. The crush-cleavage fracture: a "new" thoracolumbar unstable burst fracture. *Spine.* 1983;8:559-569.
167. Wenger DR, Carollo JJ. The mechanics of thoracolumbar fractures stabilized by segmental fixation. *Clin Orthop.* 1984;189:89-96.
168. Kostuik JP. Anterior fixation for fractures of the thoracic and lumbar spine with or without neurologic involvement. *Clin Orthop.* 1984;189:103-115.
169. Wang GJ, Whitehill R, Stamp WG, Rosenberger R. The treatment of fracture dislocations of the thoracolumbar spine with halofemoral traction and Harrington rod instrumentation. *Clin Orthop.* 1979;142:168-175.
170. Reis ND, Keret D. Fracture of the transverse process of the fifth lumbar vertebra. *Injury.* 1985;16:421-423.
171. Farcy JP, Weidenbaum M, Michelsen CB, Hoeltzel DA, Athanasiou KA. A comparative biomechanical study of spinal fixation using Cotrel-Dubousset instrumentation. *Spine.* 1987;12:877-881.
172. Gurr KR, McAfee PC. Cotrel-Dubousset instrumentation in adults: a preliminary report. *Spine.* 1988;13:510-520.
173. Aebi M, Etter C, Kehl T, Thalgott J. Stabilization of the lower thoracic and lumbar spine with the internal spinal skeletal fixation system: indications, techniques and first results of treatment. *Spine.* 1987;12:544-551.
174. Dick W, Kluger P, Magerl F, Woersdorfer O, Zach G. A new device for internal fixation of thoracolumbar and lumbar spine fractures: the "fixateur interne." *Paraplegia.* 1985;23:225-232.
175. Aebi M, Etter C, Kehl T, Thalgott J. The internal skeletal fixation system: a new treatment of thoracolumbar fractures and other spinal disorders. *Clin Orthop.* 1988;227:30-43.
176. Karlstrom G, Olerud S, Sjostrom L. Transpedicular segmental fixation: description of a new procedure. *Orthopedics.* 1988;11:689-700.
177. Olerud S, Karlstrom G, Sjostrom L. Transpedicular fixation of thoracolumbar vertebral fractures. *Clin Orthop.* 1988;227:44-51.
178. Court-Brown CM, Gertzbein, SD. The management of burst fractures of the fifth lumbar vertebra. *Spine.* 1987;12:308-312.
179. Levine A. Modular instrumentation of lumbar spine fractures. Presented at the Specialty Day, Orthopedic Trauma Association, 55th Annual Meeting of American Academy of Orthopedic Surgeons; February 1988; Atlanta, Ga.
180. Das De S, McCreath SW. Lumbosacral fracture-dislocations: a report of four cases. *J Bone Joint Surg Br.* 1981;63B:58-60.
181. Wilchinisky ME. Traumatic lumbosacral dislocation: a case report and review of the literature. *Orthopedics.* 1987;10:1271-1274.
182. Boger DC, Chandler RW, Pearce JG, Balciunas A. Unilateral facet dislocation at the lumbosacral junction. *J Bone Joint Surg Am.* 1983;65A:1174-1178.
183. Morris BDA. Unilateral dislocation of a lumbosacral facet: a case report. *J Bone Joint Surg Am.* 1981;63A:164-165.
184. Morris JM. Biomechanics of corsets and braces for the low back. In: Brown FW, ed. *Symposium on the Lumbar Spine.* St. Louis, Mo: CV Mosby Co; 1981.
185. Zoltan JD, Gilula LD, Murphy WA. Unilateral facet dislocation between the fifth lumbar and first sacral vertebrae: a case report. *J Bone Joint Surg Am.* 1979;61A:767-769.
186. Dewey P, Browne PSH. Fracture-dislocation of the lumbo-sacral spine with cauda equina lesion: report of two cases. *J Bone Joint Surg Br.* 1968;50B:635-638.
187. Fardon DF. Displaced fracture of the lumbosacral spine and delayed cauda equina deficit: report of a case and review of literature. *Clin Orthop.* 1976;120:155-158.
188. Herron LD, Williams RC. Fracture-dislocation of the lumbosacral spine. *Clin Orthop.* 1984;186:205-211.
189. Newell RLM. Lumbosacral fracture-dislocation: a case managed conservatively with return to heavy work. *Injury.* 1977;9:131-134.
190. Samberg LC. Fracture-dislocation of the lumbosacral spine. *J Bone Joint Surg Am.* 1975;57A:1007-1008.
191. Byrd JA. The treatment of L5 burst fractures with neurologic deficit. Poster exhibit presented at 55th Annual Meeting, American Academy of Orthopedic Surgeons; February 1988; Atlanta Ga.
192. Grant JMF, Sears WR. Spinal injury and computerized tomography: a review of fracture pathology and a new approach to canal decompression. *Aust NZ J Surg.* 1986;56:299-307.
193. Hearon BF, Thomas HA, Raddin JH Jr. Mechanism of vertebral fracture in the F/FB-111 ejection experience. *Aviat Space Environ Med.* 1982;53:440-448.
194. Jacobs RR. Bilateral fracture of the pedicles through the fourth and fifth lumbar vertebrae with anterior displacement of the vertebral bodies: case report. *J Bone Joint Surg Am.* 1977;59A:409-410.
195. Jacobs RR, Casey MP. Surgical management of thoracolumbar spinal injuries: general principles and controversial considerations. *Clin Orthop.* 1984;189:22-35.
196. Manaster BJ, Osborne AG. CT patterns of facet fracture dislocations in the thoracolumbar region. *AJR.* 1987;148:335-340.
197. Morgan TH, Wharton GW, Austin GN. The results of laminectomy in patients with incomplete spinal cord injuries. *Paraplegia.* 1971;9:14-23.
198. Tencer AF, Allen BL Jr, Ferguson RL. A biomechanical study of thoracolumbar spinal fractures with bone in the canal, I: the effect of laminectomy. *Spine.* 1985;10:580-585.
199. Tencer AF, Allen BL Jr, Ferguson RL. A biomechanical study of thoracolumbar spine fractures with bone in the canal, III: mechanical properties of the dura and its tethering ligaments. *Spine.* 1985;10:741-747.
200. Wilmot CB, Hall KM. Evaluation of acute surgical intervention in traumatic paraplegia. *Paraplegia.* 1986;24:71-76.

165. tomography in spinal trauma. *Spine.* 1982;7:417-431.

CHAPTER 10

Sacral Fractures

Robert G. Watkins, MD, and William H. Dillin, MD

Bony Anatomy

The pelvis is a ring structure designed to transmit force from the spine through the sacrum, sacroiliac (S.I.) joints, posterior ilium, and acetabulum to the femoral heads. It also provides insertions and origins for the muscles connecting the trunk to the legs and is responsible for the distribution of power and balance between the trunk and legs. Each lateral hemipelvis is connected through three joints: the symphysis pubis and two sacroiliac joints. The sacroiliac joint extends from the top of S1 to the top of S3.[1] The ilium connects to the sacrum through the sacroiliac joints that are synchondroses with a minimum amount of movement. The S.I. joint is supported by an anterior sacroiliac ligament and a posterior sacroiliac ligament. The sacrotuberous ligament connects the tuberosity of the ischium to the sacrum and the sacrospinous ligament connects the ischium and the ischial spine to the sacrum and coccyx. The sacrococcygeal ligament joins the sacrum to the coccyx. An obturator membrane covers the obturator foramen. The pubic symphysis is a slightly movable joint between the two pubic tubercles. The superior pubic and arcuate pubic ligaments support an interpubic disc, which is a fibrocartilage connection without a synovial membrane.

The sacrum is a flat bone with a canal that provides protection for the distal end of the cauda equina. It has both dorsal and ventral exiting foramina for the S1, 2, 3, 4, and 5 nerves. The posterior rami exit dorsally and the anterior rami exit ventrally. The sacrum articulates with the lumbar spine at L5-S1, the ilium with the S.I. joints and with the coccyx through the coccygeal joint.

Mechanisms of Injury

In most instances sacral fractures are caused by automobile accidents or falls. Transverse fractures result predominantly from falls,[2] although posteriorly directed forces on the sacrum with a flexed hip and extended knee have also been implicated as the cause of transverse sacral fractures.[3]

Lateral compression injuries result from pedestrian accidents, while shear fractures are seen in passengers injured in high-speed automobile accidents.[2] Because of the similar mechanisms of injury in high-velocity trauma, one should always be cognizant of the potential for associated skeletal injury. The possibility of thoracolumbar junction fractures should always be considered in any patient with a sacral fracture.[2]

Fracture dislocations of the L5-S1 facet joint may occur with vertical shearing. A shear compression injury can also produce a fracture dislocation of the lumbosacral joint. The stability of a bilateral SI joint dislocation depends upon the mechanism of injury and associated pelvic fractures.[4,5]

Classification of Pelvic Fractures

Among the numerous classifications of pelvic fractures,[1,6-10] the most commonly used is the Bucholz[6] classification based upon postmortem dissections and radiographic analysis. According to the Bucholz classification, Class I patients show a more obvious anterior disruption of the pelvic ring, and a less obvious, nondisplaced vertical fracture of the sacrum or tearing of the anterior sacroiliac ligament. Patients in Class II experience a disruption of the symphysis pubis or fracture of the anterior ring, with a complete disruption of the anterior sacroiliac ligament. This results in an outward rotation of the hemipelvis, akin to opening a book. Patients with Class III injuries have a complete disruption of the sacroiliac ligaments or fractures of the sacrum or ilium, producing a complete dislocation and horizontal translation of the hemipelvis.

The importance of this classification becomes apparent during initial evaluation of the patient with a fractured pelvis. It must be determined whether the patient has a stable or unstable fracture or dislocation of the pelvis. Class I injuries are nondisplaced and do not require operative intervention. Class II injuries can usually be reduced by lateral compression on the iliac crest. Class III injuries are poorly controlled with traction and bed rest[6] and are more likely to require surgery.

Huittenen and Slätis[11] classified pelvic fractures according to the mechanism of injury:

1. Minor impact injuries produce pubic ramus fracture, whereas more severe injury produces anterior and posterior ring disruption.
2. Oblique impacts produce horizontal translation of pubic disruption and posterior injury.
3. Posterior forces produce bilateral S.I. joint dislocation and pubic symphysis separation.
4. Lateral impact on the greater trochanter produces a protrussio acetabulum.

The key to proper diagnosis and treatment depends on identifying unstable pelvic fractures. Tile's definition of stability is a pelvis that can withstand normal physiologic forces without abnormal deformation.[12] The posterior osseous-ligamentous complex, consisting of the posterior and anterior sacroiliac ligaments, the iliolumbar ligaments, the sacrotuberous ligaments, and the sacrospinous ligaments,[12] is the key to whether an injury is anterior/posterior compression or lateral compression and whether the lesion is stable. Some pelvic fractures are unstable only with motion in certain directions. Preventing motion in these directions is the goal of both operative and nonoperative treatment.

Kellam et al[13] noted four signs of instability:

1. Avulsions of the ischial spine and/or the tip of the transverse process of L5.
2. Shear fractures through the cancellous bone of the sacrum.
3. A posterior gap through the ilium, S.I. joint or sacrum.
4. Vertical displacement of greater than 1 cm.[13] Denis pointed also to the instability associated with fracture of the lumbar transverse process secondary to quadratus lumborum avulsion.[2]

Separate classifications have been made for sacral fractures. Matta et al analyzed 29 unstable sacral fractures. Each patient had a Bucholz Class III unstable pelvic fracture with a sacral vertical component. He and Denis classified sacral fractures[2] into three types (Figure 1):

Class 1: The vertical sacral fracture is lateral to the sacral foramina.
Class 2: The fracture is through the sacral foramina.
Class 3: The fracture is medial to the sacral foramina and includes vertical and transverse fractures.

The Matta Class 4 is a special classification of an "H" fracture with both a transverse and vertical component. Of 29 sacral fractures, 3 patients had a Class 1 fracture, 17 a Class 2 fracture, 7 a Class 3 fracture, and 2 a Class 4 fracture.

Sacral Fractures

Denis et al identified 236 sacral fractures in a group of 776 pelvic fractures. More than 21% of patients with these sacral fractures had a neurological deficit. He classified sacral fractures into three basic categories according to the location of the fracture. Zone 1 fractures were located lateral to the sacral foramina in the ala, Zone 2 fractures occurred through the sacral foramina, and Zone 3 fractures occurred in the central canal. Fractures in Zones 1 and 2 were most likely to produce injury to individual roots, whereas those in Zone 3 were associated with a high incidence of cauda equina injury.

Sabiston et al classified transverse sacral fractures, adding emphasis to the location of transverse fractures (Figure 2). In a review of 35 cases, he found 19 with combined pelvic-sacral vertical shear fractures involving both anterior and posterior column. Eleven isolated transverse fractures occurred below S2. The mechanism of injury was a direct blow in the lower sacral area. There were five upper transverse fractures through the S2 area. The postulated mechanism of injury was indirect leverage of the spine on a fixed pelvis.[14] Displaced transverse sacral fractures are less common than vertical shear fractures. Fountain[7] found only 3% of the sacral fractures reviewed were transverse.

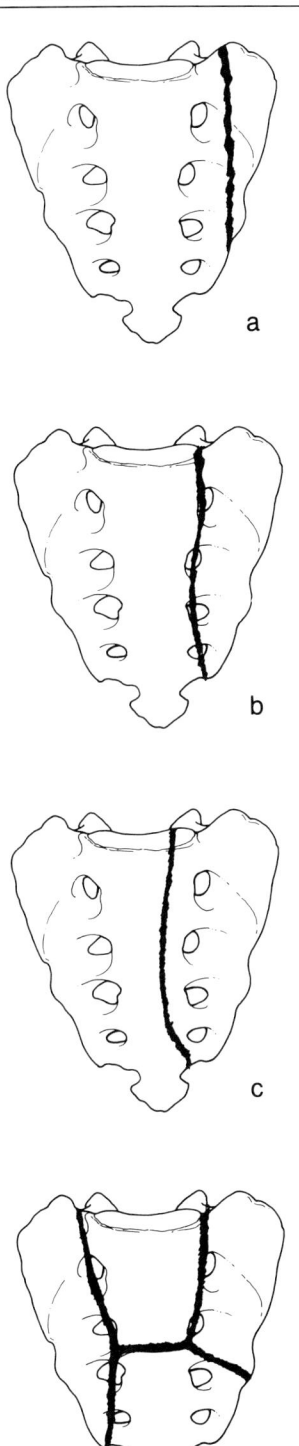

Figure 1. Classification of sacral fractures: **(a)** Class I—Lateral to the sacral foramina, **(b)** Class II—Through the sacral foramina, **(c)** Class III—Medial to the sacral foramina including the canal, and **(d)** Class IV—The "H" configuration of Matta.

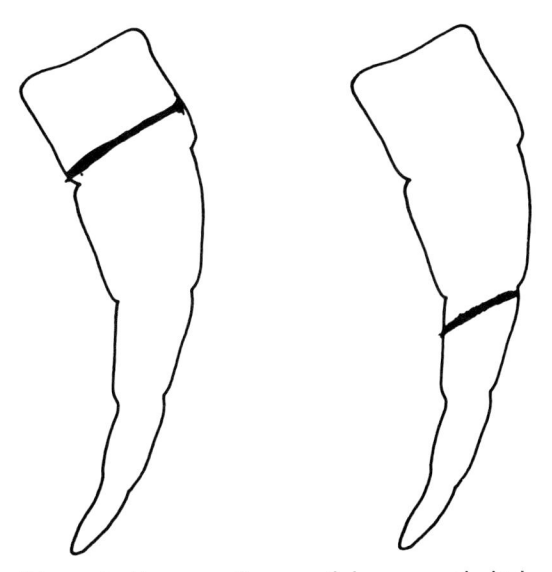

Figure 2. Transverse fractures of the sacrum, the higher level being between S1 and S2, the lower level at S4.

Radiographic Diagnosis

Sacral fractures typically occur in multiple injured patients. Reviews have shown up to a 66% incidence of multiple associated injuries including shock and hemorrhage, bladder and intraabdominal injury, and ruptured diaphragm.[15] Initial resuscitation is paramount in these patients. Only when they are stable is a more detailed diagnosis of the fractures and their relation to neurological injury carried out.

Up to 49% of sacral fractures are not diagnosed during the initial hospital stay.[2,16] Thus, an anteroposterior (AP) x-ray of the pelvis should be a standard part of the workup in the multiple injured patient, especially those with compression tenderness of the pelvis. Up to 45% of pelvic fractures will be associated with sacral fractures.[1,8] Twenty-one percent of unilateral pubic rami fractures and 66% of bilateral pubic rami fractures have associated posterior column fractures.[11] Bilateral pubic rami fractures are not only associated with a high incidence of urological injury, but also are a hallmark for a posterior column fracture.[1] Additional signs of a posterior pelvic column disruption with instability are fractures of the transverse process (Figure 3),[14] avulsions of the sacral tuberous ligament,[2] and L5-S1 facet dislocations.[17] Unfortunately, the standard AP view of the pelvis may be inadequate for properly diagnosing a sacral fracture.

The most commonly missed sacral injury is a transverse fracture at the S2 level. This produces a fracture line in the coronal plane that is easily missed on the standard AP roentgenogram. Palpation and observation of the spine, palpation and compression of the pelvis, and neurological evaluation of the patient are critical in the diagnosis of an unstable sacral fracture. Finding any pelvic fracture necessitates obtaining an inlet and outlet view of the pelvis.[1,13] The diagnosis of instability can virtually always be made with a combination of these three views. An oblique pelvic view can be included for proper assessment of the acetabulum. Anterior pelvis fractures should lead the examiner immediately to the posterior pelvis and sacrum for a thorough assessment of potential fractures posteriorly.

Neurological Evaluation

Neurological deficits are frequently not diagnosed.[1,15] Denis et al found that among patients with neurological deficits attributable to a sacral fracture, 24% lacked the appropriate specific diagnosis in the chart, and only 30% had the appropriate x-rays required to diagnose the neurological deficit.[2]

Denis showed that 5.9% of patients with fractures located lateral to the intervertebral foramina had a neurological deficit. Six of seven patients had an L5 root lesion due to proximal displacement of the ala. Twenty-eight percent of patients with fractures through the sacral foramina had a neurological deficit, but only 5% of those had loss of bowel and bladder function. The L5 nerve root also could be involved as a result of cephalad migration of both alae lateral to the sacral foramina. For S1 or S2 root lesions in patients with fractures through the bony foramina, the injury was due to disruption of the foramina. Late onset of S1 or S2 dysfunction was invariably due to bony healing, pro-

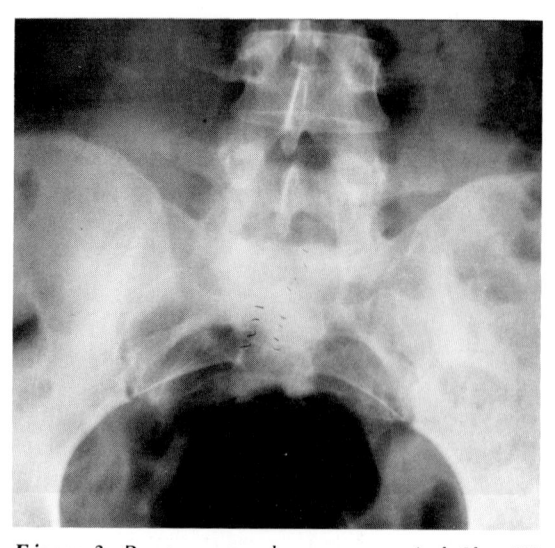

Figure 3. Roentgenogram demonstrates vertical Class III sacral fracture; note also fracture of transverse process of L5.

ducing stenosis of the sacral foramina. More than one-half of patients with fractures through the sacral canal had a neurological deficit and 76% of those had bowel and bladder impairment.[2,18]

In Matta's series, 14 of 29 patients had neurological deficits. He found that the location of the vertical unstable fracture bore no relationship to the degree of neurological injury, and felt that neurological deficit occurred as a result of traction nerve injury from vertical displacement of the pelvis.[19] Two of three patients with a cauda equina syndrome had an "H" type Class IV fracture and one had a midline split. The remaining patients had either an L5 or S1 root lesion.

An S1 or S2 root lesion is frequently seen with upper transverse fractures.[3,14] Lower segment fractures, 64% of which occur at S4, are less likely to involve isolated sacral nerve roots.[14] That does not exclude lower sacral fractures, either of the transverse or vertical variety, from producing loss of bowel and bladder function.[20] Fountain reported six cases of transverse sacral fractures, all with loss of bowel and bladder function.[7] Schmidek et al found that two-thirds of patients with transverse sacral fractures had bowel and bladder disturbances.[20] Urinary and fecal continence and sexual potency are retained in males with unilateral S2 and S3 function. Impotence and loss of sphincter function suggest bilateral injury to multiple sacral nerve roots.[20,21]

Impotence can also be caused by severe symphysis pubis disruption with injury to the prostatic urethra. In a high proportion of patients with pelvic fractures, impotence is caused by urological injury.[22] It can also result from pelvic or pudendal nerve damage, involving branches of S2-S4.[2]

Neurological injury associated with sacral fracture may occur as follows: (1) from injuries to the cauda equina within the spinal canal as a result of fracture dislocations, (2) from compressive injury within the sacral canal or at the neural foramina, (3) from traction to the lumbosacral plexus with vertical displacement of the hemipelvis, or (4) avulsion of the nerve roots from the conus medullaris.[23] Concomitant neurological injury should always be suspected in patients with sacral fractures.

Treatment of Sacral Fractures

Treatment of sacral fractures is designed to decrease the potential for neurological dysfunction and pain. The latter may result from nerve injury or musculoskeletal dysfunction. Decision making depends largely on an accurate diagnosis of the neurological and musculoskeletal injury. The treatment of a sacral fracture is inevitably interwoven with the treatment of a pelvic fracture.

Guidelines for treatment of sacral and pelvic fractures are very similar to the guidelines for treatment of spinal fractures[24] and is dependent on the following: (1) the capability of the medical facilities, (2) the condition of the patient, (3) the type and extent of neurological deficit, (4) the stability of the spine and pelvis, (5) the degree of displacement of the fracture, and (6) rehabilitation potential.

Most investigators agree that stable compression-type injuries of the pelvis can be treated symptomatically with bed rest, analgesics, and a pelvic sling.[2,4,6,9,12,13,14,25,26] Open reduction and internal fixation are more likely to be recommended for unstable Bucholz Class III injuries.[2,6,9,25] External fixation can be used to stabilize anterior disruption. With partial posterior disruption and under certain circumstances of unstable Bucholz Class III lesions,[27] Kellam has recommended sacral bars posteriorly and external fixation anteriorly, or an external fixator with double syntheseal plating and early ambulation.[13]

Fracture dislocations of the S.I. joint have been shown by numerous authors to be associated with late S.I. joint pain (Figure 4).[12,16,17,28,29] Tile showed a 60% incidence of late pain with S.I. joint injury.[12] Holdsworth showed a 44% incidence of failure to return to work compared to 13% with sacral

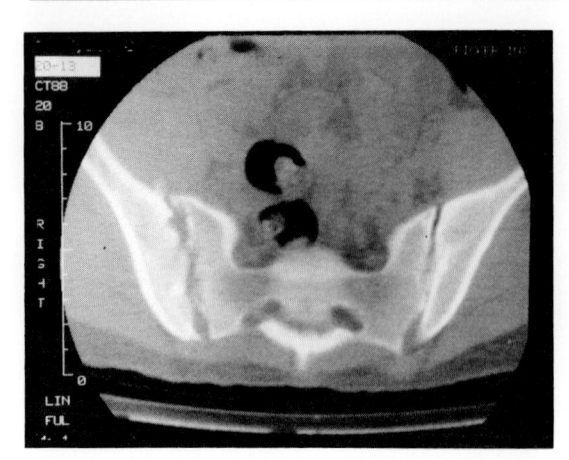

Figure 4. Malgaigne fracture dislocation of the sacroiliac joint.

and posterior ilium fractures. Raf also showed a 45% incidence of chronic low back pain, a 30% incidence of leg pain, and a 15% incidence of persistent neurological deficit with any disruption of the posterior column of the pelvis, and noted that low back pain was higher with S.I. joint injury.[29] Unstable pelvic fractures have a greater eventual morbidity as well as mortality.[13,30] Holdsworth pointed out that a symphysis pubis disruption causes significant pain for approximately two years.[28] As a general rule, unstable pelvic fractures associated with a fracture dislocation or dislocation of the S.I. joint should be treated by internal fixation including plating or screw fixation of the S.I. joint.[13,25,31]

Matta et al reported on 28 patients treated at the Los Angeles County–University of Southern California Medical Center. Eleven patients had an initial open reduction and internal fixation: four posterior, and seven posterior and anterior. Two patients had laminectomies and nine had late open reduction and internal fixation. Fourteen cases were treated with traction and bed rest. Fifty percent of the nonoperatively treated patients had a very poor result. The experience of others is similar,[32] and the tendency is for nonunions and malunions to occur with nonoperative management. The overall results in the operative cases were excellent in 21%, good in 50%, and unsatisfactory in 21%. Thirty-two percent of operated patients had no pain whatsoever and 54% had only intermittent or slight pain.

Late open reduction and internal fixation are much more difficult and dangerous. There is an average of 2,000 cc of blood loss and eight hours of surgery with the delayed cases. Neurological deficits may actually increase with delayed treatment due to scarring of the sacral roots within a malunion or nonunion. The current recommendation is for stable fractures to be treated symptomatically with bed rest and for unstable Bucholz III fractures to be treated with open reduction and internal fixation in the first week.

The techniques of internal fixation vary.[10,12,13,32] The reduction technique developed and used by Matta uses an entry point for the screw 15 cm below the posterior superior iliac crest and midway between the sciatic notch and the upper rim of the pelvis (Figure 5). The approach is through a posterior vertical incision 2 cm lateral to the posterior superior iliac spine. The incision starts proximal to the iliac crest and proceeds distal to the sciatic notch. The fracture site is exposed and reduced.

During the reduction, the sacral roots are palpated through the greater sciatic notch to ensure that compression is not being produced by bone fragments. Two 6.5 mm di-

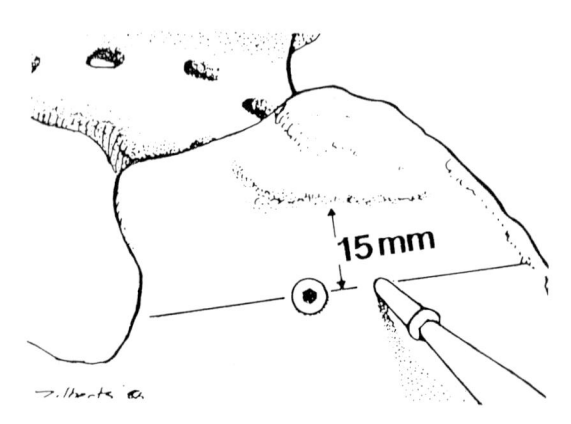

Figure 5. The insertion point for the screw used for open reduction internal fixation in sacral fractures is 15 mm anterior to the cresta gluteal line and midway between the posterior iliac spine and the sacral notch. Location of the screw in the 40° cephalad view.

ameter screws are inserted from a point 15 mm anterior to the line of the crest of glutea, and halfway between the iliac crest and the greater sciatic notch. Under image intensifier control, the screw is placed in the anterior portion of the vertebral body proximal to the S1 foramina, distal to the top of the sacral ala and anterior to the spinal canal. For long or comminuted fractures, a flexible plate may be inserted across the back of the sacrum just proximal to the greater sciatic notch. Interfragmentary screws are used in the majority of cases (Figure 6), while the double cobra plate is reserved for long fractures or very unstable fractures, or osteoporotic bone.

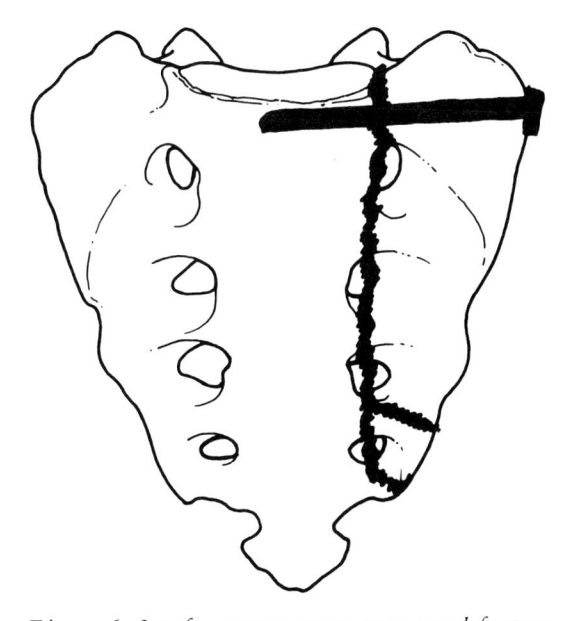

Figure 6. Interfragmentary screw across sacral fracture.

Operative Decision Making and Neurologic Deficit

The most important factor in the prognosis of the patient's neurological deficit is the severity of the initial injury.[10,26] If the initial deficit is severe, permanent disability may be unavoidable.[1] The nerve root involved is also important. For example, deficits involving the S1 nerve root tend to resolve without specific treatment. Bonnin and Denis et al both recommended conservative care for S1 root lesions due to the good prognosis in their case review.[1,2] The situation with lesions of the L5 nerve root with associated foot drop is quite different. Because 75% of patients with foot drop will have persistence of their deficit without operation, patients with a foot drop are more likely to have surgery recommended. In patients with multiple root involvement and mild bowel and bladder symptoms, resolution of signs and symptoms with nonoperative care and with only some mild hemisaddle sensory loss is the rule.

Schmidek et al felt that only 10% of sacral nerve injuries are secondary to compression and amenable to decompression.[20] The neural injury may be due to a nerve root avulsion.[23] At autopsy, nerve root avulsions have been the source of the neurological deficit in up to 40% of cases.[23] Ferris felt that neurological deficit due to a transverse sacral fracture is liable to resolve even if the patient is treated conservatively.[18,33]

If the majority of the neurological dysfunction is caused by ventral hematoma and/or ventral gibbus deformity, laminectomy is useless. Delayed treatment of the cauda equina syndrome in patients with loss of bowel and bladder and sexual function, especially those who are not improving, may lead to persistent deficit. Early reduction and decompression of cauda equina compression is felt to give the best prognosis for recovery.[2,7,25] Delay in operative intervention and conservative care may lead to additional nerve loss when the sacrum is reduced due to scarring of the nerves in the area. There may even be late neurological deterioration secondary to displacement of the fracture despite partial healing by callous and scar.[17,25]

In general, emergency operative decompression is seldom indicated. Decompression can often be achieved with nonoperative reduction, especially in vertically displaced fractures, by placing the patient in traction. This may produce a significant improvement in neurological function due to the reduction, but Matta's review shows that there is no relation between the location of an unstable vertical fracture and the degree of the neurological injury. He felt that most lesions were due to traction of roots secondary to the vertical displacement and not due to direct bone compression. If the neurological deficit fails to improve, computerized tomography (CT) scanning and evaluation of the sacral foramina for compressive lesions can be carried out.

Denis recommends the following treatment: For Class I fractures, early traction to protect the L5 root is indicated. However, if there is greater than 2 cm of displacement or more than 72 hours have elapsed since the injury, traction will not be successful and plating the symphysis and fixing the entire fracture are indicated. For Class II fractures that are stable without sciatica, nonoperative treatment, early ambulation, and non-weight-bearing on the foraminal fracture side are appropriate. If sciatica is present after six to eight weeks and, in particular, if there is severe sciatica and documented sacral foraminal loss of 50% or greater, a sacral laminectomy is indicated. Sciatica with loss of plantar flexion and a 75% occlusion of the foramina requires early laminectomy. For unstable vertical shear fractures, the treatment is immediate traction and early open reduction and internal fixation. If there is severe foraminal stenosis and deficits involving the S1 and S2 roots, early laminectomy is indicated.

On the other hand, an isolated S1 radiculopathy with severe foraminal stenosis can be decompressed late.[2] An anatomic open reduction and internal fixation of the pelvis is still the best method of neurological decompression.[2,20,25] The timing varies from within the first week[25] to 4-10 days[13] after the acute injury. However, reduction becomes more difficult with increasing time from the injury.

Decision Making in Late Displaced Pelvic Fractures

The complication rate in late displaced pelvic and sacral fractures is very high. Often, reduction of the pelvis and the sacrum may in itself produce neurological deficit as scar and bone fragments impinge on healing sacral nerve roots. When considering approaches to patients with neurological deficit in late pelvic fractures, the type and extent of the neurological deficit are important in determining the operative strategy. For example, to attempt a late major pelvic reconstruction surgery for an irretrievable neurological deficit would expose the patient to unnecessary morbidity and potential mortality. A more limited, specific decompression may be done.

Summary and Conclusions

The following steps are recommended in the diagnosis and treatment of patients with sacral fractures:

1. Resuscitate the patient.
2. Diagnose the pelvic fracture.
3. Diagnose the sacral fracture as to Class I, II, or III.
4. Determine the exact neurological deficit; consider a lumbar myelogram and contrast CT scan of the lumbar spine and entire sacrum. Even though the dural sac ends at S2, the myelogram may diagnose absent nerve roots due to avulsions and the contrast CT scan will show areas of neural compression.
5. Determine whether the fracture is stable or unstable.
6. If the fracture is stable, begin initial nonoperative treatment.
7. If the fracture is unstable, attempt a reduction in traction or lateral sling and obtain a detailed radiographic evaluation of the patency of the sacral foramina and exact bony injury to the sacrum and entire spinal column.
8. Within the first week to 10 days do an open reduction and internal fixation of the pelvic fracture.
9. If neurological deficit persists, again perform a detailed radiological

assessment to accurately diagnose neural compression.
10. If facilities for accurate open reduction and internal fixation do not exist, use traction, external fixation, limited internal fixation, and decompression by laminectomy of compressive lesions.
11. For late displaced malunions or nonunions with neurological deficit, exact anatomic detail of compressive lesions must be delineated. Late reduction of the pelvic fracture is a most demanding surgical procedure. A more limited decompressive laminectomy or foraminotomy of compressive lesions may be the wisest approach.
12. For the cauda equina syndrome with profound loss of bowel and bladder function secondary to displaced fractures of the sacrum, the fracture must first be reduced. If the ability to reduce the fracture does not exist, decompression by laminectomy is indicated.

References

1. Bonnin JG. Sacral fractures and injuries to the cauda equina. *J Bone Joint Surg.* 1945;27:113-127.
2. Denis F, Steven D, Comfort T. Sacral fractures: an important problem: retrospective analysis of 236 cases. *Clin Orthop.* 1988;27:67-81.
3. Bucknill JM, Blackburn JS. Fracture-dislocations of the sacrum: report of three cases. *J Bone Joint Surg Br.* 1976;58B:467-470.
4. LaFollette BF, Levine MI, McNiesh LM. Bilateral fracture-dislocation of the sacrum. *J Bone Joint Surg Am.* 1986;68A:1099-1101.
5. Marcus RE, Hanson ST Jr. Bilateral fracture-dislocations of the sacrum. *J Bone Joint Surg Am.* 1984;66A:1297-1299.
6. Bucholz RW. The pathological anatomy of malgaigne fracture-dislocations of the pelvis. *J Bone Joint Surg Am.* 1981;63A:400-404.
7. Fountain SS, Hamilton RD, Jameson RM. Transverse fractures of the sacrum: a report of six cases. *J Bone Joint Surg Am.* 1977;59A:486-489.
8. Mendelman JP. Fractures of the sacrum: their incidence in fractures of the pelvis. *AJR.* 1939;42:100-103.
9. Patterson FP, Morton KS. Neurologic complications of fractures and dislocations of the pelvis. *Surg Gynecol Obstet.* 1961;112:702-706.
10. Speed K. *Text-Book of Fractures and Dislocations.* 2nd ed. Philadelphia, Pa: Lea & Febiger; 1928.
11. Huittinen VM, Slätis P. Fractures of the pelvis: trauma mechanisms, type of injury, principles of treatment. *Acta Chir Scand.* 1972;138:563-569.
12. Tile M. *Fractures of the Pelvis and Acetabulum.* Baltimore, Md: Williams & Wilkins; 1984.
13. Kellam JF, McMurtry RY, Paley D, Tile M. The unstable pelvic fracture. *Orthop Clin North Am.* 1987;18:25-41.
14. Sabiston CP, Wing PC. Sacral fractures: classification and neurologic implications. *J Trauma.* 1986;26:1113-1115.
15. Peltier LF. Complications associated with fractures of the pelvis. *J Bone Joint Surg Am.* 1965;47A:1060-1069.
16. Laasonen EM. Missed sacral fractures. *Ann Clin Res.* 1977;9:84-87.
17. Matta JM, Merritt PO. Displaced acetabular fractures. *Clin Orthop.* 1988;230:83-97.
18. Byrnes DP, Russo GL, Ducker TB, Cowley RA. Sacrum fractures and neurological damage. *J Neurosurg.* 1977;47:459-462.
19. Matta JM, Anderson LM, Epstein HC, Hendricks P. Fractures of the acetabulum: A retrospective analysis. *Clin Orthop.* 1986;205:230-240.
20. Schmidek HH, Smith DA, Kristiansen TK. Sacral fractures. *Neurosurgery.* 1984;15:735-746.
21. Gunterberg B. Effects of major resection of the sacrum. *Acta Orthop Scand.* 1976;162(suppl).
22. Fallon B, Wendt JC, Hawtrey CE. Urological injury and assessment in patients with fractured pelvis. *J Urology.* 1984;131:712-714.
23. Huittinen VM. Lumbosacral nerve injury in fracture of the pelvis. *Acta Chir Scand.* 1976;429(suppl):6.
24. Watkins RG, Apuzzo M, Dobkin W. *Therapeutic Considerations in the Surgical Management of Lesions Affecting the Mid-thoracic Spine.* New York, NY: Grune & Stratton; 1985.
25. Matta JM. Operative indications and choice of surgical approach fractures of the acetabulum. *Techniques Orthopaed.* Aspen, Colo: Aspen Publishers; 1986:13-22.
26. Yngve D. Sacral fractures. *Orthopedics.* 1985;8:517-518.
27. Mears DC, Fu FH. Modern concepts of external skeletal fixation of the pelvis. *Clin Orthop.* 1980;151:65-72.
28. Holdsworth FW. Dislocation and fracture-dislocation of the pelvis. *J Bone Joint Surg Br.* 1948;30B:461-466.
29. Raf L. Double vertical fractures of the pelvis. *Acta Chir Scand.* 1965;131:298-305.
30. Dunn AW, Morris HD. Fractures and dislocations of the pelvis. *J Bone Joint Surg Am.* 1968;50A:1639-1648.
31. Slätis P, Karaharju EO. External fixation of the pelvic girdle with a trapezoid compression frame. *Injury.* 1975;7:53-56.
32. Semba RT, Yasukawa K, Gustilo RB. Critical analysis of results of 53 Malgaigne fractures of the pelvis. *J Trauma.* 1983;23:535-537.
33. Ferris B, Hutton P. Anteriorly displaced transverse fractures of the sacrum at the level of the sacro-iliac joint: a report of two cases. *J Bone Joint Surg Am.* 1983;65A:407-409.

CHAPTER 11

Special Problems in Patients with Preexisting Spine Disease

Raj Murali, MD

Preexisting spine diseases can predispose the patient to spinal injury after even trivial trauma. The more common preexisting entities are ankylosing spondylitis, rheumatoid arthritis, Klippel-Feil anomaly, osteoporosis, previous laminectomy, and spondylosis associated with a narrow spinal canal.

Ankylosing Spondylitis

The incidence of ankylosing spondylitis in the general population is one to three per thousand with young men being at greatest risk.[1] The onset of the disease is usually in the second or third decade of life. Patients usually present with early morning stiffness of the spine and diffuse pain. The sacroiliac joint is usually the first site of involvement. Some patients with extensive involvement of the cervical spine may present with chin on chest deformity due to progressive subluxation at the C1-C2 level.

Confirmation of the diagnosis is ultimately based on radiographic findings. In early cases of ankylosing spondylitis only the sacroiliac joints may be involved. However, in patients who present with spinal trauma, extensive involvement of the spine and the classical appearance of a "bamboo spine" are often present.

Extensive calcification of all the ligaments of the spine is seen, including the disc spaces[2] with associated osteoporosis and loss of normal spine curvature. Spontaneous fusion of the spine occurs over multiple segments. The fused spine is osteoporotic and tends to be inherently weak. Fractures or fracture subluxations of the spine may occur with minor injury.[3] Atlantoaxial subluxation may occur in patients where the entire thoracolumbar spine is fused. Multiple spinal fractures are also common. At times a spontaneous fracture or subluxation may occur without a history of trauma. The brittle bone heals poorly and can lead to pseudarthrosis and continued instability.

Weinstein et al reported 13 traumatic fractures and four destructive spinal lesions in a series of 105 patients with ankylosing spondylitis.[3] The commonest site of injury was the cervical region. Many of the fractures seemed to occur at an interdiscal location. This type of interdiscal fracture is quite unique to ankylosing spondylitis and other diseases associated with extensive fusion of the spinal ligaments. In our own series of eight patients complete neurological deficit was present in six.[4] The high incidence of neurological deficit is due to the severe subluxation following fracture, as the fused spine behaves like a long bone. In some cases the ossified ligaments, especially the ligamentum flavum, buckle inward compressing the spinal cord. A higher incidence of spinal epidural hematoma also occurs, probably due to increased vascularity of the epidural space.[5]

The presence of spinal stenosis in many of these patients also contributes to the high incidence of severe neural injury.

Destructive or erosive vertebral lesions (spondyloarthrosis or spondylodiscitis) are often seen on radiographs, occurring at the vertebral body end-plate.[6] Some of the lesions may be related to old unrecognized spinal fractures. The radiographic appearance may resemble bacterial discitis. Wedge deformities may also be present.[3]

The diagnosis is evident in those cases where a previous history of ankylosing spondylitis exists. However, in many patients the condition is diagnosed only at the time of the trauma, as was the case in six of eight cases in our series of patients with ankylosing spondylitis presenting with spinal fractures.

Management

In cases with only local areas of erosion or wedge compression of the spine, which usually present with local pain, healing will occur after prolonged immobilization with external orthoses. The management of patients with severe fractures, subluxations, and neurological deficits is more complex.

Middle and Lower Cervical Spine

The middle and lower cervical spine is the commonest site of injury in patients with ankylosing spondylitis.[3,7] The fracture is frequently followed by severe subluxation because of excessive leverage upon the bone fragments at the fracture site. Rand and Stern have emphasized that the normal flexibility, elasticity, and mobility of the spine are progressively lost because of the disease process. The vertebral column is transformed into a fragile segment that breaks under the forces that a normal spine can readily withstand.[7] Because the spinal ligaments are ossified and inelastic, the two fractured segments act under the forces of the cervical musculature and gravity like a long-bone fracture. These patients tend to be extremely unstable; neurological deterioration and increase of subluxation and deformities is common in spite of treatment.

The dangers of cervical traction in these patients cannot be overemphasized. The mechanical force needed to correct the deformity is quite different from that needed for the more common fractures of the spine in patients without ankylosing spondylitis. The literature contains many case reports of worsening of neurological deficit with the application of traction or during turning.[4,7,8]

The reasons for deterioration following application of cervical traction are not always clear. However, overdistraction with even minimal weights is a frequent occurrence. No more than 5 lbs of traction is generally needed to adequately immobilize the spine. While extension is generally the position of safety for cervical spine fractures, extension of the spine in patients with this condition will frequently result in increased subluxation and enhancement of the neurological deficit. Patients should therefore be placed in a neutral to slightly flexed position. The goal should be to place the spine in the same deformed position it assumed prior to trauma.

The optimum definitive management of patients after initial reduction and stabilization is controversial. In patients who are admitted with minimal or no subluxation and an interdiscal fracture, rigid immobilization in a halo vest is frequently appropriate. Bergmann has reported rapid healing of the fracture with external immobilization alone. Collar orthoses are ineffective; only a halo vest or similar device will provide sufficient immobilization to ensure healing of the fracture and prevent further deformity and subluxation. However, the halo vest provides insufficient immobilization of the fractures.

Anterior stabilization and fusion has rarely been effective as the bone is brittle and does not stay reduced. The application of anterior plates and screws is unsatisfactory because the bone is brittle and screw extrusion is likely. Posterior cervical wiring and fusion followed

Special Problems in Patients with Preexisting Spine Disease

by immobilization in a halo vest is usually the method of choice. Patients should undergo fiberoptic intubation while awake, without manipulation of the neck. A halo vest is applied, the patient is turned to the prone position, and motor and sensory examinations are performed. When it is clear that there has been no neurological deterioration, anesthesia is induced. An x-ray is taken to ascertain that the patient's alignment has not changed. Interspinous wiring and bone grafting are then performed as outlined in Chapter 8. The patient is kept in the halo vest for two to three months.

Laminectomy is not generally indicated for patients with ankylosing spondylitis. However, in patients who deteriorate as a result of extradural hemorrhage, laminectomy is the only way to decompress the spinal canal.

Some unstable patients cannot be moved from bed to operating table without hazard. In several instances, we have kept such patients in bed with cervical traction over a period of 8-12 weeks. While this admittedly old-fashioned treatment is associated with the perils of prolonged bed rest, with rigorous physical and pulmonary therapy patients can be successfully managed in this manner.

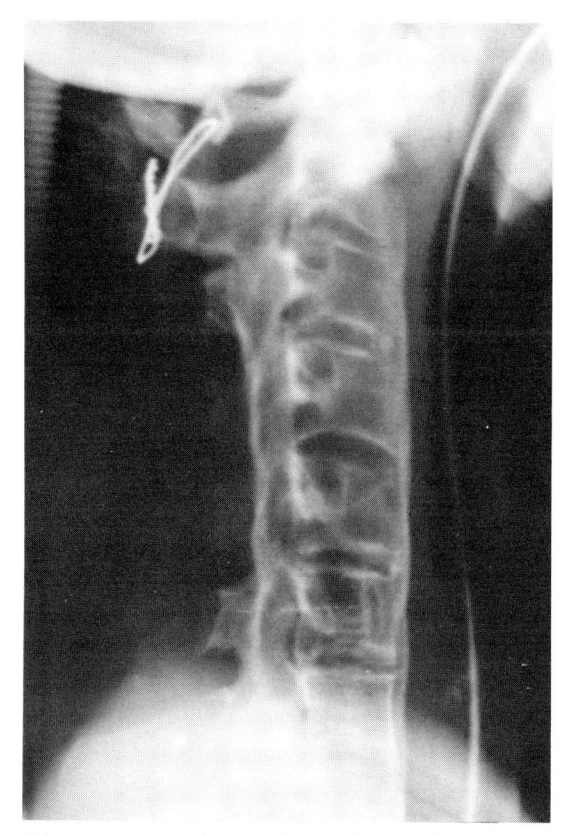

Figure 1. Lateral view of cervical spine showing ligamentous ossification due to ankylosing spondylitis and C1-C2 subluxation treated by wiring and fusion.

Craniocervical Instability

Atlantoaxial or atlantooccipital instability can be encountered in a patient with ankylosing spondylitis, although more frequently in patients with rheumatoid arthritis. The patient may present with a chin on chest deformity and no clear evidence of trauma. The mechanism, similar to that in rheumatoid arthritis, is chronic synovitis resulting in laxity and rupture of the transverse ligament. Odontoid erosion and subluxation may also be present. Basilar invagination has been reported. The patients with craniocervical instability have a slowly progressive course. They do not respond to external immobilization alone. They require reduction of the subluxation and intraoperative stabilization (Figure 1).

Thoracolumbar Fractures

Thoracolumbar fractures can occur either in isolation or coincident with a cervical spine injury. Two of our eight patients presented with both cervical and thoracolumbar fractures sustained in the same fall. Marked deformity and subluxation are common, resulting in a high incidence of neurological deficits (Figure 2). When the patient is neurologically intact, which is often the case in undisplaced fractures of the spine, treatment can be external immobilization alone. Strict bed rest with careful turning in a body cast for about six weeks usually results in good fusion.[9] However, if marked angulation or subluxation is present, intraoperative reduction and posterior instrumentation and fusion will be necessary.

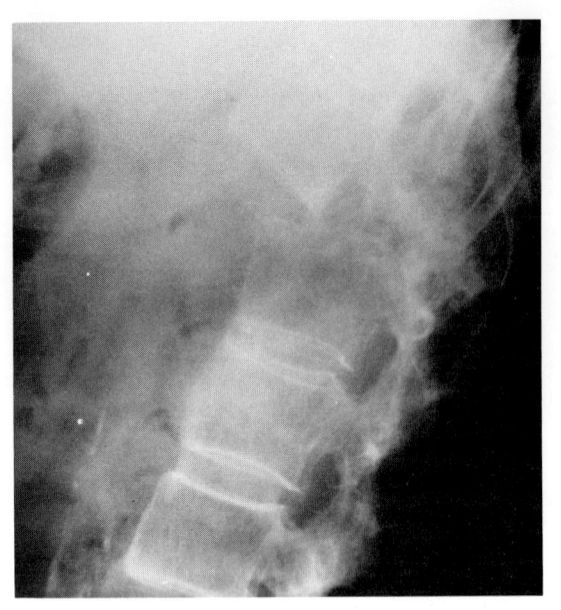

Figure 2. T12-L1 fracture subluxation in a patient with ankylosing spondylitis. Note the marked separation of the fractured segments due to the fused spine acting as a long bone.

Complications

Complications are frequent in patients with ankylosing spondylitis and spinal fractures. Most series reveal at least a 50% mortality in the presence of serious neurological deficits.[10] Three of our eight patients who presented with neurological deficits died. Respiratory complications are the commonest cause of death: patients already have decreased respiratory excursions due to a frozen rib cage, and if paralysis of respiration is superimposed severe compromise of respiratory function occurs. Associated pulmonary fibrosis may compound the problem. In thoracolumbar fractures, the fractured segment may be displaced sufficiently to cause major damage to visceral structures in the abdomen. Laceration of the abdominal aorta has been reported.[11] There is also an increased incidence of ulcerative colitis in these patients, which may become exacerbated during the stress of spinal surgery.

Prognosis and Outcome

Patients who present with severe neurological deficits have a poor prognosis. There is roughly a 50% mortality in patients with quadriplegia.[10] Those patients presenting with only a fracture, without subluxation or neurological deficits, usually heal well with rigid external immobilization alone.[12] However, great caution should be observed while treating them, as simple nursing procedures such as turning may cause a subluxation and serious spinal cord injury.

Patients known to have ankylosing spondylitis should be educated about the risks and dangers of spinal injury. They also should be alerted to report promptly to a hospital following any type of injury.

Rheumatoid Arthritis

Rheumatoid arthritis usually affects the cervical spine including the craniovertebral junction. The disease is rare elsewhere in the spine. However, sacroiliac joint involvement is common. Atlantoaxial subluxation occurs frequently. A radiological survey has revealed abnormal movement at the atlantoaxial region in up to 25% of patients.[13,14] Although the condition usually occurs in advanced rheumatoid arthritis, it can occur early in the course of the disease. The role played by corticosteroids as a predisposing factor is not clear.

Rheumatoid arthritis causes severe inflammation of the synovial structures adjacent to the odontoid process and its ligaments. This can lead to erosion and extensive destruction of the odontoid with marked ligamentous laxity. In time, such destruction, inflammation, and ligamentous laxity leads to a gradual forward slip of the entire atlas which can narrow the canal and cause myelopathy.[15] In a patient with rheumatoid arthritis and involvement of the atlantoaxial region even slight trauma can accelerate the forward slippage, resulting in severe subluxation and spinal cord injury (Figure 3). The vertebral ar-

Special Problems in Patients with Preexisting Spine Disease

examination and radiographic assessment. Computerized tomography (CT) and magnetic resonance imaging (MRI) will clearly show compression of the spinal cord due to subluxation or the formation of pannus. Severe subluxations either at the atlantoaxial region or elsewhere in the cervical spine require operative treatment with appropriate reduction and stabilization. Minor subluxation can be treated with a collar, and x-rays repeated at regular intervals to assess the progression of subluxation.

Klippel-Feil Anomaly

The classical description of Klippel-Feil syndrome is a triad of low posterior hairline, short neck, and limitation of head and neck motion. Fusion of the cervical vertebrae is a hallmark of the anomaly (Figure 4). The fusion may simply involve two vertebral bodies

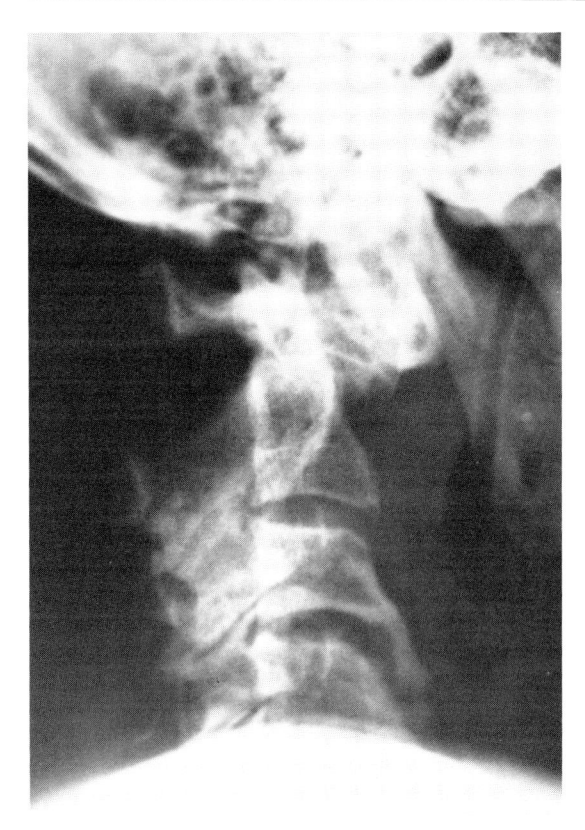

Figure 3. C1-C2 Subluxation in a patient with rheumatoid arthritis. Recent trauma resulted in further subluxation and myelopathy.

tery may be stretched and can become thrombosed.

Rheumatoid arthritis also involves the joints of Luschka which are lined by synovial tissue. Conlon noted a 60% incidence of Luschka joint involvement of the cervical spine in patients with rheumatoid arthritis.[13] Inflammation of these joints leads to the formation of a pannus, which may destroy portions of the disc and vertebra, predisposing the spine to subluxation. Trauma in these patients will result in cervical spine subluxation more readily than in patients without rheumatoid disease. Involvement of the lumbar and thoracic spine is rarer with rheumatoid arthritis, although destructive granulomatous lesions can occur in the thoracolumbar region, causing spinal cord compression.

The diagnosis of rheumatoid arthritis is readily made with a combination of clinical

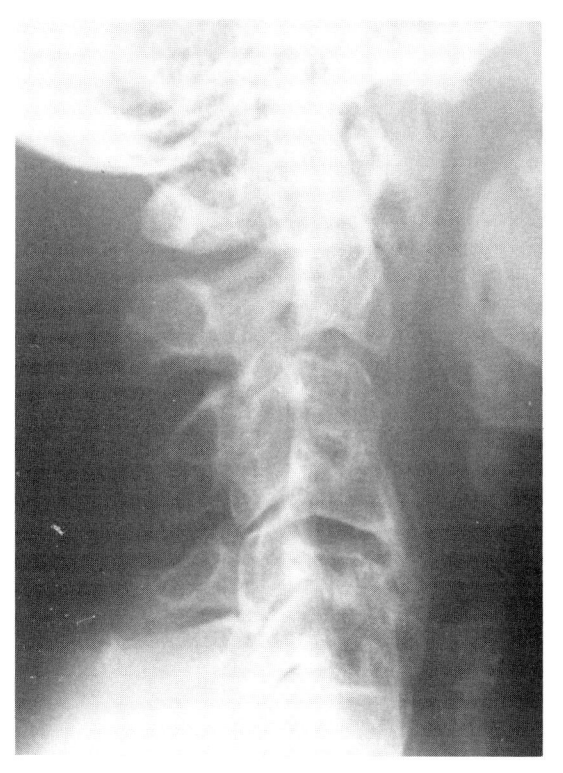

Figure 4. Klippel-Feil anomaly causing "block vertebrae" of C3-C4 and C5-C6. There is associated canal stenosis and loss of physiological lordosis.

(congenital block vertebrae) or there may be multilevel fusion and reduction in the total number of vertebrae. Flattening and widening of the involved vertebral bodies and absence of disc spaces are common. Excessive movement above and below the area of congenital fusion may result in marked spondylosis and stenosis. The patients may have other associated congenital anomalies including webbing of the neck, craniovertebral anomalies, hemivertebrae, thoracic scoliosis, and abnormalities of the rib cage.[16] The most common site of involvement is the cervical spine. Joint instability occurs above and below the level of fusion, and associated spondylosis causes a narrow canal.

Injury to the cervical spine in such a patient readily causes trauma to the spinal cord, resulting in myelopathy. Preoperatively, the patient may complain of neck pain or radiculopathy for a long period. The diagnosis becomes obvious on plain x-rays of the cervical spine. MRI or CT scan of the cervical spine clearly shows the site of spinal cord involvement. In patients with progressive neurological deficits, decompressive surgery, either anteriorly or posteriorly, accompanied by fusion, will relieve the spinal cord compression and arrest the progression of myelopathy. A high incidence of renal abnormalities occurs in these patients and renal failure may occur perioperatively, especially if the kidneys are stressed with intravenous contrast dyes.

Cervical Spondylosis

Cervical spondylosis is a degenerative disorder of the cervical spine. Degenerative changes usually start in the cervical intervertebral discs and lead to secondary changes in the surrounding bones, joints, and ligaments. As the disc spaces collapse the vertebrae settle, causing redundancy and buckling of the ligaments. The combination of hypertrophied facet joints, ligamentous buckling, osteophyte formation, and subluxation cause severe narrowing of the spinal canal (Figures 5,6). The spinal cord begins to be compressed; if trauma is superimposed the spinal cord is readily damaged.

Patients can sustain severe neurological deficits following trauma without alteration in the alignment of the bony spine. By use of myelography in cadavers with cervical spondylosis Taylor demonstrated simultaneous compression of the hyperextended spinal cord by the osteophytic spur anteriorly and the

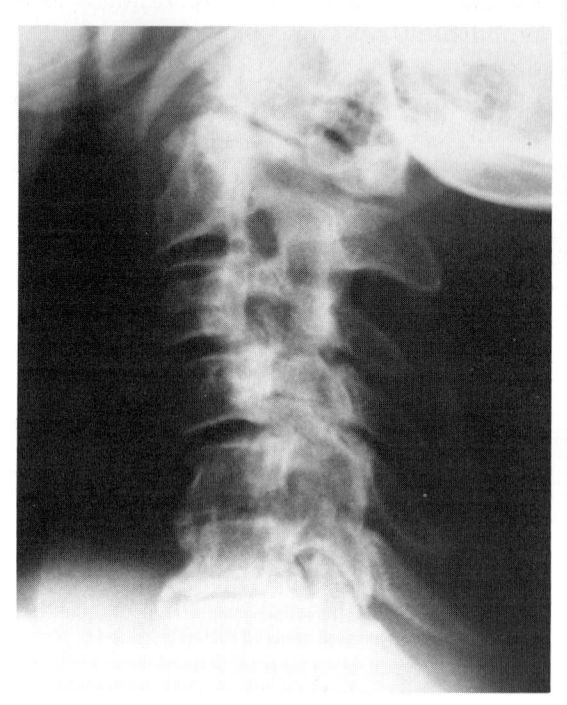

Figure 5. Lateral cervical spine x-ray showing severe degenerative spondylosis and C3-C4 subluxation.

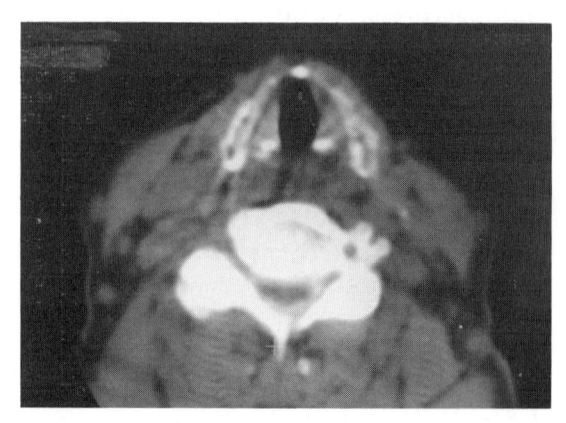

Figure 6. Same patient as in Figure 5 revealing severe cord compression from canal stenosis and ridges at C3-C4 in a postmyelogram CT scan.

buckled ligamentum flavum posteriorly.[17] Schneider et al showed that in such injuries the center of the cervical spinal cord received the major damage, resulting in an acute central cervical spinal cord syndrome[18]: disproportionately more motor impairment of the upper than of the lower extremities, urinary retention, and varying degrees of sensory loss below the level of the lesion. The cause of the trauma is usually hyperextension in an elderly individual with previous spondylosis. The diagnosis is relatively simple, with a plain x-ray showing spondylosis and MRI or postmyelogram-CT scan clearly revealing spinal cord compression. Patients may be treated with anterior cervical decompression and fusion at the appropriate levels, but there is no evidence that decompression affects outcome in patients who had no myelopathy prior to injury.

Osteoporosis

Osteoporosis is most common in postmenopausal elderly women of Caucasian descent. The spine becomes brittle, and may undergo spontaneous fracture or suffer damage after such trivial trauma as a bout of coughing (Figure 7).[19] Multiple vertebral body wedge collapses occur typically in the midthoracic spine, but may also occur in the cervical and lumbar spine. Wedge collapse fractures usually do not cause neural injury, but fracture subluxation can result if the forces are strong enough. Treatment is aimed at both correction of the recent injury and reversal of the underlying process of osteoporosis. The fractures in these patients heal poorly, and operation should be avoided if possible. Operative instrumentation is more difficult as the brittle bone does not readily hold screws and other metallic devices.

Previous Spinal Surgery

Previous spinal surgery, especially multilevel laminectomy, exposes a patient to risk of serious spine and spinal cord injuries from trauma. Multilevel cervical laminectomy, particularly in children, usually leads to the formation of angulation or swan neck deformity (Figure 8). Secondary degenerative changes occur in the intervertebral discs and facet joints, causing reduced mobility and in some cases abnormal movement or subluxation. The spinal cord could be impinged by lamina at the upper and lower end of the laminectomy.[20] The spinal cord is also more susceptible to direct injury in the presence of extensive laminectomies.

Previous anterior spinal fusion in the cervical region causes undue stress and strain on the joints above and below. Degenerative changes at these joints can result in canal stenosis, making the person more vulnerable to injury.

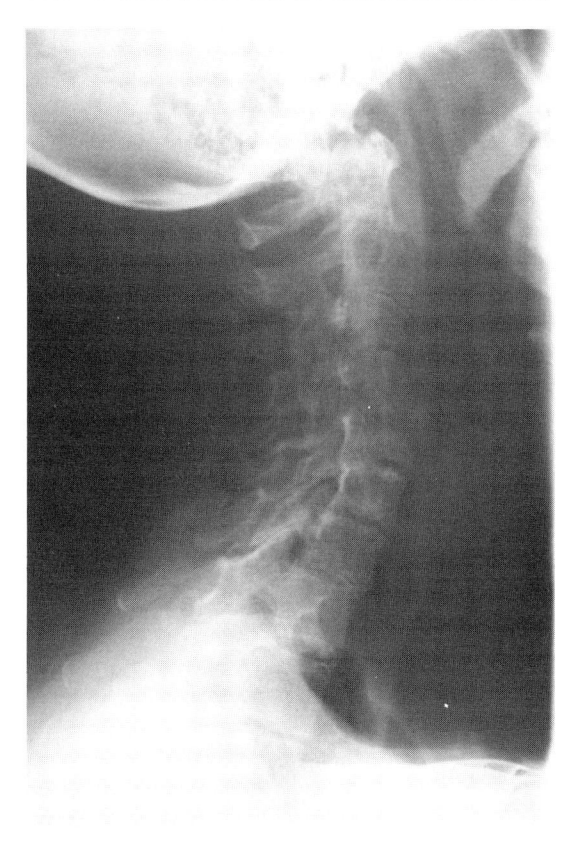

Figure 7. Lateral cervical spine x-ray showing osteoporosis, vertebral body fractures at C3, C4, C5, and multiple spinous process fractures at C2, C3, C4, C5, C6, and C7.

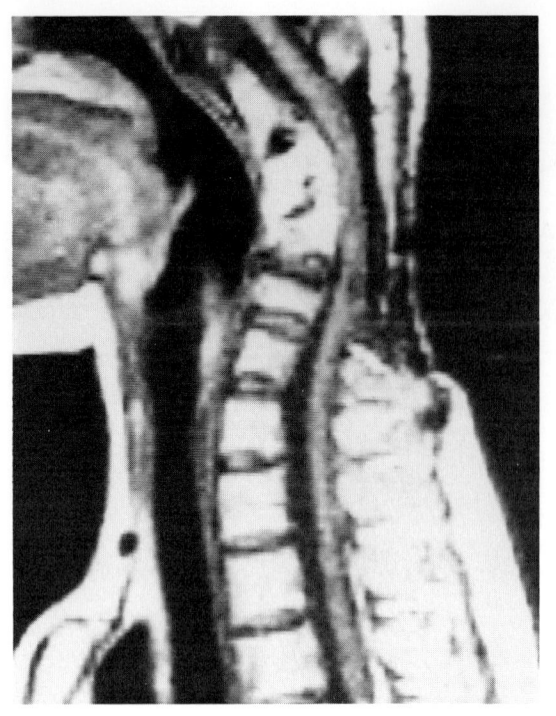

Figure 8. MRI scan of neck showing "swan neck" deformity of upper cervical spine due to previous laminectomy. Note also the spinal cord compression over the deformity.

Conclusion

A number of diseases affecting the spine make it more susceptible to trauma. Most of the diseases cause stenosis of the canal, decreased stability, or osteoporosis. Tumors such as hemangiomas of the vertebral body or metastatic tumors also predispose the spine to compression fractures either spontaneously or following minor trauma. Infections such as tuberculosis or pyogenic osteomyelitis can predispose to pathological fractures. The management of these patients is complicated and requires an understanding of the underlying pathology. After immediate treatment of the injury, the underlying pathology itself requires further investigation and treatment to prevent future injury.

References

1. Lawrence JS. The prevalence of arthritis. *Br J Clin Pract.* 1963;17:699-705.
2. Cruickshank B. Pathology of ankylosing spondylitis. *Clin Orthop.* 1971;74:43-58.
3. Weinstein PR, Karpman RR, Gall EP, Pitt M. Spinal cord injury, spinal fracture and spinal stenosis in ankylosing spondylitis. *J Neurosurg.* 1982;57:609-616.
4. Murali R, Hadani M, Rovit RL. Spinal injuries in ankylosing spondylitis. Abstracts 8th International Congress of Neurological Surgery; Toronto, Ont; 1985:71.
5. Farhat SM, Schneider RC, Gray JM. Traumatic spinal extradural hematoma associated with cervical fractures in rheumatoid spondylitis. *J Trauma.* 1973;13:591-599.
6. Rapp GF, Kerneck CB. Spontaneous fracture of the lumbar spine with correction of deformity in ankylosing spondylitis. *J Bone Joint Surg Am.* 1974;56A:1277-1278.
7. Rand RW, Stern WE. Cervical fractures of the ankylosed rheumatoid spine. *Neurochirurgia.* 1961;4:137-148.
8. Osgood C, Martin LG, Ackerman E. Fracture dislocation of the cervical spine with ankylosing spondylitis: report of two cases. *J Neurosurg.* 1973;39:764-769.
9. Guttmann L. Traumatic paraplegia and tetraplegia in ankylosing spondylitis. *Paraplegia.* 1966;4:188-203.
10. Woodruff FP, Dewing SB. Fracture of the cervical spine in patients with ankylosing spondylitis. *Radiology.* 1963;80:17-21.
11. Fazl M, Bilbao JM, Hudson AR. Laceration of the aorta complicating spinal fracture in ankylosing spondylitis. *Neurosurgery.* 1981;8:732-734.
12. Bergmann EW. Fractures of the ankylosed spine. *J Bone Joint Surg Am.* 1949;31A:669-671.
13. Conlon PW, Isdale IC, Rose BS. Rheumatoid arthritis of the cervical spine: an analysis of 333 cases. *Ann Rheum Dis.* 1966;25:120-126.
14. Meikle JAK, Wilkinson M. Rheumatoid involvement of the cervical spine: radiological assessment. *Ann Rheum Dis.* 1971;30:154-161.
15. Stevens JC, Cartlidge NEF, Saunders M, Appleby A, Hall M, Shaw DA. Atlanto-axial subluxation and cervical myelopathy in rheumatoid arthritis. *Q J Med.* 1971;40:391-408.
16. Gray SW, Romaine CB, Skandalakis JE. Congenital fusion of the cervical vertebrae. *Surg Gynecol Obstet.* 1964;118:373-385.
17. Taylor AR. The mechanism of injury to the spinal cord in the neck without damage to the vertebral column. *J Bone Joint Surg Br.* 1951;33B:543-547.
18. Schneider RC, Cherry G, Pantek H. The syndrome of acute central cervical spinal cord injury: with special reference to the mechanisms involved in hyperextension injuries of cervical spine. *J Neurosurg.* 1954;11:546-577.
19. Urist MR, Gurvey MS, Fareed DO. Long term observations in aged women with pathologic osteoporosis. In: Barzel US, ed. *Osteoporosis.* New York, NY: Grune & Stratton; 1970:3-37.
20. Yasuoka S, Peterson HA, Laws ER Jr, MacCarty CS. Pathogenesis and prophylaxis of postlaminectomy deformity of the spine after multiple level laminectomy: difference between children and adults. *Neurosurgery.* 1981;9:145-152.

CHAPTER 12

Special Problems of Spinal Stabilization in Children

Dachling Pang, MD, and Edward N. Hanley, MD

An old medical school adage holds that "children are not little adults, but have their own peculiar problems." Some of these problems can be especially challenging when treating spinal deformity or instability in children. They can be classified as follows:

1. Problems with radiographic diagnosis
2. Problems related to immediate stabilization
3. Problems with external orthoses
4. Problems related to internal (surgical) fixation
5. Problems with fusion extension
6. Problems with ligamentous instability

Problems with Radiographic Diagnosis

Epiphyseal variations, unique vertebral architecture, incomplete ossification, and physiologic hypermobility of the cervical spine may all cause uncertainty when interpreting the cervical radiograph of a child with a history of neck injury, pain, and/or stiffness. Unlike extremity injuries, contralateral companion views cannot be made for the spine. A thorough knowledge of the developmental aspects of the pediatric spine can be very helpful in the diagnosis of spinal instability and fracture.

Epiphyseal Development and Variations

Epiphyseal plates are smooth, regular, in predictable locations, and have subchondral sclerotic lines. Fractures are irregular, without sclerosis, and are frequently in unpredictable locations. Knowledge of the dates of epiphyseal appearances and disappearances is helpful in interpreting radiographic films. The first two cervical vertebrae are unique in their development; the remaining five are essentially uniform.

At birth, the atlas (C1) is composed of two ossification centers, one for each of the neural arches. The ossification center for the body is usually not calcified at birth, but appears during the first year of life (Figure 1).[1] This is why the anterior arch of C1 is usually not visible on the lateral roentgenogram in the newborn and young infants (Figure 2). Rarely, the center for the body remains absent throughout life, and the anterior ring may be incompletely formed by fusion of the neural arches anteriorly.[1,2]

The two neural arches close posteriorly by the third year, although the midline may remain cartilaginous until age 5 or 6. This is important to recognize when a C1-C2 wiring and fusion is contemplated, since the wire readily cuts through the unfused synchondrosis in the midline. The neurocentral synchondroses separating the neural arches

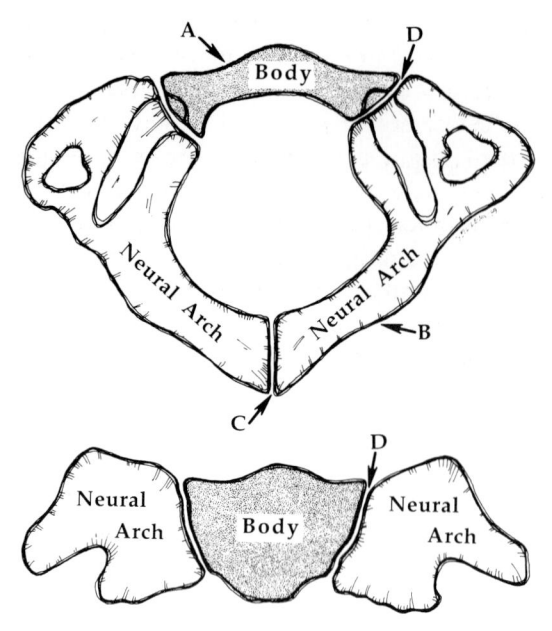

Figure 1. Diagram of the first cervical vertebra (atlas)
A. Body: not ossified at birth; ossification center (occasionally two centers) appears during first year of life.
B. Neural arches: ossification centers appear bilaterally about seventh fetal week.
C. Synchondrosis of spinous process: union occurs around the fifth or sixth year.
D. Neurocentral synchondrosis: fuses about the seventh year. (Modified from Bailey DK[1])

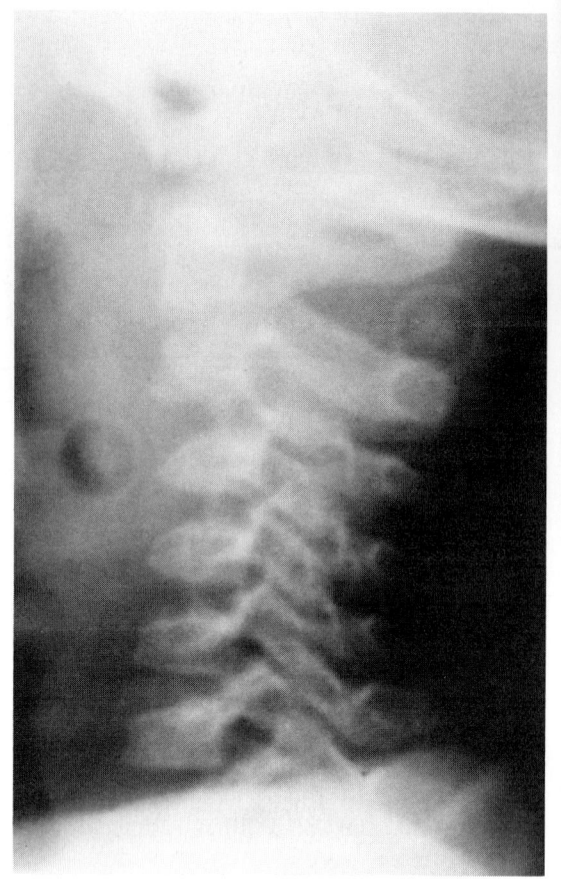

Figure 2. Lateral radiograph of a 6-month-old child. Note absence of the anterior arch of C1 before appearance of its ossification center, usually at age 1 year. The wedge-shaped anterior portions of the C3 and C4 vertebral bodies are well seen.

from the body usually close by age 7 years.[1] They are best visualized by the open-mouth view of a plain film, or with axial computed tomography (CT). These bilaterally symmetrical synchondroses should be easily distinguishable from fractures of the anterior arch.

The developing axis (C2) has four ossification centers at birth, one for each neural arch, one for the body, and a fourth for the odontoid process (dens). In the anteroposterior projection, the odontoid process surmounts the axial body in between the neural arches so that the various synchondroses combine to form the letter H (Figure 3). The odontoid fuses with the neural arches and the body between 3 and 6 years of age at the same time that the body joins the neural arches, so that no lucent line should be present in the axis in a child over 7.[3]

The odontoid-body synchondrosis, commonly known as the epiphyseal plate of the axis, does not run across the apparent "base" of the odontoid, which is generally regarded to be at the level of the articular processes; instead, it lies well below this level "like a cork in a bottle" (Figure 3). In the older child, a persistent epiphyseal line may occasionally be present and must be distinguished from a Type II odontoid fracture, but this line should be well below the base of the odontoid process where a Type II odontoid fracture would be anticipated.

The timing of closure of the epiphyseal plate also implies that shearing injury to the odontoid in children younger than 7 years

Special Problems of Spinal Stabilization in Children

does not produce an odontoid fracture, but an epiphysiolysis at the predicted site (Figures 4a,b). This distinction is important because an epiphysiolysis should be as accurately reduced as possible and a C1-C2 fusion should be carried out, whereas a Type II fracture in a young patient may be effectively treated by simple halo immobilization.

The odontoid process develops from two independent ossification centers on either side of the midline; these fuse by the seventh fetal month. A persistence of this line may be visible at birth, when the unossified tip of the odontoid is normally V-shaped. A small ossification center, known as the summit ossification center, appears at the tip at age 3 to 6 years and fuses with the main portion of the odontoid by age 12.[1,2] Its persistence is

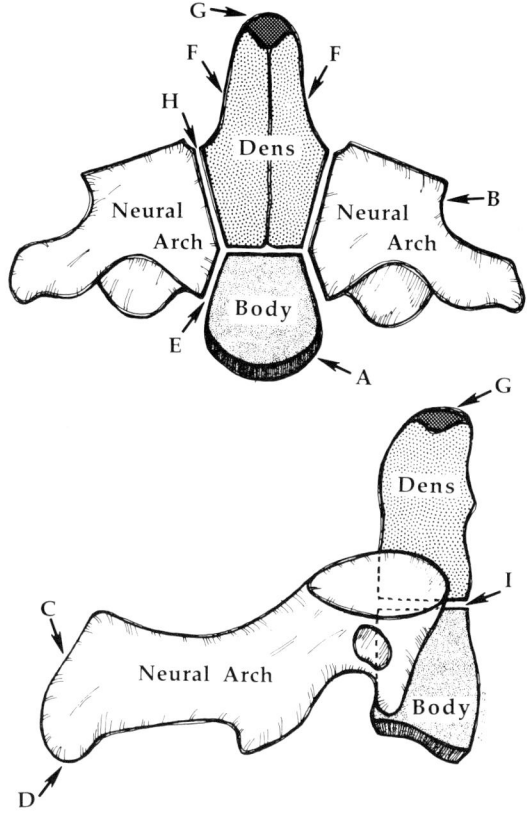

Figure 3. Diagram of the second cervical vertebra (axis)
A. *Body: one center (occasionally two) appears by the fifth fetal month.*
B. *Neural arch: appears by the seventh fetal month.*
C. *Neural arches fuse posteriorly by second or third year.*
D. *Bifid tip of spinous process.*
E. *Neurocentral synchondrosis: fuses at three to six years.*
F. *Odontoid (dens): two separate centers appear by fifth fetal month and fuse together by seventh fetal month.*
G. *Summit ossification center for odontoid: appears at four to six years and fuses with odontoid by twelve years.*
H. *Synchondrosis between odontoid and neural arch: fuses at four to six years.*
I. *Synchondrosis between odontoid and body (the "epiphysis" of the odontoid), fuses at four to six years.*
(Modified from Bailey DK[1])

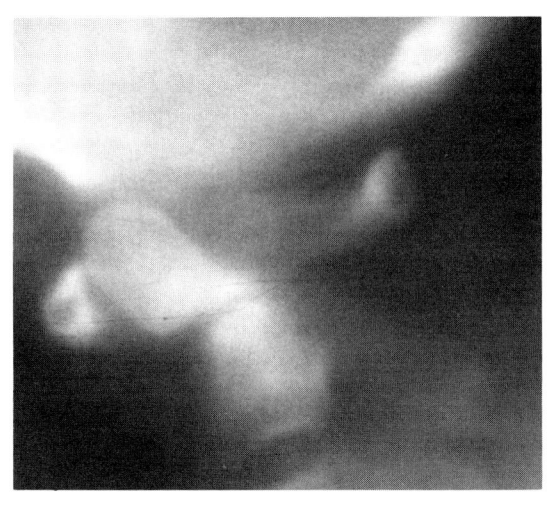

Figure 4a. Epiphysiolysis of the odontoid in a seven-year-old child. Lateral tomography.

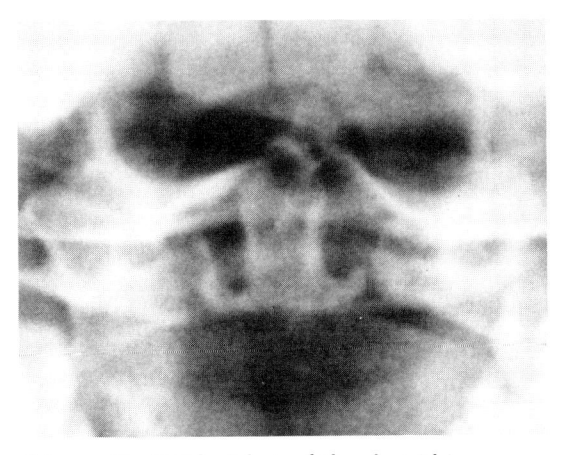

Figure 4b. Epiphysiolysis of the odontoid in a seven-year-old child. Anteroposterior tomogram showing that the separation plane corresponds to the location of the epiphyseal plate.

referred to as an ossiculum terminale,[4] whereas nonfusion of the epiphyseal plate and separation of the deformed odontoid process from the axial centrum results in the developmental form of os odontoideum.[3] As can be deduced from the timing of its appearance, an ossiculum terminale seldom appears before age 5 years, but an os odontoideum can be present much earlier.

The third to seventh cervical vertebrae ossify from three centers: one from the body and one from each neural arch. The neural arches close posteriorly in the second or third year, and the neurocentral synchondroses joining the neural arches to the body fuse from 3 to 6 years.[1,2] Secondary centers for the spines appear at puberty and unite with the spinous processes at the beginning of the third decade. Thus, the spinous processes of prepubertal children are short and stubby, whereas those of adults are large and much more robust structures. This is important when interspinous wire fusion is contemplated in young children.

In the lateral roentgenogram, the ossified parts of the vertebral bodies in young children appear wedge-shaped (Figure 2) until they become squared off at about 7 or 8 years.[1,2] Thus, anterior sliding subluxation secondary to flexion forces is much more common in young children under 8 years.[5]

Prevertebral Soft Tissue Swelling

The space between the cervical spine and the pharynx opposite the C3 vertebra has been estimated to be a maximum of 5 mm in adults and about two-thirds of the thickness of the C2 vertebra in children.[6] An increase in width of this retropharyngeal space after trauma is presumptive evidence of hemorrhage or edema from fracture or dislocation.

The retropharyngeal width is a meaningful measurement only if the lateral x-ray is taken when the child is at rest and having quiet respiration. Since the pharynx is attached to the hyoid bone, any muscle actions displacing the hyoid forward will artificially increase the retropharyngeal space. Thus, in inspiration, the pharyngeal wall is close to the vertebrae, while in forced expiration, there is a marked physiologic increase in the retropharyngeal shadow. This phenomenon is further exaggerated when the hyoid is pulled far forward during high-pitched crying, a fact worth remembering when interpreting this radiographic sign in a distressed child.

Overriding of Anterior Arch of Atlas

A mistaken impression of odontoid hypoplasia or posterior atlantoaxial subluxation may be given by the lateral extension x-ray film of a very young child, because the anterior arch of the atlas slides upward and protrudes beyond the ossified part of the dens to lie against the unossified tip. Cattell and Filtzer reported this finding in 14 of 70 normal children (20%) aged 1 to 7 years.[7]

Problems Related to Immediate Stabilization

As soon as the diagnosis of cervical instability is made, some means of immediate spinal stabilization must be instituted before further radiographic studies are obtained and while a definitive plan of treatment is being formulated. In adults, the institution of cervical traction using tongs is still the simplest and most effective method of immediate stabilization. For children, this seemingly straightforward step is difficult.

Infants and Children under 6 Years

Skull calipers are not recommended for infants and children less than 6 years of age because the skull tables are too thin. The pin pressure necessary to sustain adequate traction is liable to produce skull deformity. Even if the thickest portion of the parietal skull is chosen for the insertion site, at a point 2 cm above and 2 cm behind the top of the auricular helix, the popular Gardner-Wells tongs almost certainly would cause a "ping-pong" fracture in an infant or a depressed fracture and skull penetration in children under 6 years of age. This not only could lead to intracranial hematomas and infection, but the absence of solid pin lodgement nullifies effective traction. Even if pin fixation is adequate in some 5- or 6-year-old children, their bodies are so light that the weight necessary to maintain traction often pulls the child's head up against the head pole of the Stryker bed. In addition, these children are under extreme duress and will likely thrash about in bed. Having traction under these circumstances may actually put the cervical spine at a higher risk than if a less threatening external orthosis is used.

Thus, for children between 3 and 6 years of age whose cervical spines are unstable but do not require urgent realignment, we recommend using the halo fixation device for immediate stabilization. If a correctly sized prefabricated plastic vest is not readily available, the upright articulation bars attached to the halo ring can be incorporated in a body plaster cast. A more versatile custom-made halo vest can always be substituted later. The child can now be nursed in a regular bed, and the weight of the halo cast often imposes sufficient restriction to inhibit excessive body movement.

In any case, minor body motions and log rolling are well tolerated because the head and torso are now immobilized as one rigid unit. Halo devices designed specially for young children are available with the vertical bars adapted for posterior surgical approaches, so that elective fusion can be performed with the halo in place.

If the unstable segments in a young child are malaligned and require immediate reduction, the child should be temporarily immobilized with a Philadelphia collar while awaiting operation. The reduction can then be performed manually in the operating room under general anesthesia, with fluoroscopic and electrophysiologic monitoring, and afterwards maintained by applying the halo device *in situ*. The final position of the reduced segments may be finely adjusted by adjusting the joints between the halo ring and the articulation bars. The patient is then placed in the prone position and posterior surgical fixation and fusion can be carried out.

For infants and children less than 3 years of age, the halo fixation device cannot be used due to the fragile cranium. There is no safe and effective means of immediate stabilization if the injured segments are extremely unstable. Fortunately, unstable cervical fractures or dislocations are very uncommon in this age group, but if such injuries occur, wire and bone graft fusion with or without reduction should probably be carried out as soon as possible. An appropriate external orthosis (see below) should then be applied in the operating room.

Children 7 to 12 Years

The Gardner-Wells skull tongs can be safely used on children in this age group, but the traction protocol must be modified from that ordinarily employed for adults. These children are still too young to be expected to behave quietly with the traction device in place. Heavy sedation is usually required, partly to eliminate dangerous unruly body motions and partly to add a modicum of antispasmodic effect to the nuchal muscles to facilitate fracture reduction if needed.

In young children, the forces required for reduction and maintenance of alignment are much less than is the case for adults. In addition, the degree of instability, particularly in upper cervical injuries, may be grossly underestimated. The amount of weight used for the traction must therefore be carefully considered for children with an unstable spine that requires closed reduction. To begin traction on a child between the age of 7 and 12, each level counting from the occiput to the upper unstable segment requires 2 lbs of weight, so that a C5-C6 dislocation requires 10 lbs to start. Increments of 2 lbs can then be added depending on the type of injury and on the desired degree of realignment. Increments of 2 lbs should be used up to a maximum equivalent to 25% of the child's body weight. Each weight increment must be monitored by a lateral x-ray film. The upper cervical segments in young children are notoriously prone to overdistraction; this is particularly true in cases of atlanto-occipital dislocation.[8]

In addition, children do not tolerate the Stryker bed well. A much better bed is the Rotorest bed (Kinetic Concepts Inc., San Antonio, TX), which comes in a pediatric size. The child's entire body is fitted snugly in this bed by adjustable side panels so that he or she feels more secure and is less disposed to thrash about. Upward sliding of the child's body in response to the traction weight is checked by well-padded shoulder stoppers that extend from the headboard to the top of the shoulders (Figure 5). We find the Rotorest bed very effective in preventing skin complications in children with spinal cord injury, and its gentle rotatory motion is usually well tolerated.

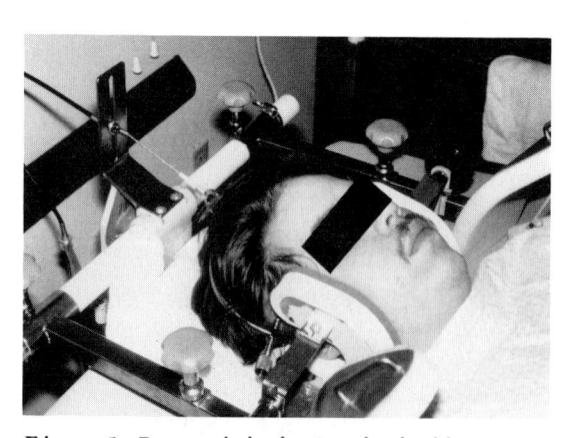

Figure 5. Rotorest bed, showing the shoulder stoppers that are fixed to the headboard. These prevent upward migration of the patient's body towards the headboard and maintain the effect of traction.

All of the above precautionary measures notwithstanding, we still recommend carrying out the definitive surgery and halo application as soon as the medical condition of the child allows.

Children 13 to 18 Years

Older children in this age group can usually tolerate skull caliper traction as well as most healthy adults. Mild sedation may be used but is often unnecessary if the Rotorest bed is available. Traction weight of 3 to 5 lbs per level is selected according to the size of the patient.

Problems with External Orthoses

The Halo Fixation Device

Of all the commonly available forms of external cervical orthoses, the halo vest or halo body cast provides the most rigid immobilization of the cervical spine.[9-11] It also permits the most precise positioning of the neck to obtain or maintain cervical alignment, and because it is the only external orthosis that does not have a chin support, it interferes less with mandibular motion and eating.[12] By allowing early mobilization of the patient, it avoids most of the complications associated with prolonged bed rest, and offers a tremendous psychological boost to the patient who can now more fully participate in a rehabilitation program. The latter consideration is especially important in children who can contrive myriad ways to sabotage the immobilization protocol if they are not allowed at least limited physical activities.

The halo vest and halo body cast are currently the orthoses of choice for most children with an unstable cervical spine.[13-15] However, the complications associated with halo application are significantly higher in children than in adults[13]; most of these are related to the thinness of the juvenile calvarium. Garfin et al determined that the thickest portions of the adult calvarium are the lateral frontal and lateral occipital areas, and recommended that halo pins be placed anterolaterally in the frontal bone and posterolaterally in the thick part of the occipital bone.[16] Ideally, the anterior pins should be placed anterior to the temporalis muscle and fossa to avoid painful mastication and skull penetration, but lateral to the midportion of the orbital rim to avoid the frontal sinus.[9]

These precautions must be strictly observed in children. The temporal fossa in children is especially thin and must never be used for pin anchorage despite its cosmetic advantage (behind the hairline). The anterior pins, however, can be moved more medially if necessary, since there is no frontal sinus in young children. These pins should also be placed immediately above the eyebrows to take advantage of the extra strength of the lateral supraorbital ridge.[13] The supraorbital and supratrochlear nerves are to be spared over the medial one-third of the eyebrow. The torque used for pin tightening in children should be reduced from the 6 inch-pounds recommended for adults to 4 inch-pounds.

We have successfully used this reduced torque on children as young as 3 years of age but would not recommend using the conventional halo device on children younger than 3 years. Recently, Mubarak et al used a low-torque multiple pin arrangement with up to 10 pins, each tightened to 2 inch-pounds torque, on a 16-month-old child and a 7-month-old infant.[17] This extraordinary new technique deserves to be evaluated for wider use in young children.

In spite of meticulous selection of pin locations at the thickest regions of the skull, a number of pins will loosen before the period of halo immobilization ends.[9,13] The frequency of pin loosening is much higher in children than in adults.[13] Some pins become loose because they were inserted at an angle to the outer table where the skull contour is sloping upwards. To prevent the resulting cephalad migration, the pins should therefore be kept below the level of the greatest skull circumference (skull equator).

Pins also may loosen because the correct degree of tightness was not achieved at the time of insertion. For instance, due to the viscoelastic properties of the skull, the pins frequently loosen 2 to 4 inch-pounds within a few minutes after the vest and uprights are attached to the halo ring, and they must be retightened to the correct torque after the vest is in place. The pins are then rechecked and retightened as necessary between 24 and 48 hours after application.

If a loose pin is discovered later than two to three weeks after insertion, the management depends on the age of the patient. Garfin et al found that with the recommended 6 inch-pounds of torque for adults, the halo pin only partially penetrates the outer table of the adult skull, and there is usually a solid margin of cortical bone to allow safe retightening.[9] Thus, for older children and adults, it is probably safe to retighten the loose pin, provided some resistance is met during the procedure.

In young children, the skull tables are much thinner, and pin loosening is also seemingly more often a forerunner of infection in children than in adults. Accelerated osteoclasis around the pin site frequently softens the bone so much that retightening can cause skull penetration and intracranial abscess (Figure 6).[18] It is advisable in these

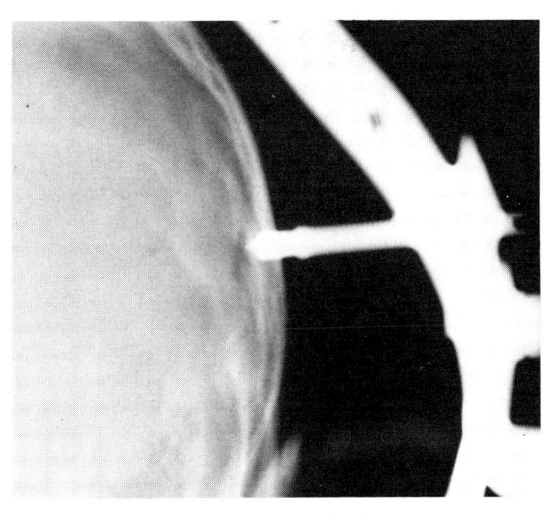

Figure 6. Tangential radiograph of the skull of a six-year-old child, showing penetration of the halo pin through both tables of the skull. The pin was retightened once after it had loosened four weeks after original application.

children to remove the loose pin and place a new one in a different site. From one to five pin changes are sometimes required before the end of the immobilization period. In several children we have treated, we were forced to prematurely abandon the halo device for other external orthoses because of repeated pin loosening.

Pin site infections are also much more common in children than in adults. Baum et al reported a 31% incidence of pin infection in children versus 6% in adults.[13] For prevention, the pin sites should be cleansed thoroughly with 10% hydrogen peroxide solution four times daily, and all scabs and crusts around the pin must be removed to allow drainage. If the infection is mild and superficial, with only slight surrounding scalp erythema and minimal drainage, and the pin remains tight, oral antibiotics may be sufficient. If the scalp is red and swollen, if the drainage becomes copious and purulent, or if the child complains of constant local pain or headaches, the pin should be removed and intravenous antibiotics should be given to prevent the dreaded complication of cranial osteomyelitis. A CT scan should be done to rule out an intracranial abscess (Figures 7a,b). At least five cases of intracranial abscess associated with halo orthosis have been reported.[18-21] Four of the five were in children. All five had associated pin-site infections, and three of the five had cranial osteomyelitis. In two children, the halo pins were tightened when found loose at some time remote from the original halo placement.

In addition to the special problems of pin loosening and infection, children immobilized with halo devices also have a greater likelihood than adults of showing slippage of the unstable cervical segments. This is partly because of unrecognized pin loosening, but children also cannot be depended upon to protect their halo rings against inadvertent stresses, most of which are related to their tossing in bed. Direct contact of the ring and posterior uprights with the bedding should be avoided as much as possible to minimize transmitted flexion stresses to the unstable

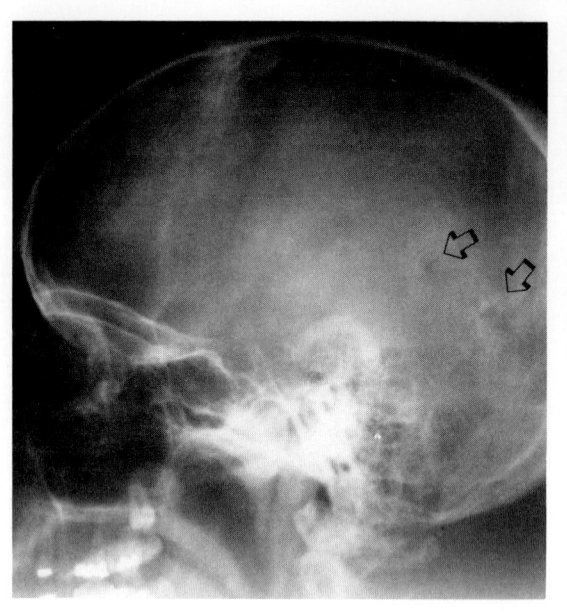

Figure 7a. Fourteen-year-old boy with halo pin site infection five weeks after pin insertion. Lateral skull radiograph showing biparietal osteomyelitis (arrows) corresponding to posterior pin sites.

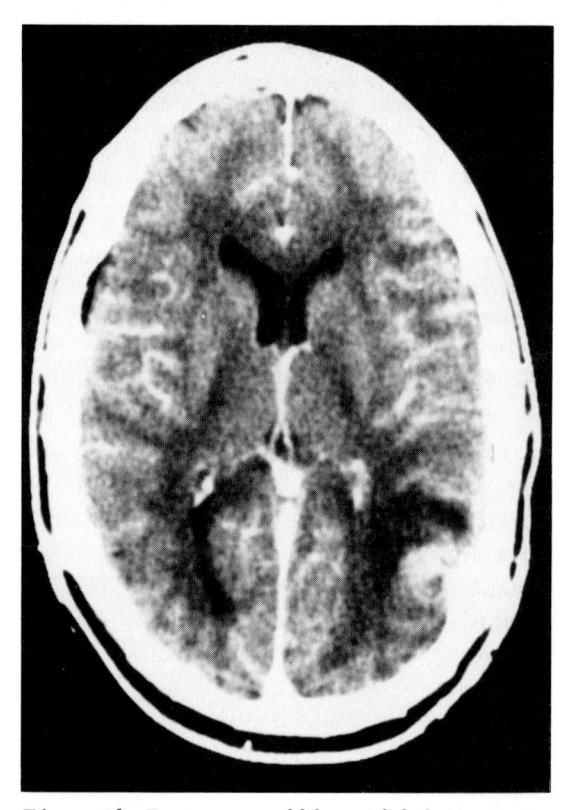

Figure 7b. Fourteen-year-old boy with halo pin site infection. CT with contrast showing left posterior parietal brain abscess.

cervical segments. We use a large wedge of foam to prop up the back of the vest so that the child can recline comfortably with the head and halo ring hanging free, while still able to watch television, read, play board games, and self-feed (Figure 8). In addition, while one well-tailored vest is usually sufficient for an adult to last the duration of treatment, children not infrequently go through rapid and drastic changes in body weight and contour, so that the original vest can become loose and ill-fitting and must be recustomized.

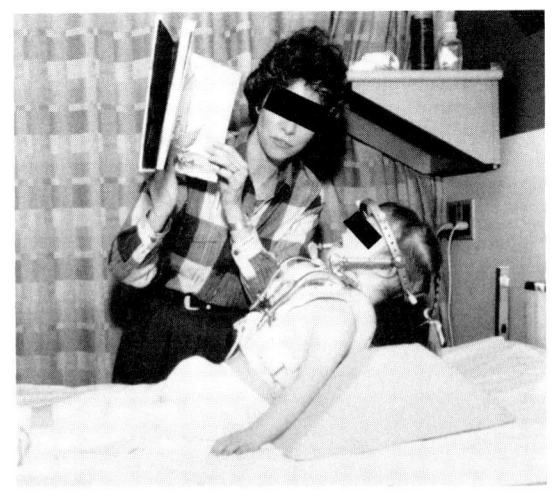

Figure 8. A five-year-old child with Down syndrome and C1-C2 subluxation, post occipital-C2 fusion. Note the large wedge foam keeping the upper portions of the uprights and the halo ring off the bed and avoiding excessive flexion stress to the neck.

Finally, children tend to be unforgiving if the head positioning is not adjusted exactly to their liking. Because most unstable injuries are unstable in flexion, it is always tempting to set the neck in slight extension, opposite to the direction of subluxation. However, children develop mechanical dysphagia rather easily when the neck is in even slight extension, and if the child's visual axis cannot command a full frontal view of his or her surroundings due to excessive neck extension, the child will simply stop walking. Thus, the preferred neck position is the "military salute" position in which posterior translation is substituted for extension. In a young child, the extra weight of top-heavy halo bars and vest shifts the center of gravity a considerable distance upward, and he or she must be patiently coached to relearn the basic skills of walking and navigating with this heavy and cumbersome burden.

Minerva Cast

We have, on rare occasions, used the Minerva plaster cast in children less than 3 years of age and in those who have failed to tolerate the halo pins. The Minerva cast is not recommended for atlantoaxial instability, because if there is adequate space for excursion of the mandible so that the patient can talk and eat, there is also space enough to allow motion between C1 and C2. We especially do not favor this device in children because the plaster cast is exceedingly heavy for a young child and essentially condemns the child to three months of bed confinement. Moreover, the impervious cast may produce dangerous hyperthermia in the infant. For children with a high cervical myelopathy and an unstable cardiopulmonary status, the Minerva cast can present great difficulties in case of a cardiopulmonary arrest.

Benzel et al have reported using a thermoplastic Minerva body jacket constructed of polyfoam (a splinting material made from a polyester polycaprolactone) and polycushion (a closed-cell foam for padding).[22] This is a lightweight modification of the classic design that purportedly solves the problems of hyperthermia and cumbersome ambulation.

The clinical trial compared this jacket with the halo vest and found that the thermoplastic Minerva jacket actually restricts intersegmental "snaking" movements in the cervical spine better than the halo vest. However, the study was flawed by the fact that the patients were first immobilized by the halo for six to eight weeks and then put into the Minerva jacket for two to three weeks before the motion x-ray films were obtained. Thus the prior bone fusions were at an advanced state of healing before intersegmental movement was tested in the Minerva jacket. Nevertheless, this new Minerva jacket deserves further evaluation for use in children.

The Guilford Brace

We prefer the Guilford brace (G.A. Guilford and Sons, Orthotic Laboratory Ltd., Cleveland, OH) when the child is intolerant of the halo device or too young for its application. This brace has padded mandibular and occipital supports that are rigidly connected to an anterior and a posterior thoracic plate. The front and back sections interlock to form a rigid metal ring below the ear level. The thoracic plates are attached to each other both over the shoulders and under the axillae by leather straps (Figure 9).

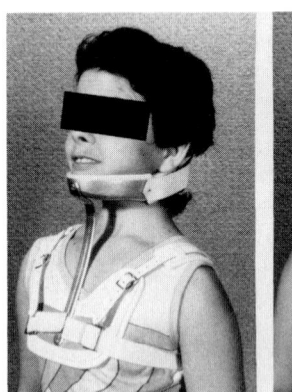

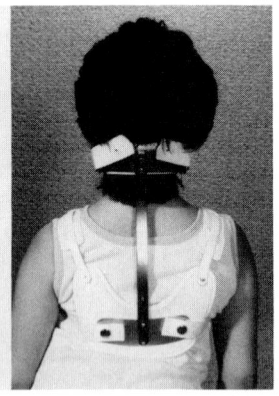

Figure 9. The Guilford brace, with solid chin and occipital supports strapped together into a rigid ring under the chin. The front and back chest plates are strapped together snugly with thoracic and cross-shoulder belts.

The Guilford brace is comparable to the rigid cervicothoracic brace in its ability to limit cervical spine motion. It is superior to most other nonhalo external orthoses in controlling flexion, extension, and rotation (in order of effectiveness), especially of the mid to lower cervical segments.[10,11] Like the other orthoses, the Guilford brace is not as effective in controlling lateral bending. Its leading advantage over most other nonhalo orthoses is that it can be custom-made within 24 hours to fit any body size down to that of a 1-year-old infant. With minor modification and deepening of the chin and occipital plates, it surpasses even the conventional cervicothoracic brace in restricting rotation, and therefore is most suitable for maintaining reduction in rotatory subluxation injuries in children.

In recent years, the Guilford brace has also been used extensively in our institution on children with spinal cord injury without radiographic abnormality (SCIWORA) syndrome. In these children, incipient ligamentous instability does not require the stringent motion control of the halo device, but unpredictable compliance with treatment necessitates something more stable and less easy to discard than the Philadelphia collar.[5,23]

Molded Body Splint

In spite of numerous trials of new products and improvisations, we continue to have problems immobilizing infants and very young children with extremely unstable cervical spines for prolonged periods. Fortunately such patients are rare, but since no external orthoses can reliably eliminate intersegmental motion in these infants, wiring and bone graft fusion often prove unsuccessful. An example is diastrophic dwarfism, in which the affected infant has ligamentous laxity at multiple segments and usually presents in the first few months of life with apnea and quadriplegic spells due to severe swan-neck deformity and multi-level subluxations. These neurologic manifestations are completely reversible as long as the neck is kept in a neutral or slightly extended position.

Because of the high failure rate, we do not attempt surgical fusion until these patients reach 3 years of age. In the meantime, the infant is immobilized in a thermoplastic back and head splint molded carefully to the contour of the thorax, head, and neck in the desired degree of extension. The thoracic section incorporates the pelvis and hip joints, and is strapped across the front with Velcro straps. The head section has a padded head-

Special Problems of Spinal Stabilization in Children

band that is strapped across the forehead to secure the head. The back slab can be fenestrated if the infant develops hyperthermia, which frequently happens (Figure 10). The

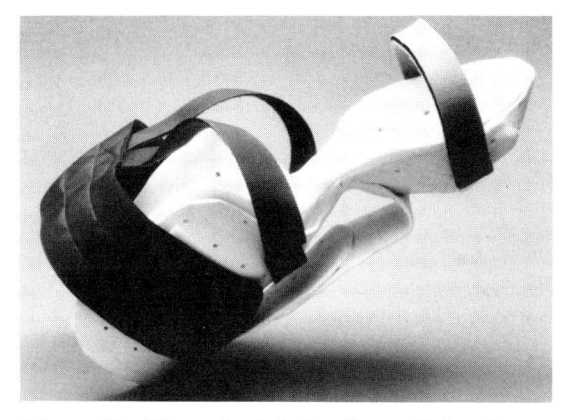

Figure 10. Thermoplastic body splint molded to the contour of the infant's neck, head, and thorax for long-term immobilization. The position of the head is adjustable, usually to slight extension. Note Velcro head and chest straps, fenestrations in the back flap for ventilation, and the flat shelf under the back section for more stable positioning on the bed or hard surface and for providing a secure hand grip for manual handling of the body splint.

diastrophic dwarfs are usually not ambulatory for many months after birth. With proper skin care by parents and nursing staff, they can be kept relatively safely in this molded body splint for up to three years (Figures 11a,b), when extensive surgical fusion carries a better chance of success.

Problems Related to Internal Surgical Fixation

General Principles

As with adult patients with unstable dislocation injuries, it is always preferable to achieve reduction of the malalignment before surgical fusion is undertaken. Spinal cord compression is thus relieved promptly and subsequent internal fixation can be performed with the least manipulation of the unstable segments. In older children, preoperative reduction can be accomplished with skull traction using tongs. In children younger than 7 years of age, reduction is probably

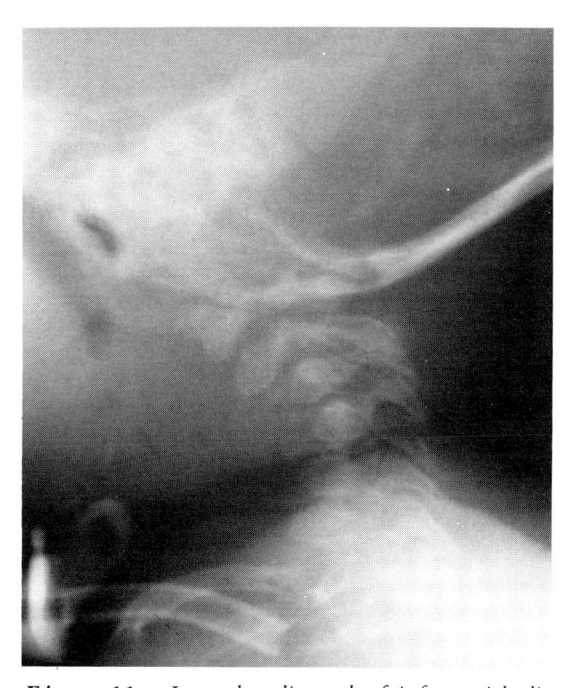

Figure 11a. Lateral radiograph of infant with diastrophic dwarfism showing multi-level severe anterior subluxation of the upper cervical spine. Infant had apnea in this position.

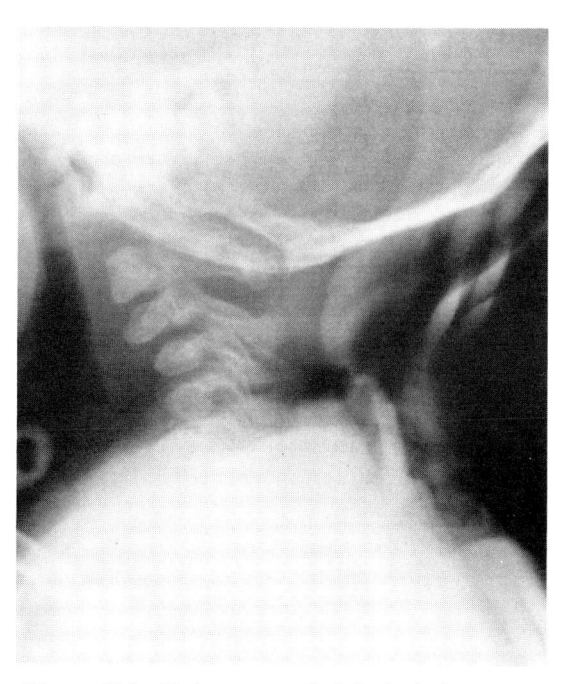

Figure 11b. Moderate reversal of the kyphotic curvature maintained by the molded body splint. Infant was asymptomatic in this position.

better attempted by gentle manual manipulation in the operating room, under general anesthesia and with fluoroscopic monitoring. If the injured segments are extremely unstable, the halo device should be applied to maintain the reduction before the surgical fusion is begun.

Many spinal cord injury centers intubate adult patients with unstable injuries while they are awake. The idea is for an alert examiner to recognize a sudden change in the patient's neurological status during the slight repositioning of the neck for intubation. This practice is not usually feasible in children, even if a potent local anesthetic spray and intravenous sedation are used. Young children, especially, tend to resist vigorously, and may jeopardize the unstable injury further.

We prefer nasotracheal intubation performed with a fiberoptic laryngoscope on children after induction of general anesthesia, and use real-time somatosensory evoked potentials (SSEPs) to monitor spinal cord function. In this fashion the endotracheal tube can be quickly and efficiently secured with minimal head movement, and the patient's neurological status can be objectively measured during intubation, halo application, and during the surgical fusion that follows.

It is our impression, and that of others, that bone-bank bone is less likely to result in successful fusion in children than autologous bone grafts.[24] In general, it is desirable to harvest bone from the child's own iliac crest. The amount of bone is obviously limited by the size of the patient, and both iliac crests may be prepared for use. We have not encountered pathological pelvic fractures at the graft site in these cases.

Permanent stability at the fusion site depends ultimately on the amount of new bone that forms and bridges the fusion surfaces of the adjacent segments. The larger the fusion surface available for new bone formation, the more exuberant will be the callous and the stronger the subsequent bony bridge. Although methylmethacrylate incorporated into a wiring construct enhances the immediate stability of the construct,[25] it also diminishes the available bony surface for new bone formation and ultimately weakens the permanent strength of the fusion site.[25] This is a particularly relevant issue in children in whom the fusion surface is already limited. Methylmethacrylate is virtually never indicated in treating children with unstable injuries unrelated to malignant diseases.

Continued micromotion between adjacent segments at any surgical fusion site is strongly correlated with nonunion. In children external immobilization with the halo vest can be associated with halo pin loosening and position slippage and cannot always provide adequate stabilization of the unstable segments. For those children who cannot tolerate the halo, other external orthoses provide even less satisfactory stabilization.[11] Thus, for children with unstable injuries, the burden of immediate stabilization rests squarely on the immediate strength of the fusion construct, much more so than for adult patients in whom the halo can be depended upon to provide more reliable external immobilization.

One should, therefore, always aim at achieving maximum *immediate internal stability* while planning the surgical fusion for children. The wire-graft fusion should be designed to eliminate intersegmental motion as much as possible, and not merely to bring the bone grafts in contact with the fusion surface. With this important principle in mind, we can evaluate the relative efficacy of several recommended fusion techniques for children with unstable cervical spine injuries.

Injuries Involving C2 to C7 Segments

Johnson et al compared the immediate stability of five posterior fusion techniques for mid to low cervical injuries by using fresh human cadaver spines divided into two-segment units fastened together by five wire-graft constructs: (1) interspinous wiring, (2) wraparound interspinous wiring, (3) facet wiring and bone graft, (4) interfacet wiring, and (5) interspinous wiring reinforced with methylmethacrylate.[25,26]

In the interspinous wiring technique, holes are drilled in the outer cortex of the spinous process adjacent to the lamina, and a loop of wire is passed through the holes in adjacent vertebrae and twisted in place. Bone grafts are wired on to the laminae.[27] This technique is probably the safest in terms of avoiding injury to the already compromised spinal cord because it does not involve manipulation inside the spinal canal. However, Johnson et al found that the interspinous wiring construct was the first of the five constructs to fail under flexion and extension stresses, mainly because the wire pulled through the drill hole in the lower vertebra.[26]

This experimental situation is similar to what we observed in children given this fusion technique. Except for the C7 vertebra, the spinous processes of prepubertal children are short and stubby. Secondary ossification centers for the spines that ultimately make them strong and robust structures suitable for interspinous wiring do not appear until puberty and are not fully ossified until the early twenties.[1,3] Even if the wire loop is made to pass around the whole spinous process and not through its drill hole, a modification thought to improve the strength of the experimental construct, the loop could easily slip off the short spinous process, or the fragile process may fracture under flexion stresses. Thus, except for the usually prominent C7 and T1 spinous processes of older adolescents, we do not recommend the interspinous wiring technique for children with unstable injuries.[26]

Like interspinous wiring, fusion techniques involving facet wiring are safe because the spinal canal is not encroached upon. The facet bone graft technique described by Callahan et al involves drilling holes in the posterior pillars of the facets, passing wires through each of these holes, and then tying these wires around struts of corticocancellous bone grafts over the row of facets to be fused on each side.[28] Johnson et al found that the strength of this technique depends entirely on the tensile strength of the strut grafts.[26]

In contrast, the interfacet wiring technique described by Johnson and Southwick involves drilling holes in the posterior pillars of the facets at two adjacent levels, passing a wire through the facet pillar above, out the facet joint at that level, and then into the hole of the adjacent lower facet pillar and out that joint.[29] Both ends of the wire are then twisted on themselves to fasten the two vertebrae together. The strength of this wiring construct is therefore dependent, not on the strength of the bone graft, but on the gauge of the wire and the thickness and strength of the facet pillars.

The interfacet wiring construct is among the strongest tested by the Johnson model.[25,26] However, we have encountered several problems when this technique is used in children. First, the thickness of the posterior facet pillar is proportional to the size and age of the child. Even in adolescents, the facets tend to be small and delicate and usually cannot sustain a large-gauge wire. On the other hand, a small-gauge wire able to thread through the delicate drill holes may break with minimal postoperative motion. In smaller children, even the drilling could chip off parts of the facet.

Secondly, the vertebral artery in children is only 1 cm lateral to the midline as opposed to 1.5 cm in adults, and it is located close to the facet pillar.[30] Vertebral artery injury is a potential risk while dissecting out the facet joints and while drilling the hole.

Finally, there is at least a theoretical disadvantage of rendering the already unstable spine even more unstable by destroying all the fibroligamentous structures surrounding the facet joints during the subperiosteal exposure.[28] As for the facet bone graft technique, the iliac crest strut grafts obtained from a child's pelvis cannot usually be depended upon to immobilize an unstable neck.

Thus, we reserve the two facet fusion techniques for those children who suffer from postlaminectomy deformity, where the only bony elements left for a posterior fusion are the facet joints.

In most other unstable injuries in children involving the C2 to C7 segments, we favor the sublaminar wiring technique. The sublaminar wire can be in the form of simple bilateral loops around both sides of the adjacent laminae, but a stronger sublaminar construct with more evenly distributed holding power involves weaving a single wire around the adjacent laminae of both sides. The wire is first looped around the lower lamina on one side, passed anterior to the upper lamina of the same side, hooked under the upper spinous process to pass anterior to the upper lamina of the other side, and finally passed around the lower lamina of the other side. The two ends can now be twisted tightly below the spinous process of the lower vertebra (Figures 12a,b). Iliac crest bone grafts are then secondarily wired to the fusion surface or tightly pressed down against it by strapping sutures strung across the deep muscles (Figures 12c,d).

This technique is slightly more complicated than the others and the wiring procedure does encroach upon the spinal canal and must be done carefully. The risk of cord injury can be minimized by using an aneurysm ligature passer to deliver a silk suture under the lamina, so that the wire can be fastened to the suture and in turn pulled around the front of the lamina. The end result is an extremely strong and stable fusion construct that produces a high rate of successful union in children. Regardless of the age of the child, the laminae are the strongest bone buttress to support the wiring and to produce immediate stability. Even in children 3 to 5 years of age, an 18-gauge Luque wire can be used without producing a laminar fracture. When the ends of the wire are twisted down

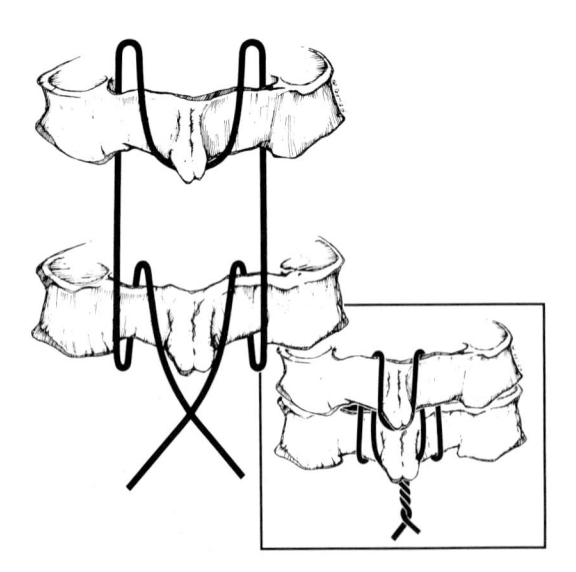

Figure 12a. Technique of sublaminar wiring. Drawing showing the single 18-gauge Luque wire looped around the lamina of the lower vertebra, then passed anterior to the upper lamina of the same side, then hooked under the spinous process of the upper vertebra before passing anterior to the upper lamina on the opposite side, then looped around the lower lamina of the other side, so that the two ends can be twisted tightly below the spinous process of the lower vertebra. Inset shows construct after wire tightening. The upper and lower laminae are approximated and held firmly together.

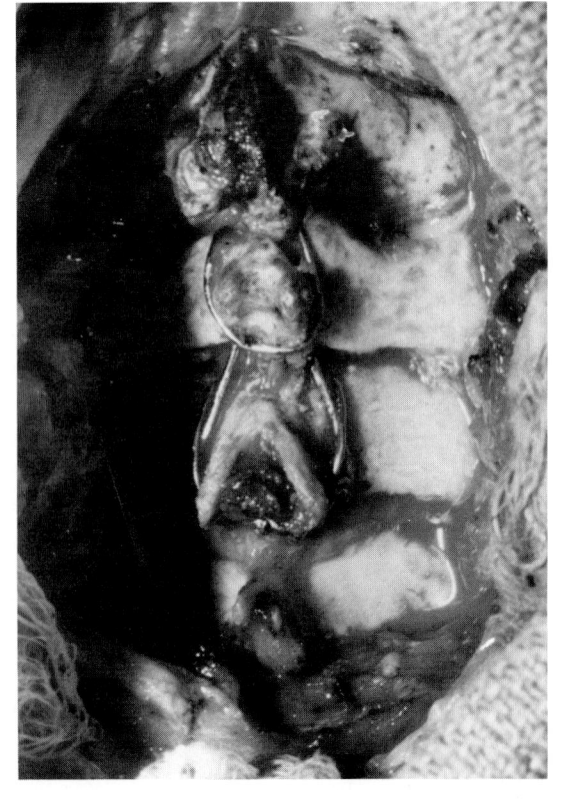

Figure 12b. Technique of sublaminar wiring. Intraoperative appearance of the sublaminar construct.

Special Problems of Spinal Stabilization in Children

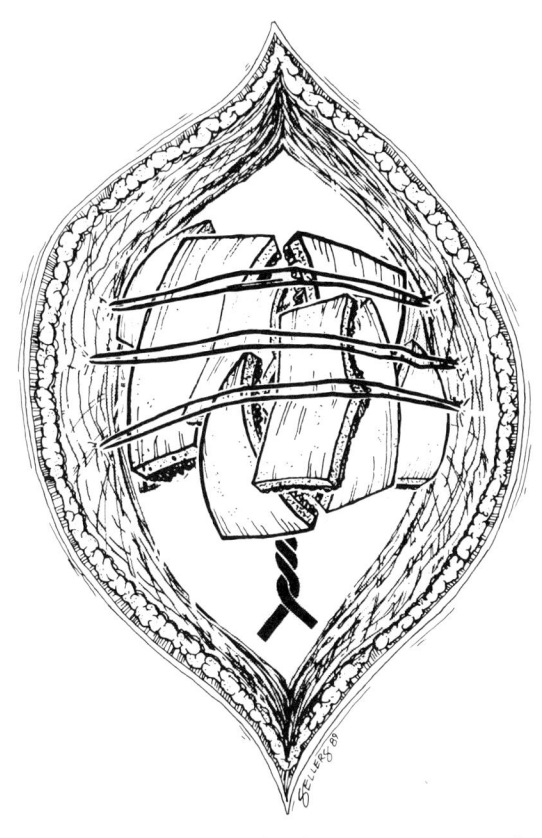

Figure 12c. Technique of sublaminar wiring. Drawing of the on-laid bone grafts being compressed against the fusion surfaces by strapping sutures strung across the deep muscle layer.

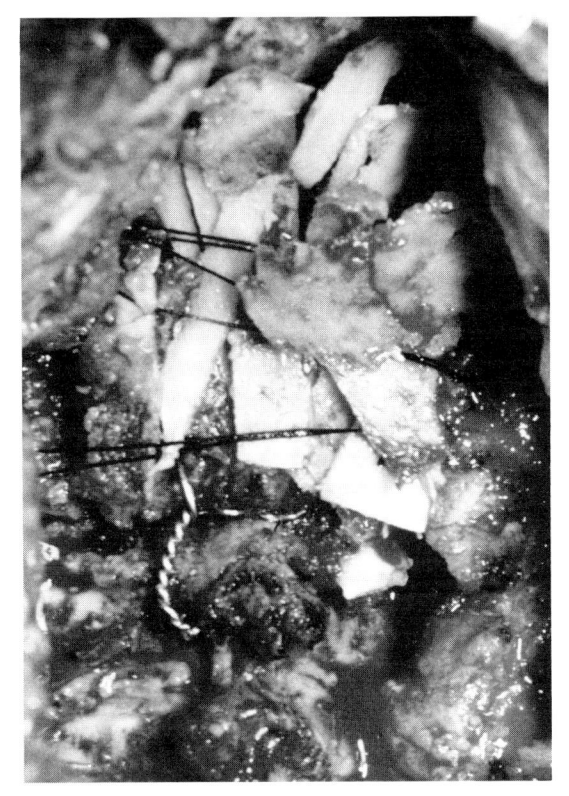

Figure 12d. Technique of sublaminar wiring. Intraoperative appearance of the on-laid bone grafts and strapping sutures.

tightly, the two adjacent laminae usually approximate each other. This eliminates almost all intersegmental motions, including extension movements; neither the interfacet nor interspinous wiring techniques can achieve this effect.[25]

Moreover, the strength of the construct is independent of the integrity of the bone graft. This eliminates the possibility of wire loosening due to graft breakage or rapid graft absorption, as could happen with the facet bone graft technique. However, even with the sublaminar technique, we have encountered problems of wire and laminar breakage in children younger than 3 years of age (Figure 13). Indeed, we are reluctant to undertake any open fusion procedure in children this young unless there are no other alternatives.

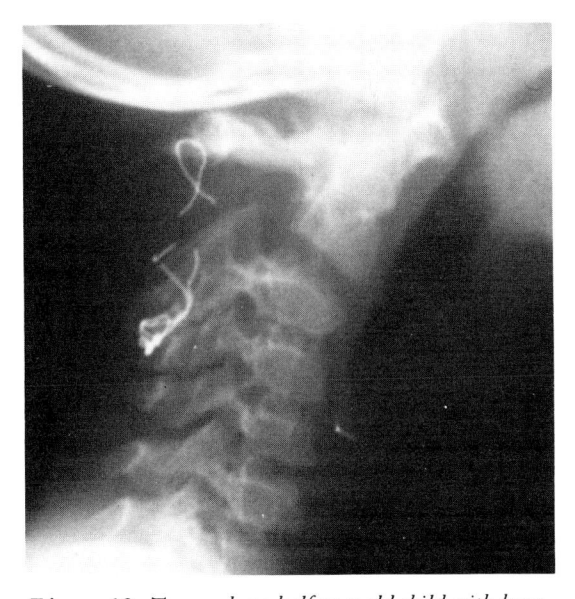

Figure 13. Two and one-half-year-old child with hangman's fracture of C2. Note broken 22-gauge sublaminar wires, absorption of bone graft, and nonunion after three months of inadequate immobilization with the halo orthosis.

Injuries Involving the C1-C2 Joint

Different fusion techniques have been recommended for the atlantoaxial articulation because of its unique anatomical and biomechanical characteristics. For example, the atlas does not have a spinous process, which precludes all interspinous procedures. There is also normally a 10° range of flexion and extension between C1 and C2, so that it would be difficult, if not impossible, for interfacet wiring to eliminate completely this plane of motion.[31,32] Because of the wide gap between the posterior arches of C1 and C2, even sublaminar wiring would not easily impart extension stability (even though flexion stability is readily accomplished) unless the two arches are actually made to approximate one another. Moreover, the inclination of the atlantoaxial facet joints and the interfacet ligaments are teleologically "suited" to a 47° range of axial rotation between the two vertebrae.[21,32] Any fusion technique must first overcome this great physiologic tendency for axial rotation before entertaining any hope of imparting immediate stability.

The Gallie method of wire fusion, which uses a single midline wire loop around the arch of C1 and then underneath the spinous process of C2, does not meet the desired objectives because it eliminates neither extension nor rotation.[33] Extension is largely unchecked because the arches of C1 and C2 rarely approximate with the single wire loop; axial rotation is only moderately restricted by the single fixation point provided by the midline loop as it continues to permit sliding motions between the two bony rings.

The Gallie fusion is particularly unsuitable for use in children because the midline synchondrosis between the two neural arches of C1 usually remains cartilaginous until age 5 or 6, and will be readily cut through by the midline wire (Figure 14). Even the newly fused arch at age 8 or 9 years may not withstand the high compression stresses exerted by the wire.

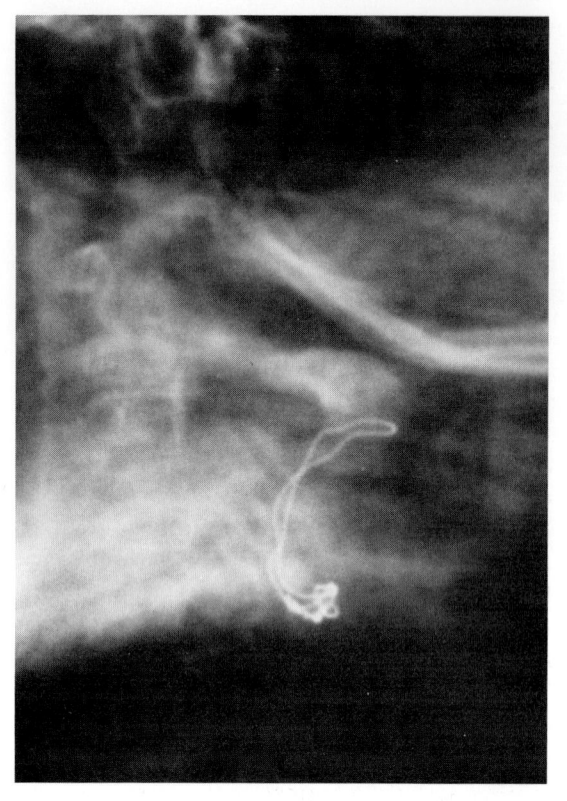

Figure 14. Lateral radiograph taken through a Minerva cast, showing a Gallie-type single-wire loop fusion of C1 and C2 in a 4-year-old child. The midline wire loop cut through the cartilaginous and mid-line portion of the posterior C1 arch, resulting in continued motion and nonunion.

In contrast to the Gallie method, the wedge compression method described by Brooks and Jenkins in 1978 offers greater biomechanical advantages.[34] In the Brooks construct, bilateral wires are passed around the arch of C1 and the lamina of C2. These wires are then tightened separately over a corticocancellous bone graft compressed against the C1 arch and the C2 lamina.

A later modification of the Brooks technique described by Griswold et al uses an almost T-shaped bone graft wedged between the C1 and C2 bony rings; the flat part of the T prevents the graft from being inadvertently displaced into the spinal canal.[35] With the modified Brooks construct, there is stability in both flexion and extension: flexion is restrained by tension in the circumferential wires, and extension is restrained by the bone graft, which serves as a buttressing block.[32] The bone graft compressed between the two posterior rings also serves as a friction block and offers stability against axial rotation.

The modified Brooks fusion is effective in adults with atlantoaxial instability and can be adapted for use in most older children. Obviously, the older the child, the stronger the posterior bony rings and the greater the immediate stability this method offers. However, it is likely that the incidence of graft resorption is higher in children than in adults. This may be related to the fact that in children, halo fixation does not provide the same degree of external immobilization as in adults, and the continued micromotion at the fusion site promotes graft resorption and retards new bone formation. Consequently, the balance of osteoclasis and osteogenesis within the graft is tipped towards osteoclasis, and the graft begins to shrink. Since the wire is wound tightly over the combined bulk of the lamina and the original graft, shrinking of the graft causes the wire loops to loosen and eventually leads to even more intersegmental motion, thereby completing the vicious cycle. The result is complete graft resorption and nonunion.

We encountered a dramatic example of this complication in an 8-year-old girl who was previously fused with the Brooks method but had rapid graft absorption and nonunion. The wire loops, lacking the bulbous wedge grafts, became loose and actually buckled forward against the spinal cord whenever the child extended her neck, causing intermittent quadriplegia and apnea (Case 1; Figures 15a-e).

Thus, in young children with atlanto-axial instability, in whom we anticipate suboptimal halo fixation, we prefer to pass bilateral sublaminar wires around the arch of C1 and the lamina of C2 and then tightly twist the wires separately beneath the lamina of C2 until the lamina and the C1 arch are just touching. This is quite easily and safely accomplished in children without compromising

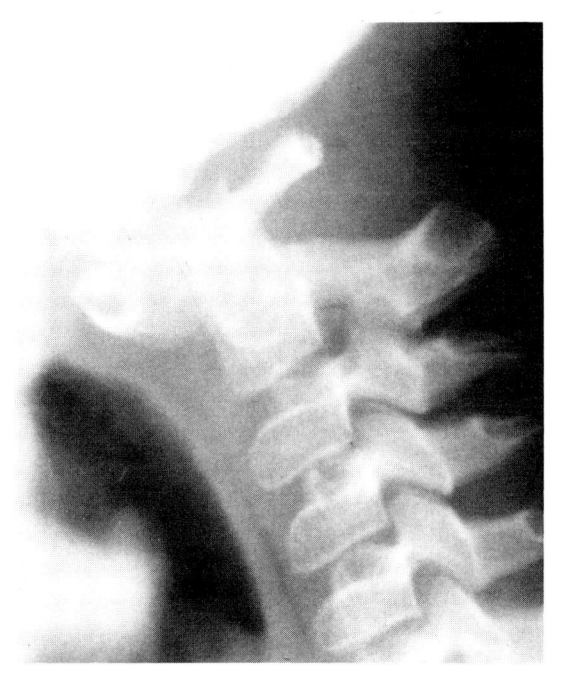

Figure 15. Case 1: Eight-year-old girl with os odontoideum presented with quadriparesis after having fallen and hit her occiput.

a. Severe anterior subluxation of C1 on C2 with an anteriorly displaced os odontoideum.

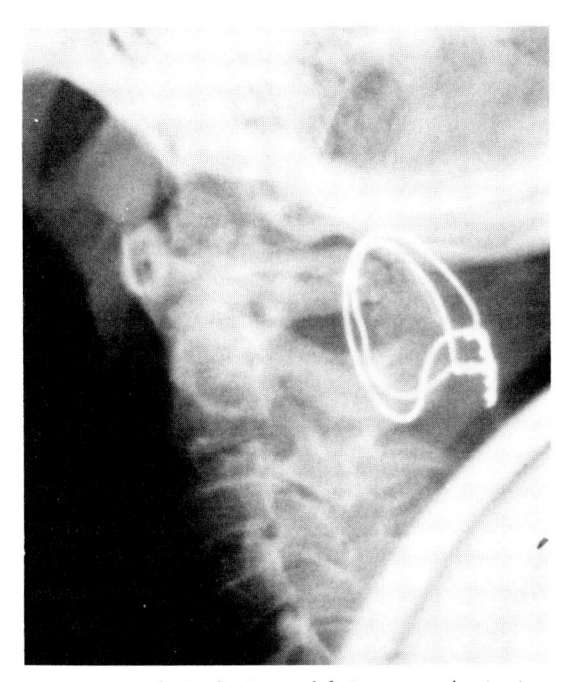

Figure 15b. Reduction and fusion at another institution with the modified Brooks method using a T-shape wedge graft and bilateral sublaminar wire loops.

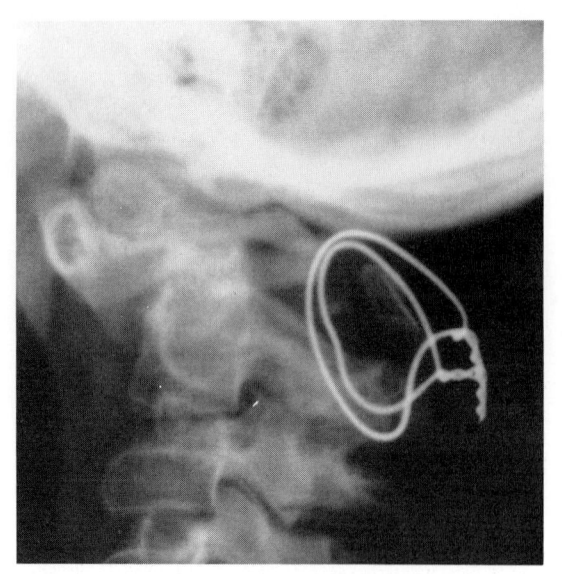

Figure 15c. Two months after Brooks fusion, showing subtotal resorption of bone graft and loosening of wire loops. This view also suggests fracture of the C1 ring by the loose and mobile wires.

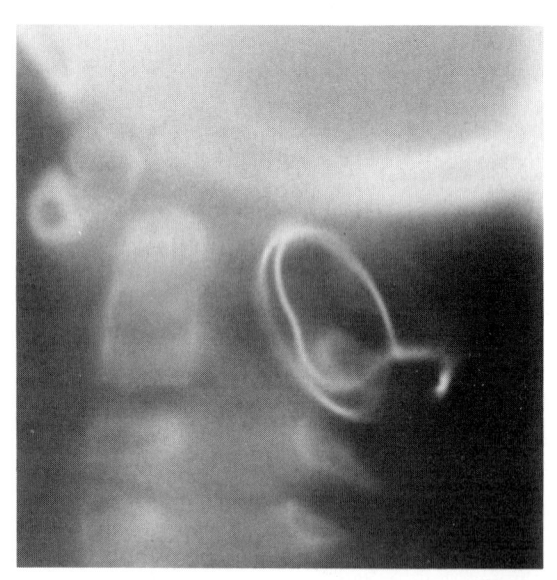

Figure 15d. After removal of halo, she began having episodic quadriparesis with neck extension. Lateral tomography shows nonunion of fusion, and buckling of the loose wire loops into the spinal canal on neck extension.

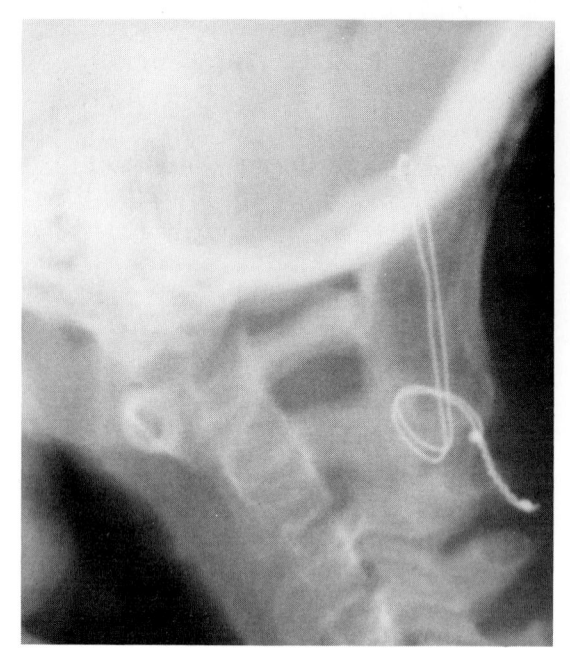

Figure 15e. Four months after second fusion with 18-gauge Luque wire loops through occipital burr holes and around the laminae of C2; the C1 ring was indeed fractured by the old wire loops, which were removed. Profuse callous and solid fusion of occiput to C2.

stability in the occipitoatlantal joint or producing much strain on the arch of C1 (Figures 16a,b). The now contiguous bony rings offer stability in both flexion and extension, and the two-point fixation provided by the double wires also increases friction between the twin bony rings and reduces the tendency for axial rotation. Autologous bone grafts are then compressed tightly against the fusion surface by additional graft-to-lamina wiring or by strapping sutures across the deep muscle layers. No matter what happens to these bone grafts, the inherent strength of the construct is undiminished, micromotion is almost completely eliminated, and fusion is almost guaranteed as long as the bony rings and wires remain intact.

Occasionally, an anteriorly dislocated C1 arch may not be reducible in spite of preoperative traction and intraoperative manipulation. This happens in some cases of os odontoideum and chronic anterolisthesis, and in several forms of mucolipidoses, in which abnormal soft tissues around the deformed and detached os prevent a perfect reduction. In this situation, wire fusion of the unreduced bony ring of C1 to C2 not only does not alleviate the spinal cord compression by

Special Problems of Spinal Stabilization in Children

the anteriorly displaced C1 arch, but further compromises the space available for the spinal cord by the presence of wires in the spinal canal. In such instances it is safer first to remove the arch of C1 to decompress the spinal cord, and then pass two wires through bilateral burr holes in the occiput and around the lamina of C2 to obtain an occipito-atlantoaxial fusion. Onlay grafts are then placed over the occiput and C2. Additional approximation of C1 and C2 can sometimes be achieved by placing lateral wires between the remaining stumps of the partially resected C1 ring and the laminae of C2 (Figures 17a-c).

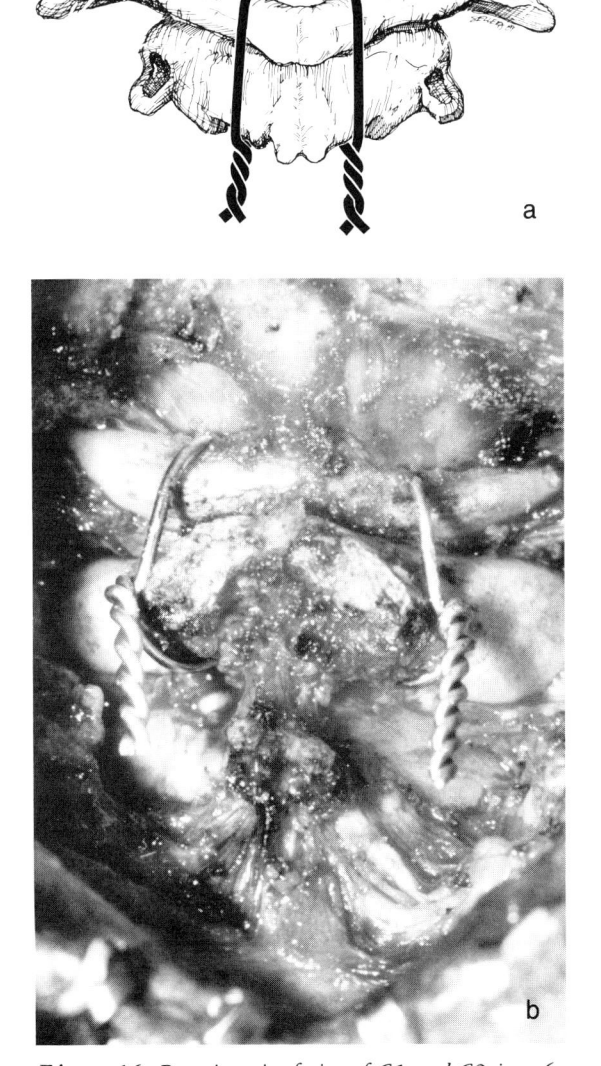

Figure 16. Posterior wire fusion of C1 and C2 in a 6-year-old child. Note approximation of the bony rings of C1 and C2 by the two sublaminar wire loops that are tightly twisted below the C2 ring.
   a. Drawing
   b. Intraoperative appearance

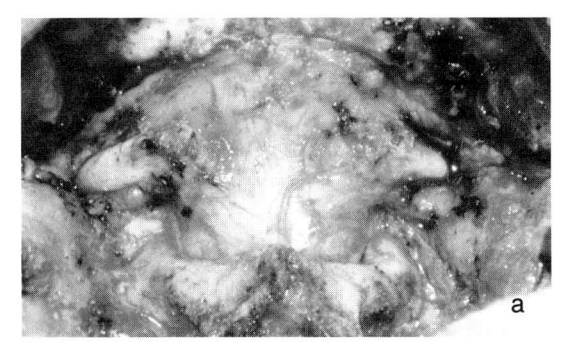

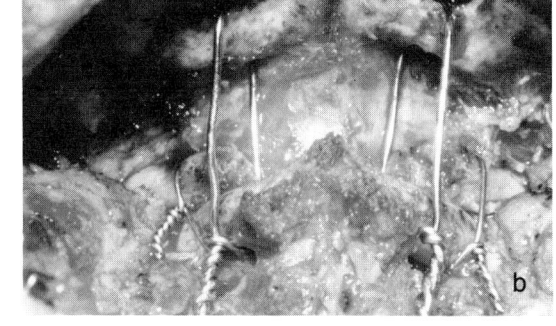

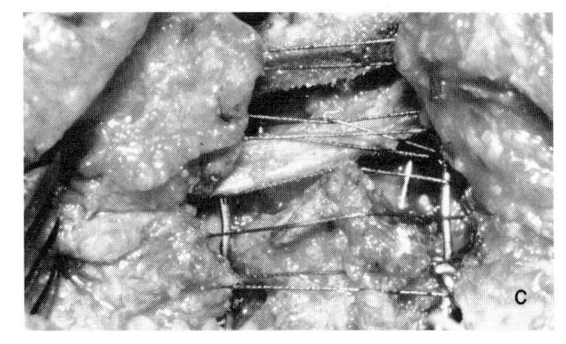

Figure 17. Posterior wire fusion of occiput to C2 in a 5-year-old child with incompletely reduced C1 anterior subluxation.
   a. Posterior arch of C1 was partially excised to relieve cord compression.
   b. Fusion with two 18-gauge wires through burr holes in the occiput and then around the laminae of C2. additional insurance of bony union was provided by two smaller lateral wires approximating the stumps of C1 and the arch of C2.
   c. Overlying bone grafts strapped down by cross sutures.

Obviously, this wiring construct does not impart much immediate stability in extension and rotation, and must therefore be supplemented by solid external immobilization with a tight-fitting halo vest.

Problems with Fusion Extension

Inclusion of one or even two adjacent levels into the fusion site may occur with posterior fusion techniques. Fielding and Hawkins reported 3 cases of overfusion in 57 posterior fusions, and 2 of the 3 patients were children.[6] The process appears to be related to a combination of (1) unnecessary subperiosteal dissection of adjacent "bystander" laminae and spinous processes and denuding of the cortical bone, (2) migration of the bone grafts away from their intended site, and (3) rigid immobilization of the entire cervical spine by the halo device. As noted by others, children have a greater capacity than adults to form exuberant callous whenever the periosteum is breached and the neck is effectively immobilized. Sometimes a formidable column of fusion is formed of six or seven consecutive vertebrae, even though the bone grafts were originally laid down to include only one or two levels (Figure 18).[3,6] Migration of bone grafts seems to be less important, for as long as the periosteum is intact, the presence of stray grafts does not promote bystander fusion.

The obvious disadvantage of overfusion is unnecessary loss of mobility in the cervical spine. There is a theoretical threat of accelerated spondylotic changes in the remaining mobile vertebral segments that are now burdened with excessive motions and stresses. The two factors are directly related: the greater the combined loss of mobility at the fusion site, the greater will be the compensatory increase in stress at the remaining mobile segments. Bystander fusion of a single level below C2 results in the loss of 8° to 17° of flexion-extension and from 8° to 12° of axial rotation, depending on the level and the age of the patient.[31,36] Inadvertent

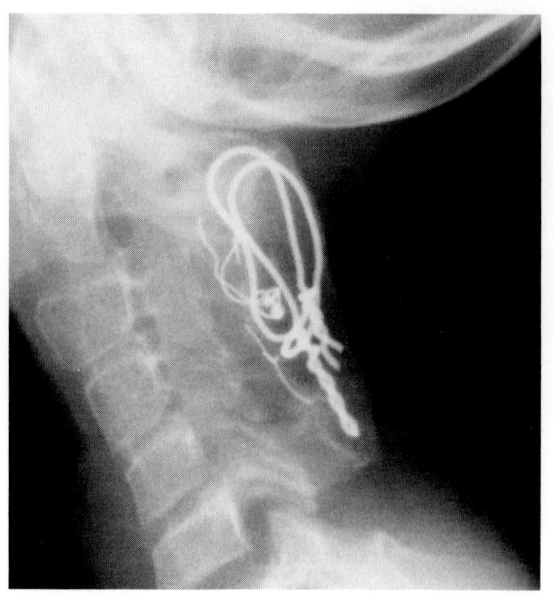

Figure 18. Lateral radiograph showing extension of fusion over six consecutive vertebral levels after intended fusion of C1 to C3.

inclusion of the occiput into an atlantoaxial fusion means a loss of 13° of flexion-extension at the occiput-C1 joint, in addition to the loss of 47° of axial rotation at the C1 and C2 joint (more than 50% of total axial rotation).[36] Both situations represent a potential handicap and should be avoided. The most effective preventive measure is still the meticulous preservation of the periosteum and other soft tissue overlying the bony surfaces adjacent to the intended fusion site.

Ligamentous Instability

When discussing posttraumatic ligamentous instability in children, it is important to distinguish between two distinct types of instability: incipient and overt.

Incipient Instability

The syndrome of spinal cord injury without radiographic abnormality (SCIWORA) is well known in children.[5,37] The spinal cord is injured without radiographic evidence of fracture or malalignment of the spinal column that would indicate severe ligamentous tear and gross instability. Yet, there had to have been sufficient intervertebral displacement at the time of impact to inflict injury to the spinal cord. This suggests that the crucial stabilizing ligaments and related fibrocartilaginous structures are flexible enough in children to allow momentary intersegmental displacement, yet maintain sufficient structural integrity to bring about subsequent recoil self-reduction of the displaced vertebra. Although these fibroligamentous structures are not completely torn, they may be sprained or even partially torn so that the involved vertebral segments are vulnerable to repeated stress: the instability is incipient rather than overt.[1,7,37-40]

The existence of incipient instability is suggested by the phenomenon of delayed neurological deterioration in a subgroup of children with SCIWORA. These children experience only transient symptoms of paresthesias or vague subjective total body weakness at the time of impact, but remain neurologically normal until hours later when, without further injury, they manifest progressive and inexorable neurological deterioration. Presumably, the stabilizing ligaments were sprained or partially torn by the initial violence, and the postimpact head and neck motions associated with normal activities were enough to cause further intervertebral displacement and delayed spinal cord injury.

Further evidence for the existence of incipient instability is also found in the syndrome of recurrent SCIWORA, in which children suffer a second and more serious bout of spinal cord injury following minor trauma days to weeks after a first episode of mild to moderate SCIWORA.[23] Invariably, these children are either inadequately immobilized or had unadvisedly discarded their neck collar at the time of the recurrent SCIWORA. The incipient instability incurred from the first SCIWORA presumably renders the spine vulnerable to recurrent stresses, so that a second bout of intersegmental displacement occurring when the spine is unprotected causes the recurrent spinal cord damage.

By definition, the incipient instability in SCIWORA cannot be demonstrated by flexion-extension views or other radiographic studies. The instantaneous elastic recoil of the flexible juvenile spine results in perfect self-reduction. The fact that dynamic x-ray study fails to reproduce the initial vertebral displacement is not surprising: most of the injured ligaments are probably not torn but only stretched, and immediately after the injury the neck is usually splinted securely by muscle spasm.[41] Even after spasm has subsided, dynamic studies involve cautiously and deliberately executed flexion and extension which cannot simulate the stresses of sudden and random neck movements in real-life activities. It is therefore entirely possible that these x-ray studies are normal, and yet seemingly tame sports can precipitate a recurrent injury when the spine has been already rendered incipiently unstable by the first episode of SCIWORA.[5]

The mechanism, clinical significance, and outcome of incipient instability in SCIWORA have been well defined. The effective treatment is cervical immobilization by an external orthosis such as the Guilford brace for three months and abstinence from all sport activities for a similar time period.[5,37] Surgical fusion is unnecessary.

Overt Instability

Unlike incipient instability, the diagnostic criteria and management of overt instability in children is not well defined. Certainly, if the x-ray shows complete disruption of either the anterior elements (the vertebral bodies, intervertebral disc, and anterior and posterior longitudinal ligaments) or posterior elements (the facets, the interfacetal ligaments, laminae, and the interspinous and supraspinous ligaments), or if one vertebral body is markedly malaligned, the implication is obvious: the spinal column is extremely unstable. However, many pediatric neck injuries exhibit radiographic findings more subtle than the extreme situations mentioned above and yet do not qualify as being normal as in SCIWORA. It is important to sort out from such "middling" findings those that represent overt instability requiring surgical fusion.

"Not-so-obvious" instability has been studied biomechanically in adults, and some useful, widely accepted guidelines have been established. Thus, for the atlantoaxial joint, the study done by Fielding et al using fresh cadaver vertebral segments indicated (1) that the atlanto-dental interval (ADI) in adults does not exceed 3 mm if all the ligaments are competent, (2) that an ADI of 3 to 5 mm implies rupture of the transverse ligament alone, (3) an ADI of 5 to 10 mm suggests additional incompetence of the alar ligaments, and (4) an ADI of greater than 10 mm exists only if all other accessory odontoid ligaments are also ruptured.[42] This led to the recommendation that an ADI in adults of greater than 3 mm be considered clinically unstable and C1 and C2 should be surgically fused.[32]

No biomechanical data are available on the atlanto-axial relationship in children, but from clinical experience we accept an ADI of 4 mm as the upper limit of normal in children under 8 years of age and recommend that an ADI greater than 4 mm be treated.[3,6] Martel and Tishler found that 20% of asymptomatic children with Down's syndrome have an ADI greater than 5 mm. They suggested that this number be accepted as the upper limit of normal in children with Down's syndrome.[43]

For the lower cervical spine, the classic biomechanical studies of White et al[48] and Panjabi et al[47] indicated that the ligaments in healthy adults normally permit very little horizontal motion between vertebrae; horizontal displacement (measured between the posterior-inferior corner of the upper vertebral body and the posterior-superior corner of the next lower vertebra) greater than 3.5 mm implies significant ligamentous rupture.[11,27] Likewise, angular displacement between vertebrae in normal adults was always found to be less than 11°. (To measure angular displacement on the lateral x-ray film, horizontal lines are constructed from two discrete points on each of the vertebral bodies. The intersecting angle at the involved level is measured and compared with the angle measured above and below the involved level.)

Extrapolating the aforementioned data to clinical situations, Johnson and Wolf recommended that for the lower cervical spine of adults a horizontal displacement between vertebral bodies of greater than 3.5 mm or an angular displacement of greater than 11° represents clinically significant instability.[15]

Exception to the 11° rule may be taken if the involved vertebral bodies have significant loss of height due to a severe compression fracture. In this case, the angulation may be falsely exaggerated and instability cannot be assumed unless there is associated wide separation of the spinous processes. When stability is in doubt and there are no associated neurologic deficits, Johnson and Wolf suggested obtaining flexion-extension x-rays to document abnormal motion and worsening of the horizontal or angular displacement. They emphasized that such studies should never be attempted in the presence of neurological deficit or when spinal instability is obvious.[43] These authors also noted that pure ligamentous injuries tend to have less predictable healing; they thus prefer surgical fusion to simple external immobilization by the halo device.

No well-established criteria exist for assessment of instability of the lower cervical spine in children. Experience has taught us to adopt different normal upper limits for both angular and horizontal displacements from those recommended for adults. For angular displacement in children, we accept an upper limit of less than 11°. We reason that since the juvenile spine is so supple and so capable of recoil, the final resting position of the dislocated segment after the impact may lie well short of its actual maximum excursion at the time of impact. The angle of displacement on the lateral x-ray film may be deceptively small, but the injury may have actually resulted in severely impaired liga-

Special Problems of Spinal Stabilization in Children

ments that will allow progression of the kyphosis.

This scenario is illustrated by the case of a 10-year-old boy who suffered a flexion injury to the cervical spine. He presented with an asymmetric central cord syndrome and a lateral x-ray in the neutral position showed a kyphotic deformity of 8° at C4 and C5, a horizontal displacement of 2 mm and a unilateral laminar fracture of C5. No dynamic x-rays were obtained for fear of aggravating the neurologic deficits, but because the angulation was less than 11°, we initially treated him with a halo vest. Three months later, when his halo device was removed, he promptly showed rapid progression of his kyphosis and required a posterior sublaminar wiring and fusion for stability (Case 2; Figures 19a-e).

This case illustrates our dilemma with an injury that by its implied violence and severity of neurological damage suggests overt instability. The neutral radiograph does not meet the 11° adult criterion for instability, yet the integrity of the ligaments could not be tested by a flexion-extension study because of the neurological deficits. In retrospect, the instability was obviously present from the

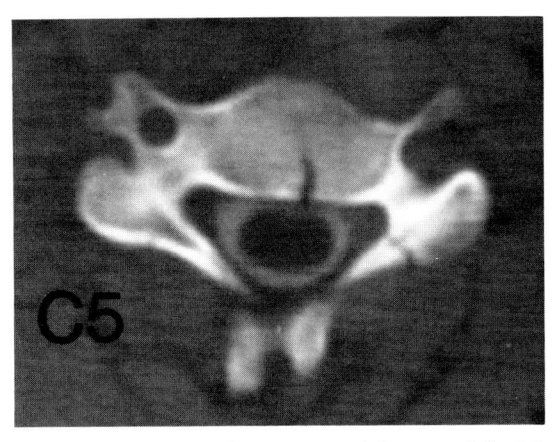

Figure 19b. CT showing vertical fracture of the C5 vertebral body and unilateral laminar fracture.

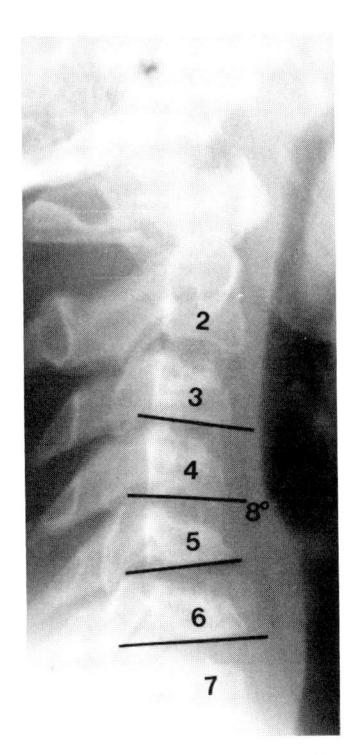

Figure 19. Case 2: Ten-year-old boy suffered a flexion injury, presented with an asymmetric central cord syndrome.
  a. Lateral radiograph showing a kyphotic deformity of 8° at C4 and C5, horizontal displacement of less than 2 mm, slight widening of the C4-C5 interspinous space, and compression fractures of the C5 and C6 vertebral bodies.

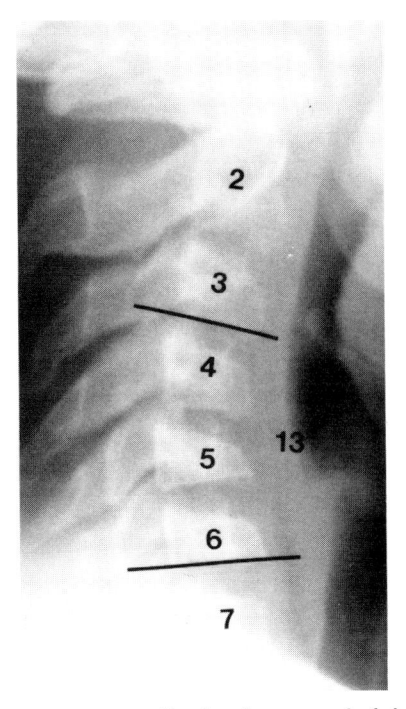

Figure 19c. Immediately after removal of the halo, lateral radiograph shows an angulation of 13°.

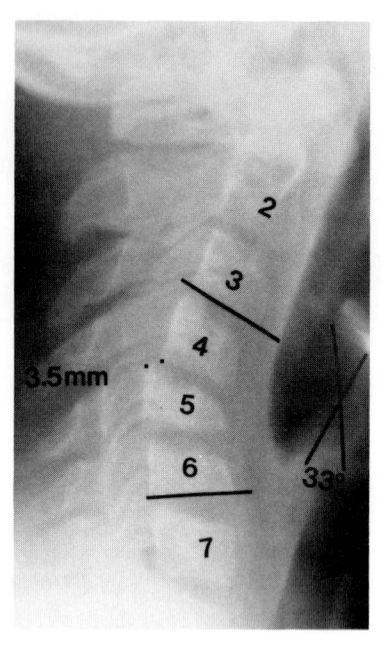

Figure 19d. One week after removal of halo, angulation increased to 33°. Horizontal displacement increased to 3.5 mm.

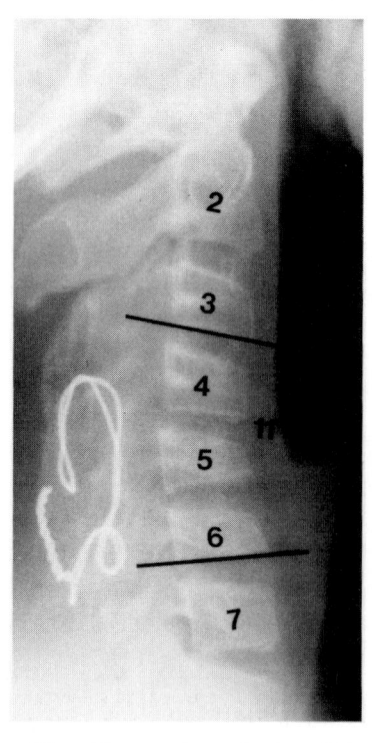

Figure 19e. After traction reduction of the kyphotic deformity, a C4-C5-C6 sublaminar wire fusion with on-laid bone grafts was successfully done to reestablish stability, with a permanent angulation of 11°.

start in spite of an angulation of only 8° on the neutral film. To avoid similar mishaps, we now recommend the algorithm seen in Figure 20.

A relatively small angle of kyphotic deformity on neutral films can belie severely impaired interspinous ligaments. However, the juvenile spine appears to tolerate a much greater degree of physiologic mobility in the horizontal plane. Radiographic surveys of large populations of normal children show that the younger the child, the higher is the fulcrum for maximum mobility and the greater the physiologic hypermobility.

In infants and very young children (under 5 years), the fulcrum for maximum flexion is at C2-C3 and C3-C4; in later childhood (6 to 10 years) the maximum fulcrum is at C4-C5, whereas the maximum fulcrum for adults is usually at C5-C6 or C6-C7.[7,39,44-46] As for the actual range of physiologic hypermobility, Sullivan et al noted a forward glide of 3.5 mm to 4 mm between C2 and C3 in 13 out of 100 normal children, and similar horizontal displacements between C3 and C4 in two other children.[46] Cattell and Filtzer observed similar findings in 19% of normal children under 8 years of age.[7] In all probability, this "pseudosubluxation" between C2 and C3, and to a lesser extent between C3 and C4, is due to elastic capsular ligaments, malleable cartilaginous endplates, relatively horizontal facets at these levels, and more marked anterior wedging of the bodies at C3 and C4.[37]

How, then, can one distinguish between physiologic hypermobility in the horizontal plane and clinical instability in the mid to low cervical segments of a child? No scientific data currently exist to support a definitive answer to this question, but the following are recommendations based on our experience during the past decade:

1. We believe that children older than 8 years are sufficiently similar to adults biomechanically that a horizontal displacement of greater than 3.5 mm at

Lateral Cervical Spine Radiograph Showing Angular Deformity

```
                                    |
        ┌───────────────────────────┼───────────────────────────┐
       ≥11°                    >7° <11°                        <7°
                                                        (with neck pain & spasm)
        │              ┌────────────┴────────────┐              │
        │         Neurologically            Neurological    Cervical Brace of Collar
        │           Normal                    Deficits           x5 Days
        │              │                        │                │
        │        Flexion-Extension              │          Flexion-Extension
        │          Radiograph                   │            Radiograph
        │         ┌────┴────┐                   │        ┌───────┼───────┐
        │        ≥11°      <11°                 │       <7°   >7° <11°  ≥11°
        ▼         ▼         ▼                   ▼        ▼        ▼      ▼
    Surgical  Surgical  Cervical Brace      Surgical  Philadelphia  Cervical Brace  Surgical
     Fusion    Fusion    or Halo             Fusion     Collar        or Halo        Fusion
```

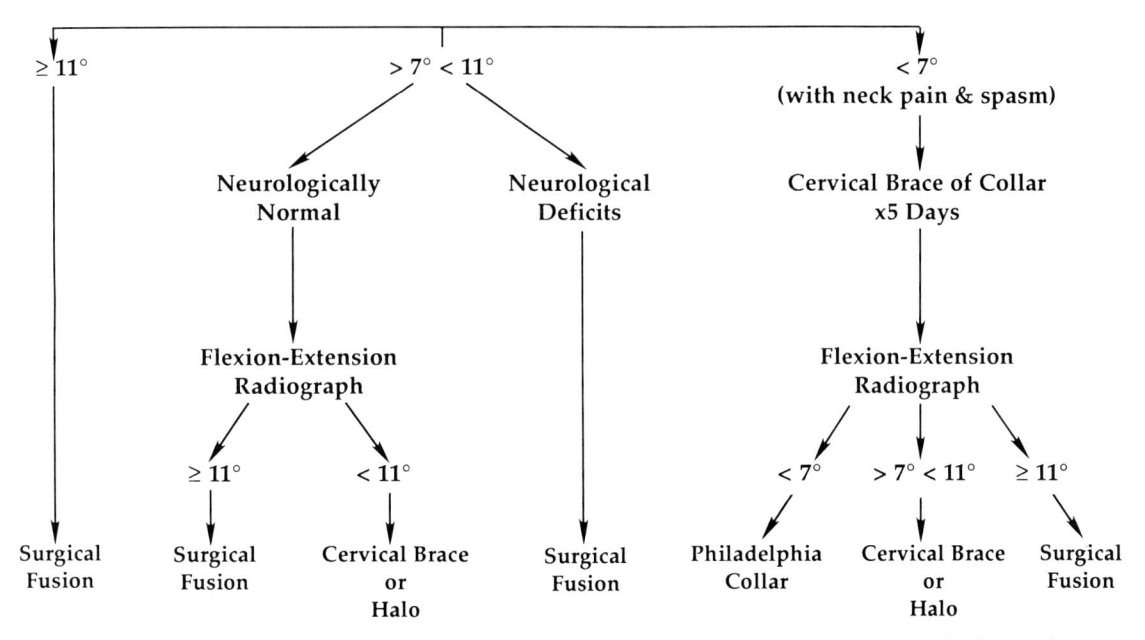

Figure 20. Algorithm of management of overt ligamentous instability if lateral radiograph shows a kyphotic deformity.

any level should be considered unstable and treated with surgical fusion.

2. Children younger than 8 years have increased physiologic mobility at the C2-C3 and C3-C4 joints, but a horizontal displacement at these levels of greater than 4 mm, with or without neurologic symptoms, should be considered to be evidence of instability.

3. In children younger than 8 years, if a horizontal displacement of 3.5 mm at the upper levels is associated with severe muscle spasm, neck pain, neurological findings, or additional abnormalities such as an avulsed spinous process or widened interspinous space, clinical instability is assumed and treated with surgical fusion.

4. Because the physiologic mobility at the C4-C5, C5-C6, and C6-C7 levels in children younger than 8 years is not significantly different from that of adults, a horizontal displacement of greater than 3.5 mm, with or without neurological deficits, implies instability and should be treated.

References

1. Bailey DK. The normal cervical spine in infants and children. *Radiology*. 1952;59:712-719.
2. Silverman FN. The neck, spine, and pelvis. In: Silverman FN, ed. *Caffey's Pediatric X-ray Diagnosis*. 8th ed. Chicago, Ill: Year Book Medical Publishers Inc; 1985:269-273.
3. Fielding JW. Selected observations on the cervical spine in the child. *Curr Pract Orthop Surg*. 1973;5:31-55.
4. Hadley LA. *The Spine*. Springfield, Ill: Charles C Thomas; 1956:62-64.
5. Pang D, Pollack IF. Spinal cord injury without radiographic abnormality in children: the SCIWORA syndrome. *J Trauma*. 1989;29:654-664.
6. Fielding JW, Hawkins RJ. Roentgenographic diagnosis of the injured neck. American Association of Orthopedic Surgeons, Instructional Course Lectures. 1976;25:149-170.
7. Cattell HS, Filtzer DL. Pseudosubluxation and other normal variations in the cervical spine in children: a study of one hundred and sixty children. *J Bone Joint Surg Am*. 1965;47A:1295-1309.
8. Pang D, Wilberger JE Jr. Traumatic atlanto-occipital dislocation with survival. Case report and review. *Neurosurgery*. 1980;7:503-508.
9. Garfin SR, Botte MJ, Waters RL, Nickel VL. Com-

plications in the use of the halo fixation device. *J Bone Joint Surg Am.* 1986;68A:320-325.
10. Johnson RM, Owen JR, Hart DL, Callahan RA. Cervical orthoses. *Clin Orthop.* 1981;154:34-45.
11. Wolf JW Jr, Johnson RM. Cervical orthoses. In: Clinical Spine Research Society, ed. *The Cervical Spine.* Philadelphia, Pa: JB Lippincott Co; 1983:54-61.
12. Prolo DJ, Runnels JB, Jameson RM. The injured cervical spine: immediate and long-term immobilization with the halo. *JAMA.* 1973; 224:591-594.
13. Baum JA, Hanley EN Jr, Pullekines J. Comparison of halo complications in adults and children. *Spine.* 1989;14:251-252.
14. Chan RC, Schweigel JF, Thompson GB. Halo-thoracic brace immobilization in 188 patients with acute cervical spine injuries. *J Neurosurg.* 1983; 58:508-515.
15. Kopits SE, Steingass MH. Experience with the "halo-cast" in small children. *Surg Clin North Am.* 1970;50:935-943.
16. Garfin SR, Botte MJ, Centeno RS, Nickel VL. Osteology of the skull as it affects halo pin placement. *Spine.* 1985;10:696-698.
17. Mubarak SJ, Camp JF, Vuletich W, et al. Halo immobilization for cervical spine instability in the infant. Abstracts Annual Meeting of Pediatric Orthopedic Society of North America. Colorado Springs, Colo: Pediatric Orthopedic Society of North America;1988:61.
18. Victor DI, Bresnan MJ, Keller RB. Brain abscess complicating the use of halo traction. *J Bone Joint Surg Am.* 1973;55A:635-639.
19. Goodman ML, Nelson PB. Brain abscess complicating the use of a halo orthosis. *Neurosurgery.* 1987;20:27-30.
20. Hoffmann GR, Merckx J, Vercauteren M. Abcès cérébral consécutif à la "halo traction." *Neurochirurgie.* 1974;20:263-266.
21. Humbyrd DE, Latimer FR, Lonstein JE, Samberg LC. Brain abscess as a complication of halo traction. *Spine.* 1981;6:365-368.
22. Benzel EC, Hadden TA, Saulsbery CM. A comparison of the Minerva and halo jackets for stabilization of the cervical spine. *J Neurosurg.* 1989; 70:411-414.
23. Pollack I, Pang D, Sclabassi R. Recurrent spinal cord injury without radiographic abnormalities in children. *J Neurosurg.* 1988;69:177-182.
24. Anderson LD. Fractures of the odontoid process of the axis. In: Cervical Spine Research Society, ed. *The Cervical Spine.* Philadelphia, Pa: JB Lippincott Co; 1983:206-223.
25. Johnson RM, Wolf JW Jr. Stability. In: Cervical Spine Research Society, ed. *The Cervical Spine.* Philadelphia, Pa: JB Lippincott Co; 1983:35-53.
26. Johnson RM, Owen JR, Panjabi MM, Bucholz RW, Southwick WO. Immediate strength of certain cervical fusion techniques. *Orthop Trans.* 1980;4:42.
27. Rogers WA. Treatment of fracture-dislocation of the cervical spine. *J Bone Joint Surg.* 1942;24:245-258.
28. Callahan RA, Johnson RM, Margolis RN, Keggi KJ, Albright JA, Southwick WO. Cervical facet fusion for control of instability following laminectomy. *J Bone Joint Surg Am.* 1977;59A:991-1002.
29. Johnson RM, Southwick WO. Surgical approaches to the spine. In: Rothman RH, Simeone FA, eds. *The Spine*, 2nd ed. Philadelphia, Pa: WB Saunders Co; 1982;1:67-147.
30. Fielding JW, Hawkins RJ, Ratzan SA. Spine fusion for atlanto-axial instability. *J Bone Joint Surg Am.* 1976;58A:400-407.
31. Jofe MH, White AA, Panjabi MM. Kinematics. In: Cervical Spine Research Society, ed. *The Cervical Spine.* Philadelphia, Pa: JB Lippincott Co; 1983:23-35.
32. White AA III, Panjabi MM. The clinical biomechanics of the occipitoatlantoaxial complex. *Orthop Clin North Am.* 1978;9:867-878.
33. Gallie WE. Fractures and dislocations of the cervical spine. *Am J Surg.* 1939;46:495-499.
34. Brooks AL, Jenkins EB. Atlanto-axial arthrodesis by the wedge compression method. *J Bone Joint Surg Am.* 1978;60A:279-284.
35. Griswold DM, Albright JA, Schiffman E, Johnson R, Southwick WO. Atlanto-axial fusion for instability. *J Bone Joint Surg Am.* 1978;60A:285-292.
36. White AA III, Panjabi MM. The basic kinematics of the human spine. *Spine.* 1978;3:12-20.
37. Pang D, Wilberger JE Jr. Spinal cord injury without radiographic abnormalities in children. *J Neurosurg.* 1982;57:114-129.
38. Aufdermaur M. Spinal injuries in juveniles: necropsy findings in twelve cases. *J Bone Joint Surg Br.* 1974;56B:513-519.
39. Townsend EH Jr, Rowe ML. Mobility of the upper cervical spine in health and disease. *Pediatrics.* 1952;10:567-573.
40. von Torklus D, Gehle W. *The Upper Cervical Spine.* New York, NY: Grune & Stratton; 1972:10-94.
41. Webb JK, Broughton RBK, McSweeny T, Park WM. Hidden flexion injury of the cervical spine. *J Bone Joint Surg Br.* 1976;58B:322-327.
42. Fielding JW, Cochran GVB, Lawsing JF III, Hohl M. Tears of the transverse ligament of the atlas: a clinical and biomechanical study. *J Bone Joint Surg Am.* 1974;56A:1683-1691.
43. Martel W, Tishler J. Observations on the spine in Mongoloidism. *AJR.* 1966;97:630-638.
44. Baker DH, Berdon WE. Special trauma problems in children. *Radiol Clin North Am.* 1966;4:289-305.
45. Braakman R, Penning L. Injuries of the cervical spine. In *Excerpta Medica.* Amsterdam:Excerpta Medica;1971.
46. Sullivan CR, Bruwer AJ, Harris LE. Hypermobility of the cervical spine in children: a pitfall in the diagnosis of cervical dislocation. *Am J Surg.* 1958;95:636-640.
47. Panjabi MM, White AA III, Johnson RM. Cervical spine mechanics as a function of transection of components. *J Biomech.* 1975;8:327-336.
48. White AA III, Johnson RM, Panjabi MM, Southwick WO. Biomechanical analysis of clinical stability in the cervical spine. *Clin Orthop.* 1975;109:85-96.

Index

Page numbers for tables, figures, and illustrations are in *boldface italics*.

A

A-O broad plates, 129, 151
Accident scene
  in general, 1-2
  initial evaluation, treatment, 2-3
  stabilization for transport, 3
  transport, 3-4
Acute injuries
  lower cervical spine, 25-28, *25, 27*
  thoracolumbar spine, 30-32, *31, 32-33*
  upper cervical spine, 28-29, *28, 29*
Age, of patient, 84, 86
Air drill, 93
Alar ligaments, 78
Alignment restoration, *139,* 139-40
Anatomy
  of flexion-dislocation injuries, 116-18, *117*
  ligamentous, 65-66
  muscular action, 66
  of odontoid process, 78-79
  osseous, 65
  pelvic, 163
  of upper cervical spine, 99-100
Ankylosing spondylitis
  complications, 176
  in general, 173-74
  management, 174-75, *176*
  prognosis and outcome, 176
Anterior decompression, 140-41, *141*
Anterior operation, 124-25
  bone grafting without plating, 128-29, *129*
  bone grafting with plating, 129-30, *130*
Anterior screw fixation, 93
Anterior wedge compression fractures, 141-42, *142*
  and posterior element disruption, 142
Anterior wiring, 92
Anterolateral fusion approach, 92
Anteroposterior (AP) radiographs, 12-13, 20-21, 26, *27,* 30, *31*

Antibiotics, 6
Aplasia, 77, 80
Apuzzo fusion modification, *91,* 91. *See also* Gallie fusion
Arthrodesis, 43
Aspiration, 2, 4
Associated injuries, 81-82
Atelectasis, 6
Atlanto-axial instability, *28,* 28-29, 38-40, *40*
  dislocation, 72-74, *73-74*
  rotatory luxation, 71-72
  transoral exposure, 93-94
  traumatic, 107-8
Atlanto-occipital
  dislocation radiology, 69-70
  instability, 37-38, *38*
Atlas-axis combination fractures, 105-6, *107*
Atlas fractures, 39, *101,* 101-2
Atropine, 3
Autonomic dysfunction, 7
Axial traction, 2
Axis fractures, *101,* 103, *103-5,* 105

B

Backboard, 13
  intermediate radiolucent, 3
BC/OA ratio, 38, *38*
Bed rest, 111-13
Beds, 5
Blood pressure, 4
Blood supply, 78-79
Body fracture, 105
Body jackets, molded, 15, 58
Body splint, 190-91, *191*
Bone grafting, 120, *121,* 126-27, *129*
  without plating, *129,* 128-29
  with plating, *130,* 129-30
Bony fusion, 92
Bracing, 52-53
  lumbosacral, *59,* 59
  thoracolumbar, 57-58, *58*
Bradycardia, 2-3, 4
  reflex, 7

Brooks fusion modification, *91,* 91. *See also* Gallie fusion
    Callahan modification, 91
Bucholz classification, 164, *165,* 167
Burst fracture, 31, 39
    classification of, 152
    decision making, 152-56, *153-56*
    in general, *148,* 148-49
    treatment, 149-52, *150, 152*

C

C1 arch fracture, *104,* 104
C1-C2 fracture, 106, *196-200,* 196-200
    fusions, 91-92
C2-C3 anterior fusion, *104*
C2 to C7 segments, in pediatrics, 192-95, *194-95*
Callahan fusion modification, 91. *See also* Gallie fusion
Callus formation, 33-34
Cardiogenic shock, 2-3
Caspar trapezoidal plates, 129-30, *131*
Cauda equina syndrome, 169
Cephalothin sodium, 70
Cervical disc herniation, 120
Cervical orthoses
    cervicothoracic, *54,* 55, *56*
    collars, 53-55, *54-55*
    halo, *54,* 56
    poster-type, *55,* 54-55
    recommended use of, *54,* 56-57
Cervical spine injuries, 13, *14*
    algorithm for instability, 44, *45*
    atlanto-axial instability, 38-40, *40*
    atlanto-occipital instability, 37-38, *38*
    lower, 25-28, *25, 27*
    middle, lower, 41-44, *42*
    neural arch of axis fractures, 40-41
    suspected, 11-12, *11-12,* 21
    upper, 28-29, *28-29,* 99-103, *101, 103-5,* 105-9, *107-9*
Cervical spondylosis, *178,* 178-79
Cervicothoracic orthoses, 55, 57
Chance fracture, 144
Children. *See* Pediatrics
Chin lift, 2
Cine recordings, 21
Clamps, interlaminar, 92-93, 127
Cloth tape, 3
Cloward fusion method, 128
Collars, 53-55, *54-55*
Combined C1-C2 fractures, 86, 88
Combined instability, 20
Compression-burst fractures, 122-23, *122*
Compression injuries, 25, 30-31, *31,* 43-44
Compressive flexion
    anterior wedge compression fractures, 141-42, *142*
    and posterior element disruption, 142
    three-column injury, 142
    treatment, 142-43, *143*
Computerized tomography (CT) scanning, 5, 7-9, 13, 19-21, 23, *24,* 26-29, *27,* 31, *31-33, 35,* 73
    coronal reformatted, *29*
    -myelography, 23
    and odontoid fractures, 82
Confused, combative patient, 2, 5
Congenital anomalies, 80
Conradi's syndrome, 100
Contiguous spinal injury, 136
Corset, lumbosacral, *59,* 59
Cotrel-Dubousset instrumentation, *150,* 150
Coupling, 67
Cranial pin site care, 61
Craniocervical instability, *175,* 175
Craniovertebral junction (CV), *68*
Cricothyroidotomy, 2
Crutchfield tongs, 84

D

Decompression, 8, 122, 139
    alignment restoration, *139,* 139-40
    anterior, 140-41, *141*
    laminectomy, 140
    in middle burst injuries without neurological injury, 154-55
    posterolateral, 140
    in upper burst injuries, 153-54
Decubitus ulcers, 6
Deformities
    chronic fixed facet, 120-21, *120-21*
Denis type classifications, 144
Diazepam, 9
Disc disruption, 26
Disc herniation, 20
Dislocation
    and atlanto-occipital radiology, 69-70
    lumbosacral, 156-57
    and occipito-atlantal instability, 67-68, *68*
Displacement, 86, *88*
Distraction, 53
Distractive extension injuries, 156
Dopamine, 4, 10
Down's syndrome, 88, 100, 202
Dural tear, 23

E

Emotional support, 7
Epiphyseal development, variations, 181-84, *182-83*
Euthermia, 5
Extension injuries, 25, 123-24

Index

F

Face shield helmets, 2
Facet
  dislocations, 43, 118-20
    bilateral, 26
  fusion, 127
  subluxations, 116-19, *116-17*
Fiberoptic bronchoscope, 4
Fixation points, 52, 53, 54, 58
Flexion-compression injuries, 121-22
Flexion-dislocation injuries
  chronic deformities, 120-21, *120-21*
  facet dislocations, 118-20
  facet subluxations, 116-19, *116-17*
  operative stabilization, 119
Flexion-distraction injuries, 1, 143-44, *144*
Flexion-extension views, 19, 21, *22*, 28, 29, 34, *45*, 202
Flexion injuries, 25, *203-4*, 203-4
Flexion-rotation injuries, 25
Flexion-teardrop fracture, 26
Fluid compression, 53
Fluoroscopy, 21
Foley catheter, 4, 6
Force, application of, 52
Four-poster brace, 54-55, *54-55*
Fractures, 143
  anterior wedge compression, 141-42, *142*
    posterior element disruption, 142
  of atlas, *101*, 101-2
  of axis, 103, *104-5*, 105
  of combination atlas-axis, 105-6, *107*
  compression-burst, 122-23, *122*
  healing, 23
    age of, 86
    combined C1-C2, 86
    displacement, 86, *88*
    location on odontoid, 86
    nonunion rate, *85*
    preexisting pathology, 87
    stable vs. unstable, 138-39
    type and nonunion rate, *87*
  sacral, 163-71, *165-66, 168-69*
  of third cervical vertebra, 107
  three-column injury, 142
Fusion, 3, 23, 71
  anterior wiring and bony, 92
  anterolateral approach, 92
  extension, 200, *200*
    in pediatrics, 200
  facet, 127
  Gallie, 90-91, *91*
    Apuzzo modification, *91*, 91
    Brooks modification, *91*, 91
    Callahan modification of Brooks, 91
  occipital-C2/C1-C3, 91-92
  pediatric, 192-200, *194-200*

G

Gallie fusion, 90
  Apuzzo modification of, *91*, 91
  Brooks modification of, *91*, 91, 196-97, *197-98*
    Callahan modification, 91
  in pediatrics, *196*, 196
Gardner-Wells tongs, 7, 9, 12, 13, 84, 101, 119, 185
Gastrointestinal system, 6
Gelpi retractor, 93
General care, 5-7
Glasgow Coma Scale, 10
Glucocorticoids, 11
Glycopyrolate, 3
Guilford brace, *190*, 190. See also Two-poster Guilford brace

H

Halifax clamps, 127
Halo orthoses, 33, *54*, 56-57, 61, 84, 89-90, 108, 185
  for lower cervical spine, 113-15, *115*
  in pediatrics, 186-89, *187-89*
Hangman's fracture, 79, 86, 103, *104, 195*, 195
Hard collar, 11-12
Harrington rods, *139*, 139-40, *143*, *145*, 145-46, 149-51
Headache, 7
Head and spinal cord injury, 10
Heparin, 6
Holdsworth classification, 136
Hospital course, 113
  combined head, cord injury, 10
  imaging studies, timing of, 7
  initial evaluation, resuscitation, 4-5, *11-12, 14-15*
  MRI, myelography, early surgery, 8
  multiple level injuries, 10
  nursing, general care, 5-7
  patient transfers, 8
  pharmacologic treatment, 10-11
  specific treatments, 11-15
  tongs, traction, 9-10
Hyperflexion
  -compression injuries, 1-2
  -distraction injuries, 1
Hypertension, 7
Hypoplasia, 77, 80
Hypotension, 2, 3
Hypovolemic hypotension, 2

I

Imaging
  acute injuries, *25*, 25-29, *27-29*
  introduction, 19
  stability defined, 19-20
  subacute injuries, 32-35, *33-35*

Imaging continued
   techniques of, 20-21, *22*, 23, *24*
   thoracolumbar spine, 30-32, *31-32*
   timing of studies, 7
Incipient instability, 200-201
Initial evaluation, 2-3, 4-5, *11-12, 14-15*
   resuscitation, treatment, 2-3, 4-5, *11-12, 14-15*
   stabilization, 81-84, *82-83*, 101
Inotropes, 3
Instability
   craniocervical, *175*, 175
   of lower cervical spine, 41-42, *42*
   of lumbar spine, 46-47, *47*
   at occipito-atlantal dislocation, 67-68, *68*
   pediatric ligamentous, 200-205, *203-5*
   sacrum, *47*, 47-48
   in thoracic, thoracolumbar spines, *45*, 46, *46*
   traumatic atlanto-axial, 107-8
Interfacet wiring, 193
Interlaminar clamps, 92-93, 127
Interspinous ligament injury, 26
Interspinous wiring, 125, *126*, 193
Intraabdominal injuries, 4-5
Intubation, 2, 4

J

Jacobs locking rods, 150
Jason brace, 89-90, *90*
Jefferson fractures, 25, 29, 39
Jewett brace, 57
Jumped facets, *116-17*

K

Kendricks Extrication Device, 3
Klippel-Feil syndrome, *177*, 177-78
Kostuik-Harrington distraction rods, 151-52, *152*, 154

L

Laminectomy, 140, 175
   multilevel cervical, 179, *180*
   rolls, 70
Lap belt, 1
Lap-belt injuries, 31
Late displaced pelvic fractures, 170
Lateral cervical spine radiograph, *205*
Lateral displacement, 39
Lateral film, *25*, 25-26, *27*
Lateral flexion injuries, 144-45, *145*
Lateral radiographs, 12-13, 20
Lerman Minerva cervical orthosis, *55*
Ligamentous anatomy, 65-66
Ligamentous disruption, 20-21, 23, *24, 27, 28, 68*, 70

Ligamentous instability
   incipient, 200-201
   overt, 201-5, *203-5*
Ligaments, 78
Los Angeles County—University of Southern California Medical Center, 168
Lower burst injuries, *155-56*, 155-56
Lower cervical spine
   and ankylosing spondylitis, 174-75
   bed rest, traction for, 111-13
   compression-burst, 122-23, *122*
   extension, 123
   flexion-compression, 121-22
   halo vest immobilization, 114-15, *115*
   specific, 116-21, *116-17, 120*
   surgery, 124-25, *126*, 127-31, *128-31*
Lumbar spine, 46-47, *47*, 135
Lumbosacral spine
   dislocation, 156-57
   instability, *47*, 47-48
   orthoses, 58
      brace, *59*, 59
      corsets, *59*, 59
      spicas, *59-60*, 59-60
Luque wiring, 151, *198*
Luschka joints, 177

M

Magnetic resonance imaging. *See* MRI scanning
Malgaigne fracture dislocation, *168*
Malibu collar, *55*
Management guidelines
   anterior wiring, bony fusion, 92
   anterolateral approach, 92
   decision-making factors, 84, *85*, 86-87, *87-88*
   stabilization, 84, 92-93
   nonoperative, 89-90, *90*
   operative, 90-92, *91*
      vs. nonoperative treatment, 84, 88-89
   transoral exposure, 93-94
MAST. *See* Military anti-shock trousers
Matta classifications, 164, *165*, 168
Mechanical instability, 20
Methylmethacrylate (MMA), 92, 128-29
Methylprednisolone, 11
Middle burst injuries, 154-55
Middle cervical spine and ankylosing spondylitis, 174-75
Military anti-shock trousers (MAST), 2
Milwaukee brace, 58
Minerva jacket, *54*, 56-57, 61, 89
   in pediatrics, 189-90
Molded body splint, 190-91, *191*
Morbidity, mortality, 113
   of odontoid fractures, 81
Motion range, 66

Index

Motion, spinal, 52
MRI scanning, 7-8, 13, 19-20, 23, *24*, 28, 67, 73
Multiple-level injuries, 10
Muscle relaxants, 9
Muscular action, 66
Myelography, 8, 13, 20, 23

N

Naked facet, 26, *27*
Naloxone, 11
Nasotracheal intubation, 2, 4, 70
National Collaborative Spinal Cord Injury Study, 10, 11
Neo-Synephrine, 10
Neural arch of the axis fractures, 40-41
Neurogenic urinary retention, 4
Neurological deficit of sacral fractures, 169-70
Neurological involvement, 68
Neurological outcome, 112-13
　evaluation, 166-67
　of flexion-dislocation injuries, 118-19
Neurologic instability, 20
Nicoll classification, 136
Noncontiguous spinal injury, 136
Nonoperative management, 84, *85,* 86-89, *87-89*
　orthotic devices, 89-90, *90*
　thoracolumbar spine injuries, 137-38, *138*
Nonunion rate, 85
　amount of displacement and, *88*
　fracture type and, *87*
Nursing care, 6-7
　autonomic dysfunction, 7
　bed choice, 5
　emotional support, 7
　gastrointestinal system, 6
　nutrition, 6-7
　physical, occupational therapy, 7
　pulmonary care, 5-6
　skin care, 6
　urinary system, 6
　venous thromboembolism, 6, 7
Nylon seat-belt webbing, 3

O

Oblique films, 5
Oblique radiograph, 13, 21
Occipital-C2 fusions, 91-92
Occipito-atlanto-axial complex
　biomechanics of, 66-67
　dislocation, 67, *68*
　presentation, 68-70
　treatment, 70-71
Occupational therapy, 7
Odontoid agenesis, 77
Odontoid fracture, *22, 29,* 29, 39-40, 106

Odontoid process
　anatomy, 78-79
　embryology, 77
　fractures, 79-80, 82-83, 87-88
　　Type I, 79, *80, 87,* 88
　　Type II, 79-80, *80, 82-83, 87,* 88
　　Type III, *80,* 80, *82,* 87
　initial diagnosis, assessment, 81-84, *82-83*
　management options, 84-90, *85, 87-90*
　operative management, 90-94, *91*
　pathology, epidemiology, 79-81, *80*
　pediatrics, *183,* 183-84
　radiograph, 13
Operative management
　anterior, 124, 128-30, *129-30*
　anterior wiring, bony fusion, 92
　anterolateral approach, 92
　compression-burst fractures, 122-23
　flexion-dislocation injuries, 120
　fusion methods, 90-92, *91*
　newer methods, 92-93
　pediatrics, 191-200, *194-200*
　posterior, 124-28, *126, 128-29, 131*
　thoracolumbar spine injuries, 138-41, *139, 141*
　timing of surgery, 90
　transoral exposure, 93-94
　upper cervical spine, *108-9,* 108-9
　vs. nonoperative, 84, *85,* 86-89, *87-89*
Opioid antagonist naloxone, 11
Oral intubation, 2
Orotracheal intubation, 2
Orthoses
　bracing, 52-53
　cervical, 53-56, *54,* 57
　complications of, 60-61
　in general, 51-52
　lumbosacral, 58-60, *59-61*
　thoracic, 57-58, *58*
Os odontoideum, 77, 80, 100, 107
Osseous anatomy, 65
Ossiculum terminale, 77
Osteoporosis, *179,* 179
Overt instability, 201-5, *203-5*

P

Parasite shadows, 23
Paraspinal spasm, 44
Pathology
　classification of odontoid fractures, 79-80, *80*
　congenital conditions related to C1-C2 instability, 80
　injuries mechanisms, 79
　preexisting, 87
Patient
　age, 84, 86
　management algorithms, 11, *11-12, 14-15*
　transfers, 8

Peak expiratory flow rate (PEFR), 6
Pediatrics
    common odontoid fractures of, 79
    external orthoses and, 186-91, *187-91*
    fusion extension, *200,* 200
    immediate stabilization, 184-86, *186*
    internal surgical fixation, 191-200, *194-99*
    ligamentous instability, 200-205, *203-5*
    radiography and, 181-84, *182-83*
    spinal cord injury without radiographic abnormalities, 100-101
Pedicle, 151
Perched facets, 26-27, *27*
Peritoneal lavage, 4-5, 13
Pharmacological treatment, 10-11
Philadelphia collar, 41, *54,* 54-55, *55,* 56-57, 127, 185, 190
Physical therapy, 7
Pin site infection, 187-88, *188*
Ping-pong fracture, 185
Plain film. *See* Radiography
Plates, posterior, 127-28, *128*
Plating, 93
    anterior cervical, *130,* 129-30
Pneumonia, 6
Poikilothermia, 3
Posterior operation, 124-25
    constructs using methylmethacrylate, 128
    facet fusion, 125-27
    interlaminar clamps, 127
    interspinous wiring, 125, *126*
    plates and screws, 127, *127*
    sublaminar wiring, 125
Posterolateral decompression, 140
Poster-type brace, *55,* 54-55
Preëxisting spine disease. *See specific types*
Prevertebral soft tissue, 26
    swelling, 184
Previous spinal surgery, 179
Pseudoarthrosis, 146
Psychotherapy, 7
Pulmonary care, 5-6

Q

Quadriplegia, *25,* 113, 115, 197-98, *198*

R

Radiography, 7, 9, 12-13, 19, 20-21, *24*
    of atlanto-occipital dislocation, 69-70
    lateral cervical spine algorithm, *205*
    of odontoid process, *82-83,* 82-84
    pediatrics, 181-84, *182-83*
    sacral fractures, 166, *166*
    of upper cervical spine, 100-101

Radiolucent backboard, 3
Reflex bradycardia, 7
Regional Spinal Cord Injury Center, 140
Regurgitation, 4
Rheumatoid arthritis, 88, 100, 176-77, *177*
Rotary dislocation, 72-74, *73-74*
Rotary subluxation, 40
Rotation, 66-67
    -flexion dislocation, *147,* 147-48
Rotational injuries, 27, 31
Rotobed, 5, 6, 8, 9, 12, 13
Rotorest bed, 186, *186*
Roy-Camille plates, 112-13, 123, 127, *127,* 146
Roy-Camille screws, 122, 127, *127*
Rule of thirds, 39

S

Sacral fractures
    anatomy, 163
    classification, 163-65, *165*
    injury mechanisms, 163
    late displaced, 170
    neurological evaluation, 166-67
    operative management, 169-70
    radiographic diagnosis, *166,* 166
    treatment, 167-69, *168-69*
Sacrum, *47,* 47-48
Sagittal reconstructions, 26-27, *27*
Sagittal translation distance, 41-42, *42*
Sandbags, 3
Scalp injuries, 3
Scoop-sled stretcher, 3
Screw fixation, 93
Screws, posterior, 127-28, *127-28*
Shear-type fracture/dislocation, 145-47
Shock, 2
Skin care, 6
Skin flushing, 7
Skull calipers, 184
Sleeve principle, 53, 58
Smith-Robinson fusion method, 128-29
Soft collar, 3, 53-54, *54,* 56
Soft tissue, 26
SOMI brace, *54,* 54-55, 57, 89, 106
Spicas, *59-60,* 59-60
Spinal cord injury without radiographic abnormality (SCIWORA), 200-202
Spinal motion, 52
Spirometry, 6
Spondylitis, 21
    ankylosing, 173-76, *175-76*
    cervical, *178,* 178-79
Stability, 19-20, 43
Stabilization, 8
    children 7 to 12 years, 185-86, *186*

Index

Stabilization continued
    children 13 to 18 years, 186
    infants, children under 6 years, 184-85
Stable fracture, 138, 149
Starling mechanism, 3
Sterno-occipito-mandibular immobilization. *See* SOMI brace
Stokes litter, 3, 101
Stretch test, 42
Stretcher scoop-sled, 3
Stryker Frame, 5, 9, 12, 13, 185-86
Subacute injuries, early treatment, 32-35
Sublaminar wiring, 125, 146, *194-95*, 194-95
Subluxation, *24*, 25, *25*, 27, *27*, 31, 40
Swan-Ganz catheter, 4
Swan neck deformity, 179, *180*
Sweating, 7
Swelling, of prevertebral soft tissue, 184

T

Teardrop fracture, 122, *122*
Third cervical vertebra, 107
Thomas collar, 54
Thoracic orthoses
    braces, 57-58, *58*
    corsets, 57
    Milwaukee brace with molded body jackets, 58
Thoracic spine, 44-46
Thoracolumbar junction, 135-36
Thoracolumbar spine injuries, *12*, 12-13, *15*
    acute injuries, 30-32, *31*
    and ankylosing spondylitis, 175, *176*
    classification of, 136-37
    clinical features of, 44-46, 135-36
    nonoperative treatment for, 137-38, *138*
    operative treatment for, 138-41, *141*
    specific, 141-156, *143-45*, *147-48*, *150*, *152-56*
Thoraco-lumbosacral orthosis (TLSO), 58
Three-column concepts, 136-37
Three-column injury, 142
Tomography, 7, 23, 34
    multidirectional, 73
Tongs, cranial, 53. *See also specific tongs*
Torsional flexion, 147-48
Tracheostomy, 70
Traction, 9-10, 13, 32-33, *34*, 70, 111-13
    and ankylosing spondylitis, 174
Transcutaneous oxygen saturation, 6
Transfers, of patients, 8
Translation, 67

Translational fracture/dislocation, 145-47
Transoral fusion approach
    operative technique, 93-94
Transport, 3-4
Trendelenburg position, 2, 4
Trippe-Wells tongs, 84
Two-column concepts, 136-37
Two-poster Guilford brace, 54-55, 57

U

Unconscious patient, 2, 5
Unilateral facet dislocation, 26
University of Michigan Medical Center, 47
Unstable fracture, 139
Upper burst fracture, 152-54, *153-54*
Upper cervical spine injuries
    anatomy of, 99-100
    evaluation of, 100-101
    specific, *101*, 101-3, *103-5*, 105-8, *107*
    surgical techniques for, *108-9*, 108-9
Upper thoracic spine, 135
Urinary system, 6

V

Venodyne Stockings, 6
Venous thromboembolism, 6
Vinke tongs, 84
Vitamin C, 6

W

Warfarin syndrome, 100
Wedge compression fractures, 141-43, *142-43*, 196
White-Panjabi stretch test, 12
Wilmington jacket, 58
Wilson frame, 70
Wire fusion, posterior, 198-200, *199*
Wiring, *108-9*, 108-9
    interspinous, 125, *126*
    sublaminar, 125

Y

Yale orthosis, 55

Z

Zielke instrumentation, 151
Zone fractures, 165